Training Mission Two

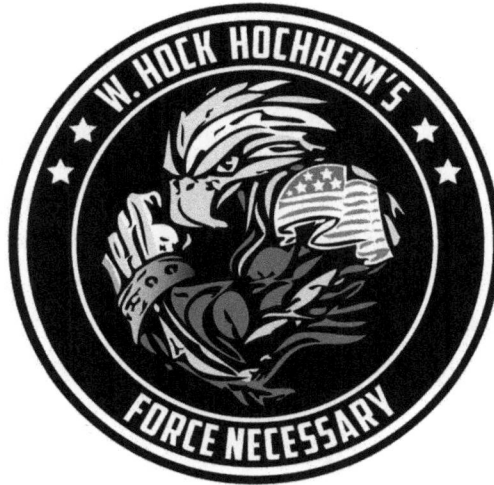

Hardcover ISBN: 978-1-932113-80-8
Paperback ISBN: 978-1-932113-67-9
Digital ISBN: 978-1-932113-33-4
Copyright 2003 and 2021
Published by Lauric Press
www.ForceNecessary.com
All rights reserved.

Other Titles by W. Hock Hochheim
Fightin' Words
Knife Combatives
Impact Weapon Combatives
Footwork and Maneuvering
My Gun is My Passport
Last of the Gunmen
Rio Grande Black Magic
American Medieval
Blood Rust
The China Alamo
Be Bad Now
Fighting Words
The Great Escapes of Pancho Villa
Training Mission Series 1-5

TABLE OF CONTENTS

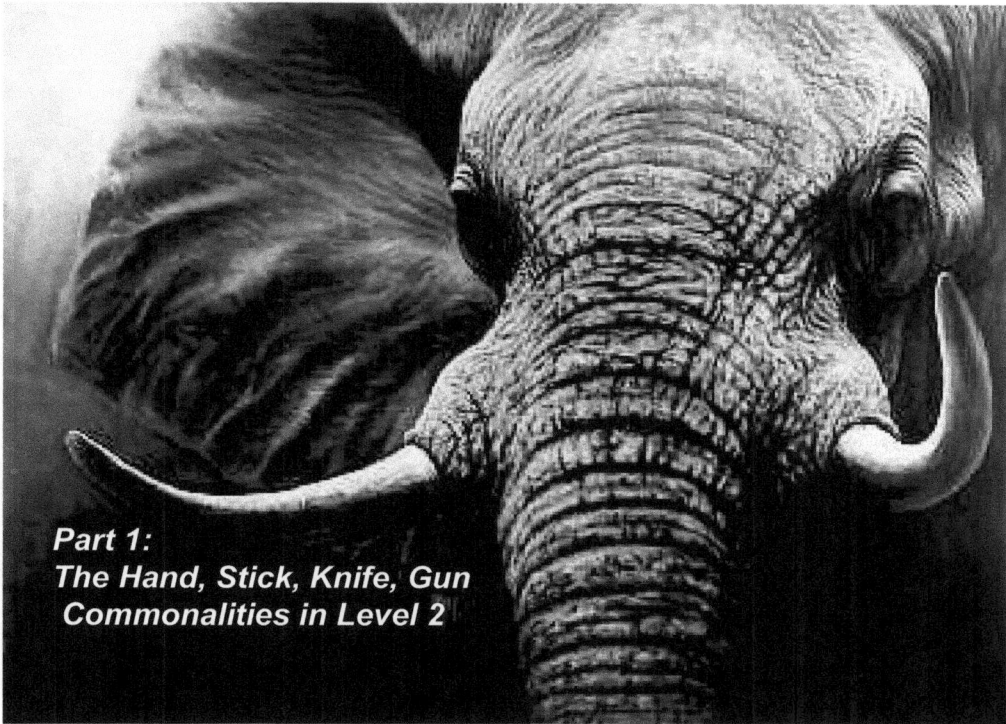

Part 1:
The Hand, Stick, Knife, Gun
Commonalities in Level 2

CHAPTER 1: STOP 2 –"CAUGHT RED HANDED" HANDS ON FINGERS, HANDS,

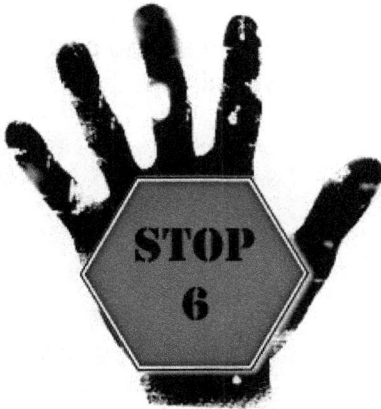

In *Training Mission One* we covered the *Stop 6*, the six common collision, stopping, sticking points of a typical fight, or arrest. And, we also covered *Stop One* of the Stop 6, which includes all the pre-crime, pre-confrontation, pre-contact, information and advice. This included stress weapon quick draws from visual and audio cues.

Stop 2 is about the hands and grabbing. In *Training Mission Two* we get closer in to the enemy, "catching him" or he "catches us" in the first possible contact range and the grabbing of weapons in our hands. We are "tangled" up.

The parameters of the *Stop 2* study progression are when two aggressors reach for each other, either one at a time, or both at the same time and if they catch fingers, hands, wrists, even the stick, pistol or long gun of each other. (It's a pretty grim accident to grab a knife blade, but it does happen.)

In *Stop 2* we are still standing (or perhaps seated). The ground? The floor/ground is the 6th Stop of the Stop 6. These grabs also happen down on the ground, but that is religated later to *Stop 6* of this progression and subsequent *Training Mission* books. And as an early reminder, we are not saying that all fights always unfold in *Stop 1, 2, 3, 4, 5 or 6* order. This is just a training progression we use to organize education.

I use the term "caught red-handed." The expression originates from England. It's a straight forward description of having blood on ones hands after the execution of an attack, or being caught in an animal poaching hunt. If you know your Robin Hood, you know the King didn't like his deer poached. I also use the term "tangler" because we are now entangled. In this level of study, we will grab, and we will counter these grabs.

Incoming! His or yours. Your hands go up and then his hands go up, or vice versa. A common reaction, virtually a reflex action. This type of grab "collision" is seen often in arrests and anytime when people of various skill levels get first involved in a grabbing or respond to a shoving match, or when one wants to prevent another from pulling a weapon, or using a pulled weapon. The grabs might be incidental and accidental to the fight.

The *Stop 2* entanglements are:
- fingers in fingers.
- hands on fingers.
- hands on hands.
  * palms on palms.
  * palms on back of hands.

- hands on wrist areas and low forearms.
- hands on holstered, sheathed weapons.
- hands on his weapon, stick/club, long gun, handgun and the infamous "other."
- *Stop 2* weapon retention and for our purposes here, a quick introduction to disarms, as disarms will appear in great detail is later Stop 6 studies.

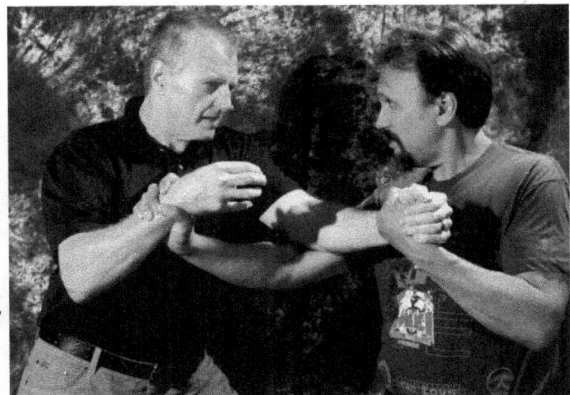

What's Stop 2 look like?

1: *Entanglements. Fingers into fingers.*
   It is unlikely all 20 fingers will blend and mesh perfectly. If it does? The strong one will win the twist or push-pull, bending match. More than likely it will miss-match.

   Mirror Hands (same-side)
   - right hand into the left hand - "single mirror hand grab."
   - left hand into the right hand - "single mirror hand grab."
   - both hands, same side - "double mirror hand grab."

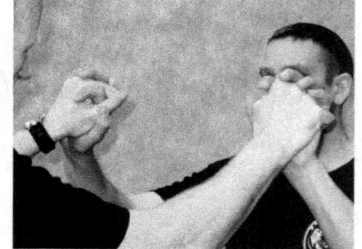

20 fingers perfectly tangled? Unlikely. In which case, the "strongest guy" usually wins.

   Cross hand grabs: His or your hand cross his body.
   - right to right - "single, cross hand grab."
   - left to right - "single, cross hand grab."
   - both hands - "double, cross hand grab."

2: *The list of palm/full-hand grabs on fingers, hands, wrists and sticks, pistols and long guns.*

   - on fingers.
   - on palms.
   - on the backs of hands.
   - on wrists.
   - on holstered, sheathed, carry site weapons.
   - on hands pulling weapons.
   - on weapons being pulled.
   - on weapons drawn.
   - on a knife blade? This has and can accidentally happen. Training to grab the blade of a knife? No.
   - (It would be common in some knife classes for the instructor to walk around and suddenly grab a trainee's knife blade, ripping the knife from the hand, as a surprise grip test.) It's just a test.

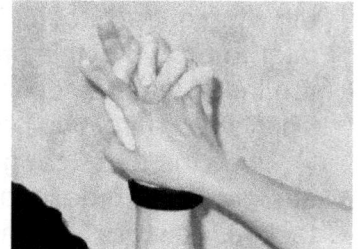

Probably, a few fingers will be mixed-match and tangled.

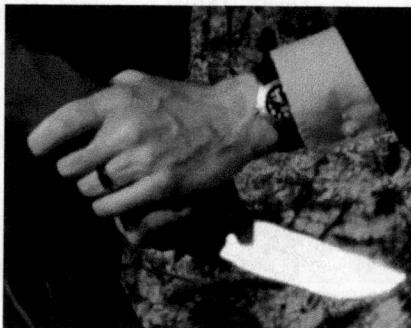

Wrist grab.

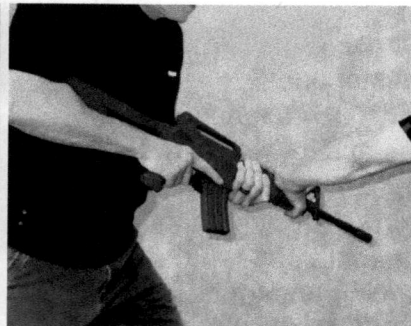

Gun grab.

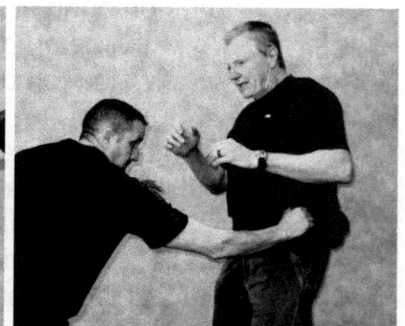

Gun or baton in holster grab.

3: Heights of Grabs, High, Low, Mixes, Crossed

These are what we call "in the clutches of," (unarmed and stick) and "death grips of" (knife and gun). Heights matter. It changes the arm position and angles of grips, wrists and arms.

- classic, double, high hand catches.
- classic, double, low hand catches.
- mixed high and low hand catches.
- cross hand, double catches.
- accordions, as the torsos move in and out and arms stretch out. This may lead to a chest to chest collisions, bites and other problems.

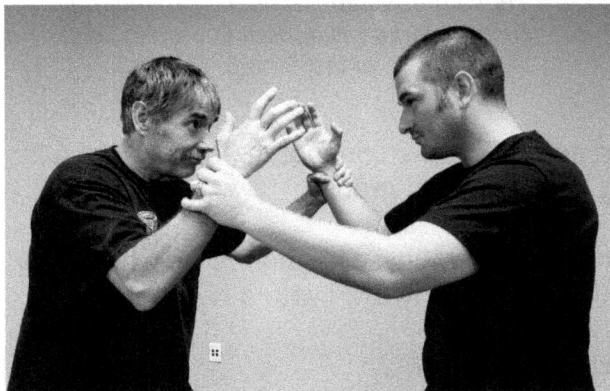
Heights - Classic high catches.

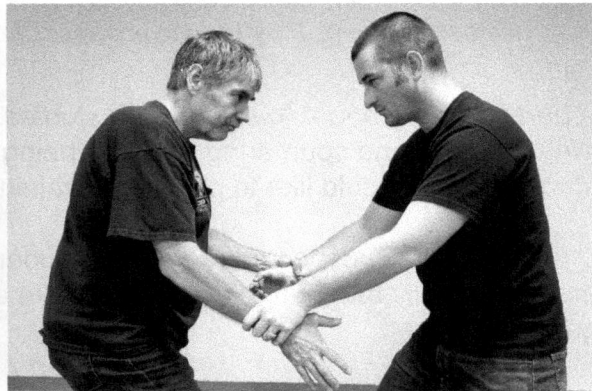
Heights - Classic low catches.

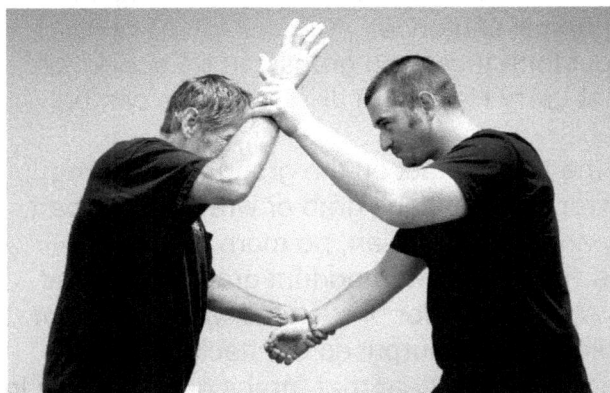
Heights - Classic mixed, high with low catches.

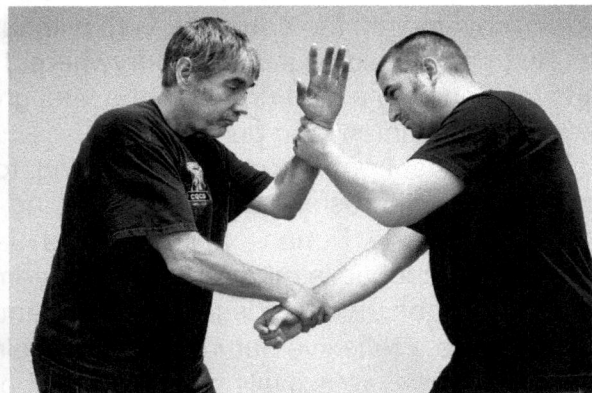
Classic mixed, cross hand, high with low catches.

In this book, this *Stop* and with these hand, stick, knife and gun levels we acquire grabs and we counter these grabs (plus there are deeper, requirements of the unarmed level.) Follow-ups and finishes officially come later but practitioners can experiment with them in training. *Training Mission Two* will cover weapon retention and review weapon disarming.

Study these grabs and releases. They are basics. They aggregate as the *Training Missions* and *Stop 6* program progresses. For example, if someone grabs a hand, and the *other* hand grabs a throat? That is also a *Stop 4* problem. The isolated, digestible skills developed here in *Stop 2* will be used later in *Stop 3 through Stop 6*.

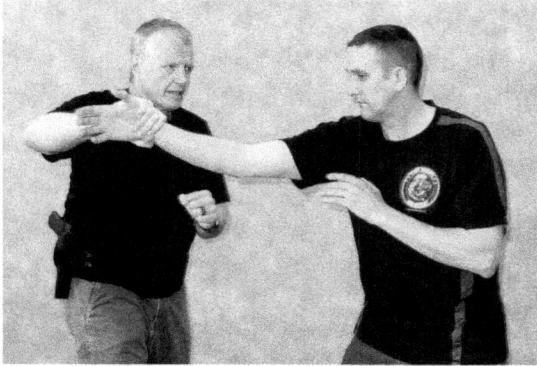
Let beginners begin. They have to start somewhere. They have to progress.

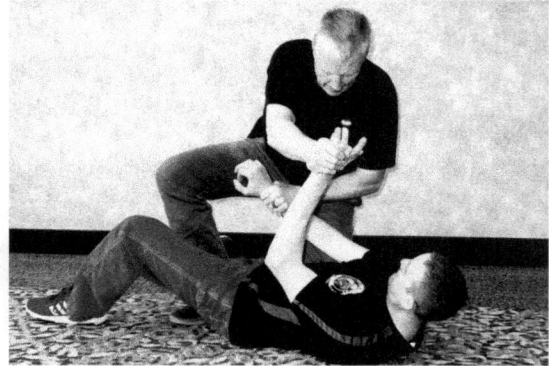
These grabs happen on the ground, but such material will appear in the 6th Stop of the Stop 6.

A early warning about "dissing" grab studies.
With the grab and countering the grab being a central *Stop 2* concept, before we get fully started here, I would like to clear up a training point on hand grabs.

Are grabs disrespected? By some modern instructors, yes. The manner in which they are traditionally taught makes it appear like a fight is going to start with a hand-on-wrist grab...

"Fights don't start this way!"

...the complainers complain and therefore never or barely cover the catch and escape subjects as a result. Whether they realize it or not, traditionalists are only showing the basic movements, the noun and verb without the full sentence.

But, grabs inside fights are everywhere. I put forth that hand grabs can be accidental and incidental to a fight (to quote the late, great Larry Hartsell of JKD) or grabs can be very much on intent and purpose.

Grabs exist from first contact, standing, to the last contact on the ground. Grappling involves hand grabs and arm wraps and leg wraps. If you can't grab or wrap a body part, you can't grapple. Period. No more jujitsu, Japanese or Brazilian, no more Catch, no more of the countless other grappling systems. THAT is how important grabbing is. And escaping grabs therefore is just as important. Also, a number of systems will advise that people have a reflexive nature to put up their limbs when surprised or attacked. These lifted hands may reflexively grab or be grabbed. Yet, I still hear that "grabs don't happen in *real* fights."

Yes, I frequently read, see and hear from self defense naysayers who make fun of basic, self defense classes, especially when they introduce grabs and counter to grabs. In those classes, trainers are showing rank beginners - virgins if you will - how to escape being grabbed in the most simplistic manner. These are ignorant/new people being grabbed in these simplistic manners, sometimes for the first time in their lives. They are taught to get out of the grab. Their stances are terrible. The grab is static. They look con-fused, or maybe even amazed. They might even giggle. They're new people for God's sake. And to us, it looks unreal. But, it's like teaching a non-athletic person to catch a foot-ball or throw a baseball. They are not in a situational throw in the 9th inning of the World Series. This is new to them. Of course it doesn't look like a real Saturday night bar fight. They first must learn how to hold and throw a ball. You have to start somewhere. It has to be introduced in a very, slow, isolated, non-realistic manner.

All sports, all martial arts and martial materials are introduced in this simplistic manner. A progression ensues. Early on, all these first steps and drills appear to be, "dead drills," to quote other, ignorant martial instructors and complainers.

While that simple wrist grab may actually happen. Kidnappers, rapists and terrorists grab and then pull their victims away to capture them. Police grab to restrain and/or handcuff. The big mission of learning grabs and escaping grabs is to absorb the big, overall concept and use that the grab, escape/counter concept is in every mixed-weapon, mixed-range, situation from standing to the ground.

You might complain that the trainers do not explain the big point I am making here. That would be a valid complaint. Or maybe trainers fail to explain that self defense cannot be taught in one fun, little session. That's another valid complaint. But, perhaps the accused trainer did indeed explain these though, and you-the-naysayer have no idea if they did or did not, after seeing the out-of-context, short video clip or seeing a still photo set you are complaining to the world about. Continued training is the key.

In the world of hands, sticks, knives, pistols, long guns and expedient weapons, grabbing, controlling and then escaping such grabs (and the limb wraps of upcoming *Stop Four*), from standing on down to the ground, is vital knowledge.

Continued, consistant training is the key, but people have to start somewhere. Let's not ridicule them for starting.

A So-Called "Wrist Grab" Point
Getting more of the hand than wrist alone has more potential verus weapons as in restricting hand movement. You might be able to manipulate or even freeze the hand, especially when he holds a pistol and tries to twist his gun hand in and shoot you with it. If he holds a knife he might with a freer hand sneak the blade up or down and stab or slash your grip, or with more tricks, the rest of your body.

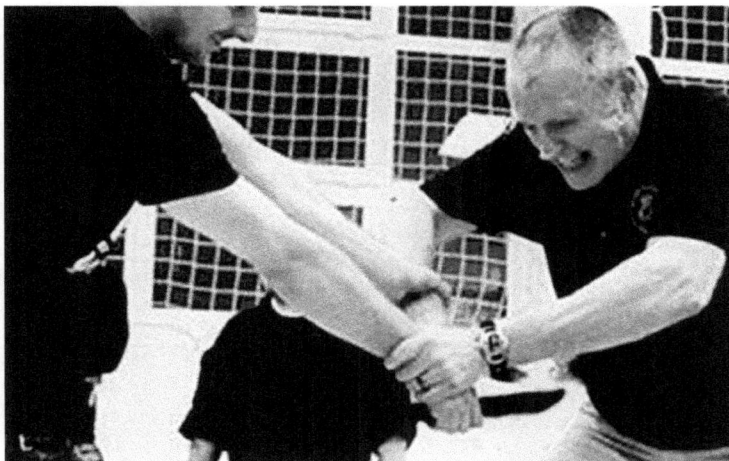

Unarmed grapplers like the hand control for potential follow-ups.

Fighting is chaotic. You may well have tried to grab the hand, or mostly the hand, but in the mess of movement, you only got the wrist. There still might be the chance to slide your hand down to the preferred shared wrist-hand split. Experiment.

Clutches and Death Grips.
For the purpose of doctrine organization and the *Force Necessary* training courses, the *Stop 2* problems are frequently called here:

   1: In the Clutches Of - When the limbs are grabbed in unarmed fighting and stick fighting. This is dangerous of course, but not as dangerous as...

   2: Death Grip Of - When the limbs are grabbed in knife and gun fighting. One mistake and it could be dead.

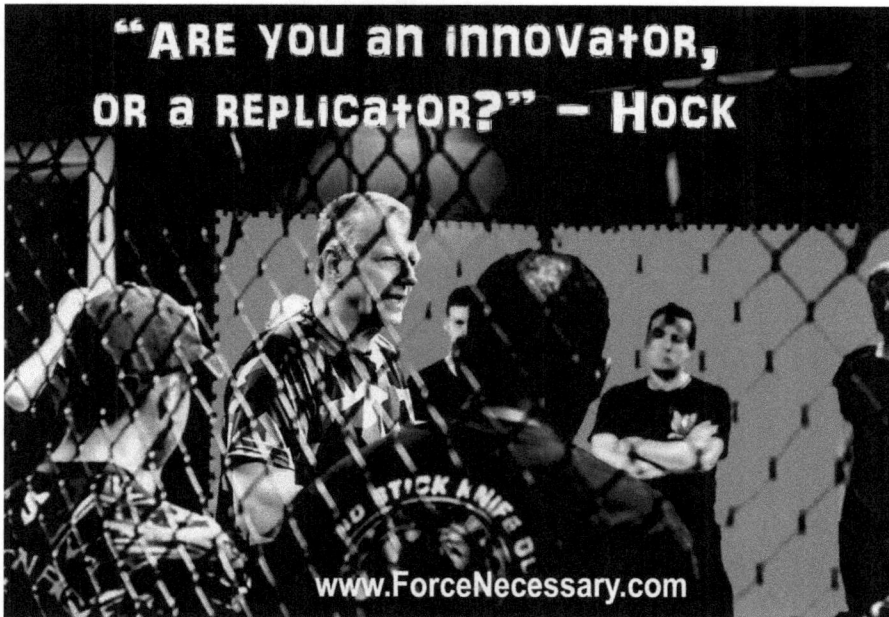

"ARE YOU an innovator,
OR a REPLICaTOR?" – HOCK

www.ForceNecessary.com

*Either way is a fine thing, providing you know your goals
and know what you want to be. Just know.*

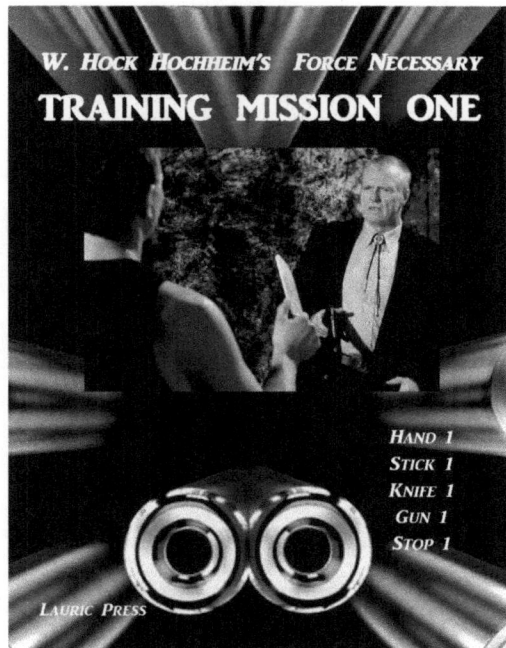

W. HOCK HOCHHEIM'S FORCE NECESSARY
TRAINING MISSION ONE

HAND 1
STICK 1
KNIFE 1
GUN 1
STOP 1

LAURIC PRESS

*Mandatory reading...
The* Traning Mission One *book.*

Chapter 2: The What Question

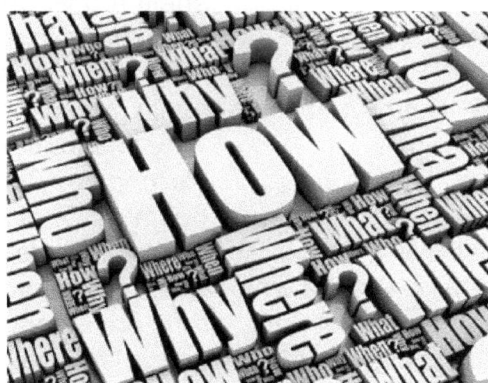

In *Training Mission One* we introduced the *Who, What, When, Where, How and Why* questions, not just for the survival aspects, but also for life in general. And then, we took a specific look at the *Who* question. Here in *Training Mission Two* we explore the second question, the "what" questions, both big and small. You must continually collect intelligence information to make accurate answers as much as possible.

What can happen to you in Paris?

Paris? One of my favorite examples of collecting intelligence information that might be lead to great preparation is about tourism in Paris, France. Just about every tourist review on Paris warns travelers of the constant scams and cons of pick pockets and various gypsy tricks, too long to list here. I was briefed on this before a trip and was confronted with these *exact* problems when there, every single one, and thanks to the warnings, avoided trouble. I have yet to meet a Paris tourist who hasn't run across the same con man problems during their visits, too. The intelligence information was excellent and consistent.

Each location, neighborhood, city and country has its problems, and it behooves each of us to collect intelligence on them. Unlike Paris, this is not easy at times, and I am not suggesting such an obsessive investigation on quick, pass-through locations and events, unless one is warranted by common sense.

The "What" of It All

- *What* can really happen to you in your home or travels? Take a hard look at your life and circumstances, and try to learn and figure out what bad things could happen to you. You could be a victim of a list of crimes or all sorts of accidents, be they car wrecks or faulty stairwells, etc.

- *What* will happen in the actual event? Exactly. Start with probable events on down to improbable events, and examine each one. What is he doing in the actual event? Exactly. What are you going to do? Exactly.

- *What* weapon will you have? Will you have a weapon? If so, what weapon? Will "he" have a weapon?

- *What* training course will you take to prepare?

- *What* happens when you become "adrenalized?"

- *What* happens when you get hurt?

- *What* other outcomes might have happened?

- **What** should have happened instead?

- **What** will this cost me? (Laywer's fees?)

- **What** is normal/abnormal? "Hey! What's wrong with this picture?"

What's Normal Looking?

My friend, former police chief/SWAT commander and 101st Airborne Mike Gillette was hired by the world's largest amusement park company to do a counter-terrorism, security survey on their parks. Mike traveled to them, lived at each one for a brief time and dressed as any normal civilian would. He spent days walking around and observing people and the grounds. During these times, numerous park attendees would approach him asking for directions. Gillette is a very friendly fellow and would graciously help them as best he could, but each time he grew more curious about, "Why are all these people stopping me for questions?"

Finally, a couple with children approached him for directions and Mike asked, "Just a question, though, why did you ask me?"

"Because you are the only guy walking around not looking like you are having any fun!" the dad said spontaneously. Gillette was not smiling or happy on his inspections, just seriously walking around inspecting things. He was an abnormal vacationer.

This is a great story about peoples' inherent observation and detection powers.

Store detectives watch for customers who don't shop "normally," like normal shoppers examine merchandise, but rather are too busy looking around for people, not products, to see if they are seen stuffing away items into their clothing.

Another favorite of mine is hearing stories about the old "amish-like" religions, and the sects where a young man reaches a certain age and then must journey into the real world, perhaps to witness the "horrors"

of the techno, big city and outsiders. This sheltered life, his uneducated subconscious and conscious mind is quite vacant for trouble beyond some deeply inset, virtually genetic, human fears.

Genetic, human fears? Experts from *Psychology Today* say - "Are you afraid of heights? Or closed spaces? Or snakes, bugs, and rats? Are you afraid of the water? Well, you're not alone. Our prehistoric ancestors had the very same fears, which is why you are alive today." Our sect traveler has never quite seen these types of "human" snakes before.

A study of the obvious leads to spotting the unusual. People go about their everyday lives, spotting things odd and unusual, even if it never reaches their conscious mind.

"So, stay alert!" Are you a bit sick of being told that? Be alert for rapists? Be alert for terrorists? "See something, say something?"

"Oh! Ahhh, okay," the populace says, your squad says, your family says. Then you move on with your day never really knowing what that phrase truly means or what precisely you should be alert for. What to exactly look for?

"No worries," some leading experts say, "you've been anointed with the 'gift of fear!' That ESP! That magic Spidey Sense. You just tingle when you mingle with the scoundrel."

Then the concealed bear trap snaps shut on your ankle, and you're in it. The bombing. The mass shooting. Whatever. While our brains are natural spotters of the unusual and the abnormal, we need more tips, help and hope to avoid the bear traps than just "icky" feelings about pending danger.

One of the key, built-in radars we have in life is spotting the abnormal. Military experts now call it "pattern recognition." We record the normal. That helps spot even the tiniest things that doesn't fit properly. Much has been written and studied about this subject in the minutest detail, pages of psycho-techno-jargon and pontification, even just in the last 5 to 10 years. I can steer you to these sources. There are hundreds of examples and stories. The military research is so full of such dense jargon it is almost unreadable.

To save time here, I will simply cleave it down to a few sentences. In our business, our world of safety, crime, and war, we want to spot suspicious people, criminals, and enemy soldiers/terrorists. And we need to spot their dangerous deeds and plans aforehand!

As stated, first, you must become a student of the normal to be a spotter of the abnormal. You might think this is a new discovery by some self-defense instructor, but it's not. It was explained to me, for example, about 45 years ago in the Army's military police academy. They ordered us to study the neighborhoods we patrolled, so we could become "students of the usual," so we could spot the unusual. Abnormal-normal, usual-unusual. Same-same.

"Become 'students' of the usual, so you can spot the unusual."

Your brain does a lot of this automatically, and I have written about these neural functions in blogs, articles and books. The "sub-committees" in the brain send messages to the conscious, main "committee." It helps greatly if you'll add some effort to the cause. You must educate yourself with relevant details. Educate the subconscious and conscious of your brain. In shorthand, this time-and-grade-process equals the vital term "experiences" of *all* sorts.

But whatever source, you can't spot the abnormal in its domain, be it the woods, the jungle, the desert, the streets, etc., and their inhabitants without first being a student of the normal.

Yeah, we have a low-running radar system. Yeah, it's like a gift. But it's not enough to loosely call it a gift. Not by a long shot. You must couple this with intelligence information you glean on the usual, the unusual, and what we police folks call "MO", the method of operation – of the people we watch for. Do this, and you are breathing life and depth into that shallow term ..."stay alert."

"Sensemaking!" It's a movement from many avenues of study and think-tankers since the 1970s. American organizational psychologist and theorist, Kerl E. Weick is a pioneer of the contemporary SenseMaking movement, with several books including SenseMaking in Organizations.

In the last decade the US military has co-opted the civilian term to define it as "A motivated continuous effort to understand connections (which can be among people, places, and events) in order to anticipate their trajectories and act effectively."

I am amazed at the very brief, concise military definition. They are usually so dense and jargon-heavy, as to create an impenetrable language.

The phrase, "anticipate their trajectories" is one way of trying to predict the situational actions of others. Can you anticipate the trouble you might get into, when taking action to protect yourself? Can you think checkers or chess? I know its easier said than done, but I like to suggest

"fight like checkers, think like chess."

What is winning?

You find yourself in a 6-man foot patrol in the Mekong Delta during the Vietnam War. You suddenly are confronted by an entire battalion of North Vietnamese. Do you stay, fight and...win? What if you are surrounded by a gang armed with chains and knives on a supermarket parking lot? Must you win, win, WIN, as so many "Win Instructors" declare and pound into your psyche with their courses? No. Everyone's definition of winning is different.

It is small-minded, inexperienced, immature and plain wrong for instructors to preach this "must always win" mentality to everyone, every time. Their perspective isn't from a high enough altitude to see these win messages spread across the board to police, military and citizens, all the while creating a generic, confusing and dangerous message. Missions are different. Daily life is different. Citizens, soldiers and cops have different goals. Even so, for all these groups, we share the temporary solution that discretion may be the better part of valor, at times. Live now to fight another day when there is a chance to win.

To a police officer winning usually means arresting the suspect, or at times, just staying alive. To a citizen it usually means escaping a crime or escaping injury, or possibly confining a criminal until the authorities arrive. For the officer or citizen, this may also mean killing a criminal. If you are in the military, winning means winning. Both small and big battles. And it may mean also winning the hearts and minds of the populace around you. Winning may also mean escaping to fight another battle another day. A prisoner of war wins by escaping, not stopping and fighting every guard and soldier along the way in hand-to-hand combat.

Who are you and what is winning, surviving, escaping to *you*? We all share these same possibilities and goals in the situational combat of crime and war. I warn you to be leery of these Win-Only courses and

Win-Only teachers. Their altitude and perspective are unsophisticated, short and low bar. Their message is dangerous. Crime and combat are not like a Sunday football game. In real life, even a tie or yes, even a loss, can be a win. Here are some ways to "win," or to "finish" a fight:

1) Escape from the opponent (using the "Orderly Retreat" concept).

2) Threats, demands and actions to make the opponent surrender and/or desist and leave.

3) Less than lethal injury to the opponent. Injure and/or diminish to a degree that the opponent stops fighting and chasing you.

4) Control arrest, contain and restrain. Capture and escort the opponent. Or, you detain/capture the opponent and await the proper authorities.

5) Lethal methods. We fight criminals and enemy soldiers. Sometimes we kill them.

What do we do to the people and personnel when we fight them? To have some sort of finish to our fight, to situationally win.

1) We chase them off, or -
2) We escape, or -
3) We wound them, or -
4) We capture them, or -
5) We kill them.

What is the winning attitude? What are the steps to winning? Is it a desire? A winning attitude? A winning mindset? I often preach the story of the two baseball pitchers, pitching in a baseball's World Series. Both pitchers have an incredible desire to win. They possess the winning attitude. They can recite positive winning speeches.

   * Pitcher One desperately wants to win. As he looks at his catcher's signals, as he prepares to throw, and throws, he's thinking about winning the game. He needs the money for his new house, his family. His kids need braces. He needs a better contract for next year. He MUST win.

   * Pitcher Two desperately wants to win. Maybe for all the same reasons, or more that are better or worse, he wants to win. As he looks at the catcher's signals, he prepares to throw. But he thinks about his grip on the ball. His feet positions. The right elbow angle, the best wrist twist. He is thinking about the steps toward winning, to the point of even forgetting about the game and the World Series game and all the ramifications. He is in the moment, the process of pitching the best pitch. This is my prescribed suggestion for "winning." It's about the best pitch. Baseball and fighting?

   I cannot remember from whom or when a professional kickboxer inspired me to think about this process as it was back in the late 80s. The idea of shutting everything else out, and taking and doing the steps to win. I worked on this idea in terms of police work. There were times when I was faced with full-out fighting people bigger, faster and stronger than me. Kidnapping? Bar fight? Road Rage? Etc. Some even have an imaginary perception of how they will handle gun. Knife? MMA?

   What are your preconceived notions about fighting? Your first fight? Your next fight? I use to complain that so many of these modern fighting systems inadvertently train for a fight in "the bar," or on the sidewalk or parking lot right outside the bar? Or, that cursed dark alleyway out back of the bar? Roadhouse movie world? Bars. Bars. And bars. How many training videos were shot right inside bars? Young guys teaching other young guys how to fight in bars and they just automatically assume/gravitate to the barroom setting. Meanwhile a soldier in northern Afghanistan has another location in mind.

What is the perception of your next or first fight? This may be the most important essay I've ever written. I am an old police detective from a time when Community Oriented Policing was going to save the world and cure cancer. One of the main points of said movement was that the "perception of crime" was just as real to citizens as the real crime was. Look at how the murder rates in small parts of Chicago, Baltimore or St. Louis effect the opinions of outsider people on those entire states. In other countries, those tiny jurisdictions effect the opinion of the USA. Usually the perception of crime was/is always way higher than the real McCoy.

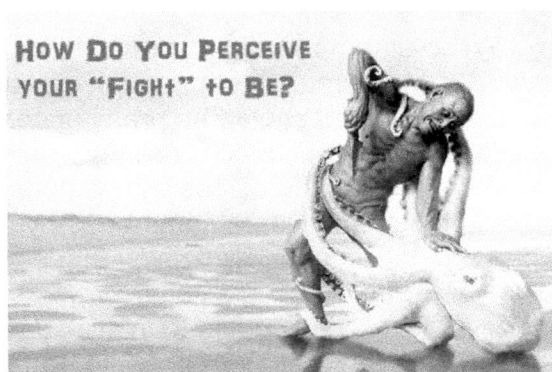

HOW DO YOU PERCEIVE YOUR "FIGHt" tO BE?

How you perceive your next or your first fight will be how you train. Will your perception be wrong? How wrong?

So, police then not only had to fight real crime, but had to have an advertising and public relations campaign against the perception of crime.

Fact was and is, in the big picture, most people in the USA and other civilized countries will never be victims of crime. But people have fear and a perception of their future crime problem. They imagine a home invader? Rapist? Mugger? Mass shooter. Crazy guy? Serial killer?

Perception, as defined – "a way of regarding, trying to understand, or interpreting something; a mental impression." Mental impressions and being impressionable. I recently watched the very first episodes of the 80s "TJ Hooker" cop show, just for sheer nostalgia. I was already a street cop and detective when TJ was on prime time TV. On patrol in a giant squad car prowling residential streets, Hooker lectures his rookie partner – you know, that skinny kid with the weird hairdo – the shame and horror of Los Angeles, how people cowered and hid in their houses, fearing the crime on the streets. That was 1981! They were scaring the BeJesus out of you way back then. Of course that was dramatic, but the fear idea fed and still feeds people.

Gun instructor and ex-cop Tom Givens reports that through the years his shooting students have had over 60 gun encounters in parking lots (Memphis is a little crazy by the way) so an emphasis on shooting live fire AND SIMS (simulated ammo), in and out of, and around cars should be pretty important. Parking lots are indeed melting pots of all kinds of people and places with various temperaments, and where some bad guys do go to hunt. Records even show that one in every five vehicle accidents occur on parking lots too. Parking lots then are super-duper dangerous? But then, once again, in the big picture, if you compare say, Walmart's total sales/customers, (in the millions) to its parking crimes and accidents

each year, their parking lots are still pretty safe places.

We see crazy reports on the news about road rage. But look at the millions of cars in the USA taking billions of trips each day, compared to road rage incidents. Road crime and even vehicle accidents stats in comparison tell us the roadways are pretty darn safe too. Domestic and family violence/disturbances are way too high, but in comparison to the big picture of 340 million people in the USA? Not too bad (as far as we officially know).

Wrong training place? Wrong training people? Wrong training mission? How deep was that paranoid perception of criminals? Has that perception changed? Many perceptions about fighting against bad guys are subliminally shaped by books, movies, TV and even personal fantasy projections. Same with fights. One old friend named Ted for example told me back then, "I wanted to fight like Seagal. I turned my car into the first martial art school I drive by every day and signed up."

But, Ted pulled into a Tae Kwon Do school and very quickly realized he was financially contracted to the wrong place with wrong people, the wrong system for his mission. He had no "who, what, where, when, how and why" going for him. No one there was doing "Seagal-Fu" as in the movies. My point being is that Ted started something out of ignorance. What did he want and what did he need?

Remember back when Chuck Norris or Claude Van Damme would kick a bad guy down? The bad guy would crash and the Chucks and the Claudes would just stand there, in a poster-boy, fighting pose, bouncing up and down, waiting for the serial killer or hit-man to...stand back up! Waiting to continue the fight. Art imitates life and life mimics art. How many people in real fights actually, waited for bad guys to stand back up?

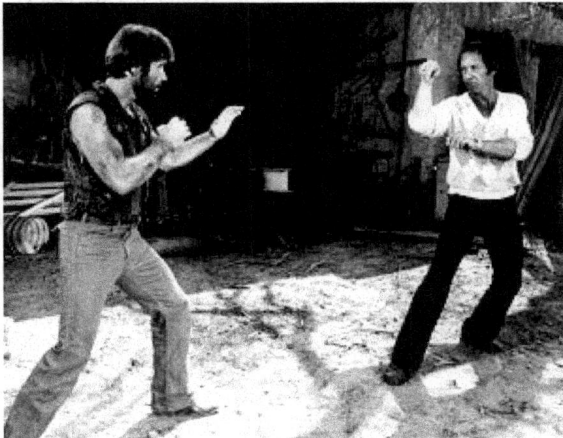

Do you think your next fight will be like a movie fight or a sports match, with a lot of stand-off posturing?

That became a perception about fighting. And when we prepare, we perceive. You are still left with these guesses, your perceptions and mental impressions of your future fight. We now watch crazy, reality, video clips on YouTube and perhaps they do help the real perception of the wacky chaos that will most likely occur in a fight, and not leave us with some Chuck Norris, karate fight scene in our minds.

Come what may? We learn the "come what may" via collecting good intelligence info on crime and war where you are and where you are going. So, we train to fight the fight we perceive and who, what, where, when, how and why we perceive it will happen. Who will you really be fighting? What will it be like? Where do you perceive your fight will be? When will this happen? How will it unfold? Why are you there? Why are you still there? Will things happen as fast as you think? Slower? Sporty Non-sporty? Indo artsy? Slinky Systema? Crazy? Hand? Stick? Knife? Gun? Will it start with an interview or ambush? How do you perceive your fight?
Come...what...may?

One of the five universal critical thinking questions taught in classes is, "What are the assumptions?" What do you assume?

We had a champion black belt in one of karate school I attended decades ago, who got into a fight….in a bar…and lost. He came to class and told the school owner,

"I was in a fight last night and it wasn't anything like I thought it would be."

If you are in a non-sport class, your student should return to you and say instead,

"I was in a fight last night and it was just like you told me."

Perception is the running guts of training though isn't it? We martial folks, civilians, police and military train for the perception of what we think our "fight" will be like. If you are sport fighting, you know exactly who, what, where, when, how and why about your scheduled fight. You have a darn good perception of the "Ws." Even if you are a soldier, you have some good perceptions about what might happen.

What you need versus ***what*** you want. Studying the training process in order that I mention in the photo to upper the left has become much easier now than in decades past when a person (such as me) had to slog through six or more arts and systems to filter out the real core, generic survival, offensive and defensive material, while adorned in a bevy of different uniforms, rules, hero worship and system worship. Wants and needs. It comes down to a series of "who, what, where, when, how and why" questions.

What you need versus *what* you want. Studying the training process in order has become much easier now than in decades past when a person (such as me) had to slog through six or more arts and systems to filter out the real core, generic survival, offensive and defensive material, while adorned in a bevy of different uniforms, rules, hero worship and system worship. Wants and needs. It comes down to a series of "who, what, where, when, how and why" questions.

  * What's the subject and what will it teach you?
  * What materials? What do I REALLY need? Want? Art? Science? Both?

Hand. Stick. Knife. Gun. Standing through ground. The laws of your land. Savvy. Awareness. Studies of crime and war. It's been an evolution I too have been part of, evolving and teaching for 25 years now. A movement. My personal suggestion and advice is one of common sense. Try and get those foundational defense, offense survival stuff first and then move off to more confining hobbies later. Needs first. Then wants.

"Fighting first, systems second!" Remember my quote for three decades now? I have used it for 24 years since I emancipated myself from all systems. But, like a college counselor ordering a college kid to take all the college courses in precise order - 101, 102, 103 - and then they simply can't do that because of filled classes and scheduling, a student takes what he or she can at the time. You too, may have trouble completely doing all unarmed and mixed-weapon combatives first and then arts second. While it is easier these days for you to get right to what you want than in the past, you may have to do this training side-by-side? Generally people are busy with life and can only chip away at this training stuff, anyway. Do something rather than nothing. Get off the couch. Do something.

Again, I always say I want people to be happy. Just know where you fit into the big picture. If you told me,

"Yeah Hock, I completely understand what you are saying, but I just want to do traditional _____. I love the culture and the country of _____."

Terrific. Okay, I am thumbs up with you. Unlike the aforementioned Ted, you get the big picture and can articulate it. Just know the big picture of "needs and wants." Or, one might add to that "love" list,

"Hock, I also just enjoy developing the overall personalities of children and being a positive staple in my community."

Fantastic. Okay. Go for it. All martial arts do have abstract benefits. And there are some established, "martial-artsy-named-sounding" schools that really try to get survival theories and materials in the curriculum.

So...dance in some kung fus? Throat punch in some combatives? Art? Science? Nuts and bolts? Investigate and figure out what you really need and what you really want to do. Use the "W's and "H" questions. The choices and opportunities are more clear and obvious than ever before.

Finally, a litmus test question - look at it this way. Speaking of college, if you were sending your daughter off to a big city college, would you want her to know, so-called "traditional karate?" So-called "Brazilian wrestling?" So-called "stick dueling?" Or, so called "unarmed and mixed-weapon, combatives?" What does she really NEED to know?

Want what you need?
Or, need what you want?

The "**What's** It Gonna' Take," Game
Here's another important "what," in the who, what, where, when, how and why. WHAT is it going to take? It's a mental prep game I have been suggesting for years and one I used for decades as a cop to make best use of spare time. You can play it anywhere there are people around you. It doesn't matter where you are, a sports event, a ghetto, Rockefeller Center, a supermarket or a POW camp. See someone and pick one out. Ask yourself, "What is it going to take to put this person down and out" of a potential fight.

You should inspect and evaluate that person's size, strength and endurance. Then mull over some options you might have to take the person down and out. I hope this will include cheats, fakes and distractions when possible.

This kind of mental, crisis rehearsal can be used for any kind of potential situation. In police work since the 1970s we used this idea for patrol time. Instead of mindlessly driving around, our smarter trainers suggested we crisis-rehearse various incidents at various locations on our beat.

What happens next? And that is perhaps the consummate "what" question. The *"what happens next"* continuum. Big and small what worries:

    * If he moves this way or that way, what do you do?
    * If he decided to do _____, what will you do?
     * What happens next? (After the fight.)
           - did you fight and get arrested?
           - did you just get sued?
           - did you fight, get arrested *and* get sued?
           - did you get home safe, or back on the military base safe
             and unhurt?

What is safe and safety where you work? You should investigate.

What is guarded and what is not?
What are common hazards at a construction site?
What are common safety hazards in a facility?
What are different types of workplace safety?
What are examples of administrative controls?
What are hazard controls?
What are hazards in a confined space?
What are occupational health hazards?
What are safeguards?
What are the steps to becoming a safety manager?
What are ways to stay awake at work?
What are workplace safety requirements?
What does a safety professional do?
What does emergency egress mean?
What is a confined space?
What is a hazard?
What is a job safety analysis?
What is a risk assessment?
What is composite risk management (CRM)?
What is process safety management (PSM)?
What is the difference between a job safety analysis?
What is the goal of a risk assessment?
What is the hierarchy of hazards?
What is the role of PPE in workplace safety?
What's inside the first aid kit?

What's left? Continue developing and asking the what and what-if questions.

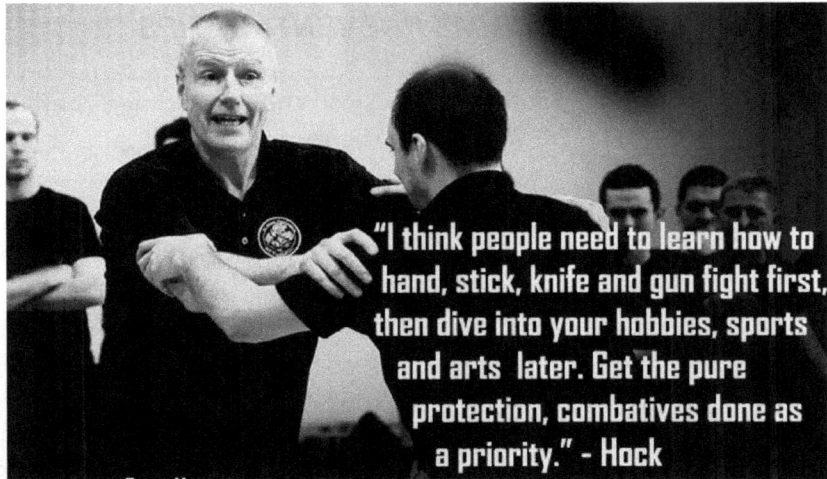

"I think people need to learn how to hand, stick, knife and gun fight first, then dive into your hobbies, sports and arts later. Get the pure protection, combatives done as a priority." - Hock

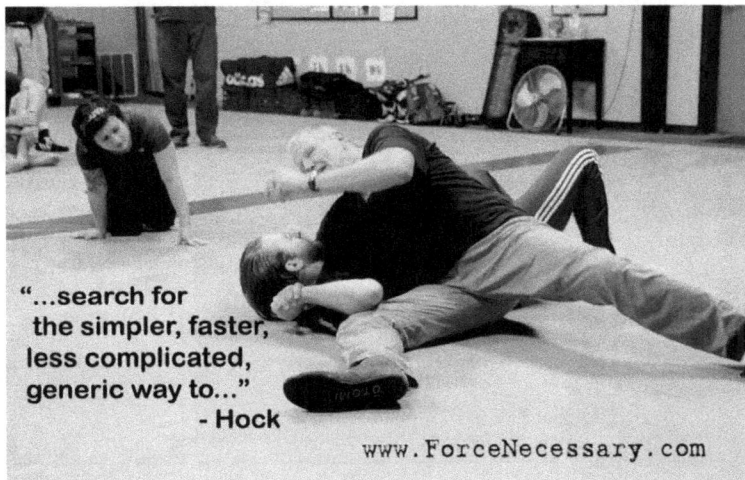

"...search for the simpler, faster, less complicated, generic way to..." - Hock

www.ForceNecessary.com

Fighting is checkers not chess. Lessons learned come from arts, sports, war and crime. Decipher. Filter.

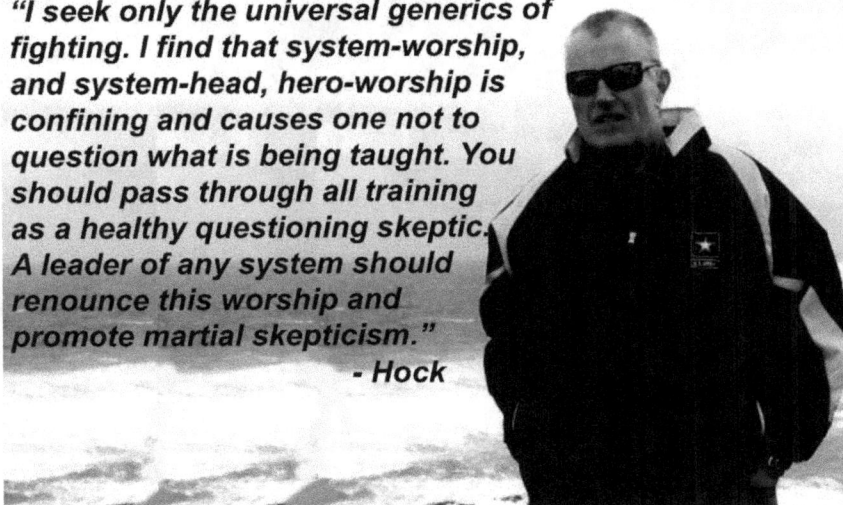

"I seek only the universal generics of fighting. I find that system-worship, and system-head, hero-worship is confining and causes one not to question what is being taught. You should pass through all training as a healthy questioning skeptic. A leader of any system should renounce this worship and promote martial skepticism." - Hock

GENERIC CRIME PREVENTION TIPS

Vehicle Theft Prevention:

- Lock your vehicle
- Do not leave keys or fob in the vehicle (Nearly 40 cases involved had keys left behind)
- Do not leave valuables in plain view or in the car at all!
- Park in well-lit areas
- Do not leave personal identifying papers in your vehicle
- Consider theft prevention devices
- Do not leave the vehicle running unattended if you can't lock it or engage the alarm.

Personal Safety Tips When Walking at Night:

- If possible don't walk alone during night hours.
- Walk in groups whenever you can-there is always safety in numbers
- Let a family or friend know your destination and your estimated time of arrival or return
- Stay in well-lit areas as much as possible
- Walk on sidewalk whenever possible
- Always be aware of your surroundings. If you are wearing headphones, don't turn up the volume so high that you cannot hear outside noises
- Cell phones can be a distraction or a target for theft.
- Wear bright clothing

Package Theft Prevention:

- Have your package delivered to your work
- Have your package delivered to the home of a relative or friend that you know will be home
- Have your package held at your local post office for pickup
- Take advantage of "Ship to Store" option that many stores offer. Amazon offers a "locker" feature that allows you to pick up your package from a secure location
- Request that your package has signature confirmation upon delivery
- Ask your carrier to place package in an area out of plain view

Suggested reading....

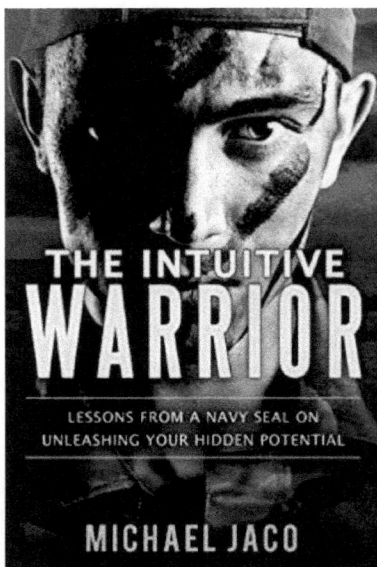

THE INTUITIVE WARRIOR

LESSONS FROM A NAVY SEAL ON UNLEASHING YOUR HIDDEN POTENTIAL

MICHAEL JACO

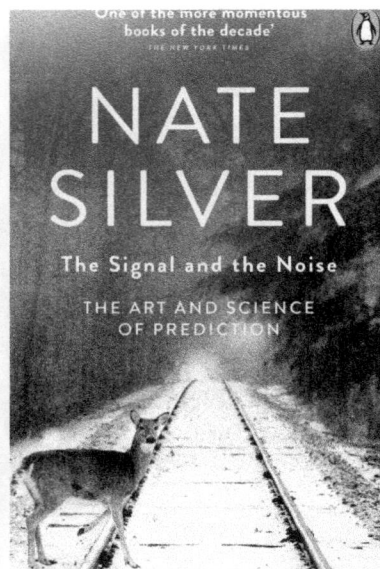

'One of the more momentous books of the decade'
THE NEW YORK TIMES

NATE SILVER

The Signal and the Noise

THE ART AND SCIENCE OF PREDICTION

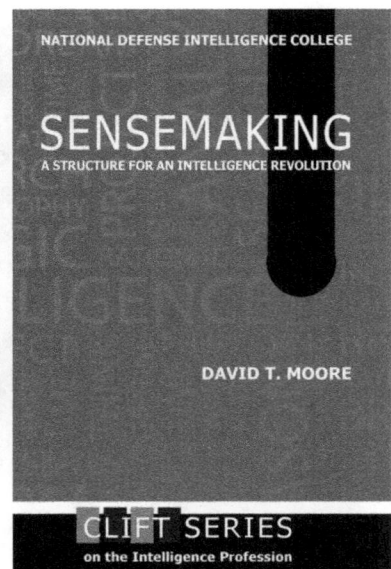

NATIONAL DEFENSE INTELLIGENCE COLLEGE

SENSEMAKING
A STRUCTURE FOR AN INTELLIGENCE REVOLUTION

DAVID T. MOORE

CLIFT SERIES
on the Intelligence Profession

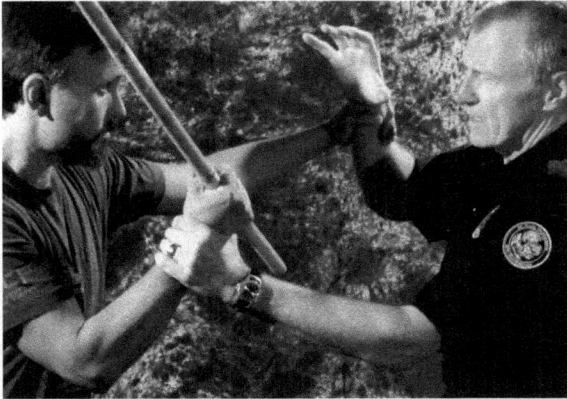

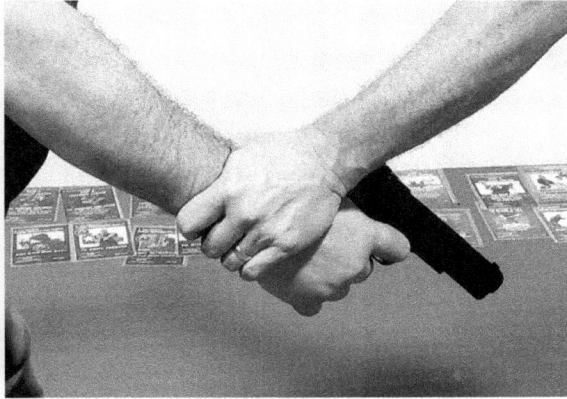

A "death grip" is defined as an extremely tight grip. But before you can grip, you have to grab. You have to catch. *Stop 2* covers the hand, stick, knife, gun catches and grabs on fingers, hands, wrists, and weapons. And importantly, their counters, escapes. The *Death Grip* grab I teach is related to Stop 2 progression is made of two components:
  1: the grab/catch and,
  2: the subsequent grip of your opponent's wrist area, hand and weapon itself.

You might have a great catch but a weak grip. You might have a tremendous grip but a weak catch. In all of the *Stops*, 2 through 6, a catch and grip is not a catch or grip without using your thumb. Your life depends on this, especially with a knife and pistol. All martial and even various sports training requires much catching skills and as much overall, hand gripping strength as you can muster. Exercises and drills that directly or indirectly increase such are vital. Almost all people immediately get this idea.

"If your grips fail, all your technique goes out of the window. It becomes hard to execute anything." - BJJ Coach Lawrence Griffith

All people get this? Well, not all. Decades ago, various, yet small group of famous martial artists would suggest not using your thumb in a capture of an opponent's limb. I stood in numerous seminars in the 1980s and 1990s hearing some martial instructors say this. Their small point usually being that your thumb or hand could be caught in some kind of lock and you would be supporting that capture with your full grip. As one famous JKD guy use to say,

"Rule of thumb? Don't use your thumb."

Huh? At first I mindlessly accepted that martial arts advice. But when I gave it a mere second thought? No. The bigger point? Minutes later when trying to stop and grip a stick or knife attack, I watched these same instructors all unconsciously demonstrate full hand grabs on the wrist or forearm. They fully grabbed limbs (and clothes) 99 percent of the time. I would see in seminars, mine and others, an unchallenged, playful catch or stop with just a curved hand, sometimes called a "monkey paw" with the thumb beside the fingers. NO! This no-thumb-helping move stops almost nothing and an attacker can move but an inch and instantly swoop under the curved hand to hit, stab or shoot. The proper, c-clamp thumb grip, stops this. Look at grabs in the UFC fights. Thumbs used.

Today, once in a while, I still hear this no-thumb, advice echoed around the world. It is down-line lineage advice and it takes a little "mental slap to the brain" to shake them out of it. Not using your thumb to grab is a thinking disorder mistake. When doing throws and takedowns you use your full grip. In ground fighting you use your full grip. And, these naysaying instructors ignore their own advice 99 percent of the time. (They too, have to fully grab at times and don't even realize they are violating the no-thumb rule.)

The Four Ways
In *Training Mission One* and all the courses, I list the four ways a human limb attacks you, hand, or with holding a stick or a knife, as they relate to catching as in not hurting your hand, and maintaining a grip after the catch.

> **1: A thrusting motion.**
> **2: A hooking motion.**
>   (Delivered either as a-)
> **3: A hit and retract, or...**
> **4: A committed lunge.**

It will always be hard to catch a thrust or hook, sure, but all kinds of untrained and trained people do in crimes and fights, when fighting trained and untrained people. But more importantly, look at the last two on the list. The hit and retract and committed lunge.

The hit and retract is a natural counter to a grab as it snaps back, and very difficult to seize. We have drills for that.

Some notes on the Catch and Subsequent Grip Alignment. Many experts tell us to align with the forearm as much as possible. The palm strike, when thrusting, is called the palm heel strike because it can align with the forearm.

In karate and various striking systems, they tell us to align the top two knuckles with the forearm. Folks suggest getting a pistol grip that aligns with the forearm, even though we can't always shoot that way. In an Army gym decades ago, a power lifter told me to bench press using the bar on my palm heels as much as possible. You push a car with your palm heels, not your fingers. It is a good idea to practice for that sort of alignment with a catch, to save your thumb from hyper-extensions and worse. Other steps like this are accomplished in sports and you can develop this movement too. We have drills for this.

In upcoming, *Stop 2* segments we cover the hand, the stick, the knife and the gun, catch and grab specifics, pros and cons. And their counters/escapes! Need we list all the exercises for grip strength here in this introduction essay? I hope not, because so many exercises develop it. Simple weight lifting improves your grip strength, even though you think you are working some other body part. Just search around for the strength experts and exercises.

"The trouble is, grip training often requires equipment that's not available in mainstream gyms. No worries, serious hand training isn't out of reach. Anyone can build a tremendous grip without devoting a whole lot of extra time to it, or relying on any equipment beyond a basic pull-up bar." - Al Kavadlo, TNation

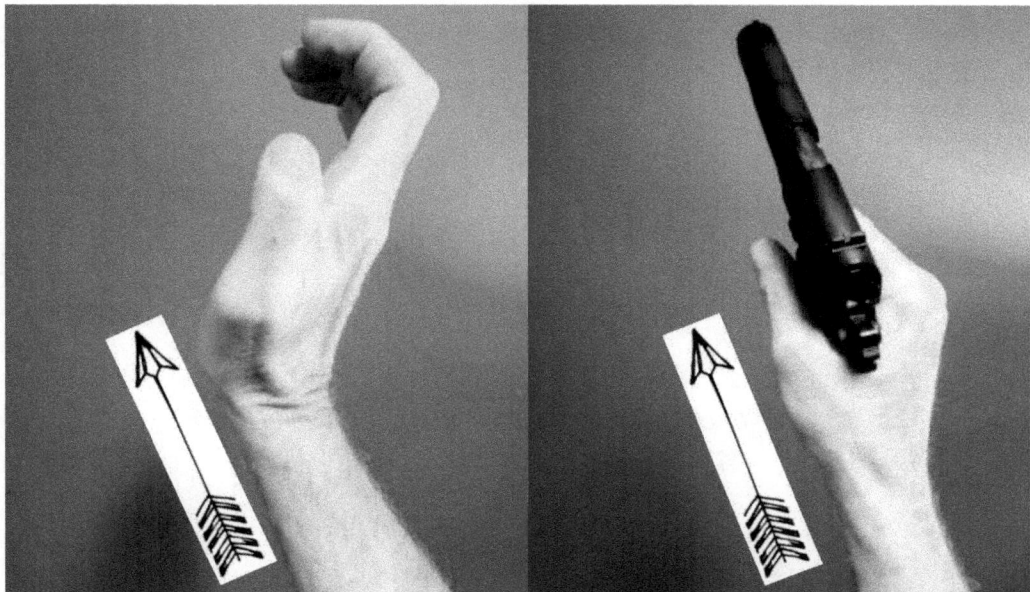

Heel-palm and forearm alignment. Palm strikes, pistols, punches, bench presses, car pushing, etc. We are even often mindlessly advised to align the handgun with our forearms, even though many possible shooting positions won't allow for this and require a bent wrist.

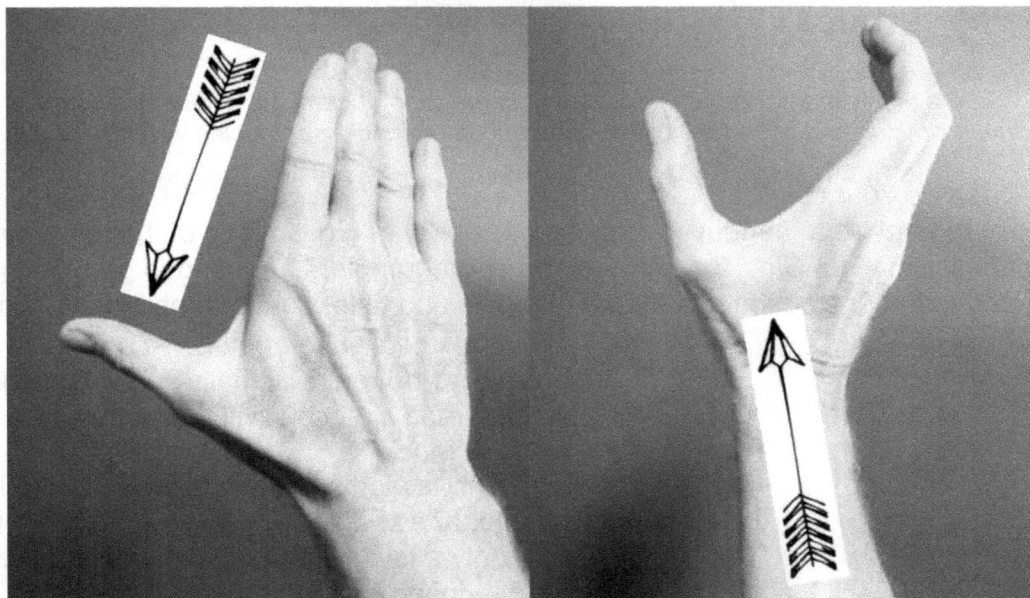

A "flagging thumb" can be injured in a catch/grab attempt. Try catching with forearm alignment.

Death grips on retaining your weapons and those grips on his weapon bearing limbs
Before we detail the specific stick, knife, pistol and long gun retention tips of holding your weapons with a strong grip, I wish to mention it generically here in the opening common-alties section because it is important. I don't think this is mentioned enough in training. Grips and grabs are often held poorly and haphazardly in practice, which carries over to reality use. A strong grip on a weapon can simply stall and/or stymie a weapon disarm. A strong grip can be a fundamental counter to a disarm.

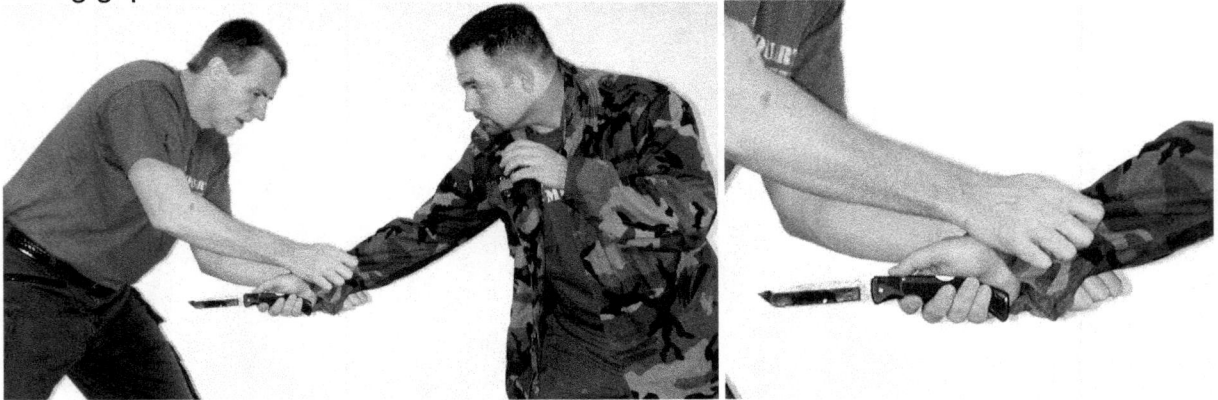

You think you got something, but you didn't.

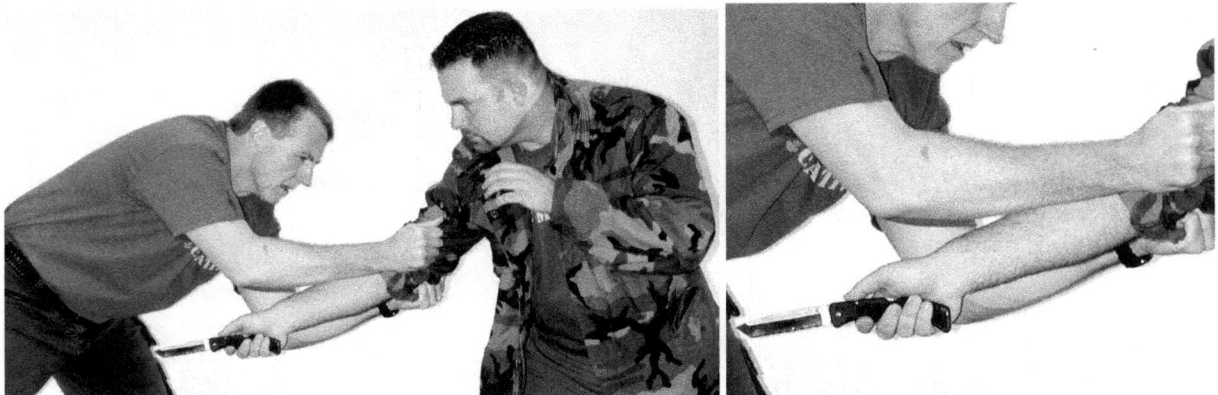

This is a highly dramatized demonstration. In the case of grabbing a knife limb, and getting too much clothing and not enough flesh and bone, there might be troubles with the loose clothing.

How "Deep" is Your Grip?
It is easy to forget the maneuverability and flexibility of the clothing of the opponent when grabbing his limb in a *Stop 2* depth. Art and sport grapplers are used to grabbing gi-uniforms and experiencing the movement, the give and take a uniform and in the *Stop 2*

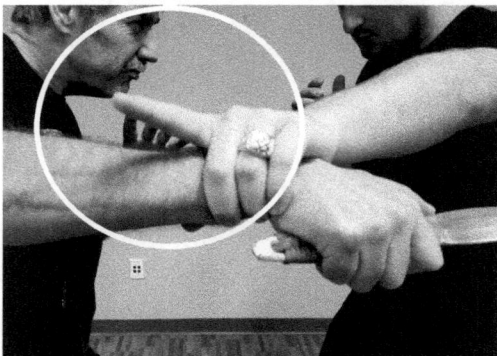

situation, the sleeve of the wrist and forearm area. Are you really, actually seizing/catching the limb? Or the clothes? Will the clothes move? If so, how much?

There is also an utterly ridiculous, stupid, unsafe, artsy habit of gripping aggressive limbs with only a few fingers. It's play-acting. If you are lucky enough to grab an aggressive limb? Save your life and USE ALL YOUR FINGERS!

CHAPTER 4: SUBJECT TO GRABS? OVER-EXTENSIONS AND FADE-AWAYS

Grabbing limbs and getting limbs grabbed. It's *Stop 2,* shop-talk. In *Training Mission One* we covered the four ways a hand strikes (and a foot kicks too!) This includes a hand holding a stick or a knife, delivering an attack. Review this yet again here!

> 1: A thrusting motion. Any straight line attack, hand, foot, stick or knife.
> 2: A hooking motion. Any attack off of a straight line to a complete hook, hand, foot, stick or knife. (Delivered by...)
> 3: A hit and retract. The attack goes out and efficiently returns back to as covered and balanced a structure as possible, hand, foot, stick or knife.
> 4: A committed lunge. The attack goes a little or a lot off-balance, providing extra power but extra exposure. Or, the attack lands and fades off to 12, 3, 6 or 9 o'clock quarters, and does not efficiently return to cover or balance, hand, foot, stick or knife.

A thrusting attack or a hooking attack can be delivered via a hit and retract, or via a committed lunge. If your hand, limb or weapon is "out there" too long? It is subject to a grab. A hit and a quick retraction gets the hand back. A committed lunge tends to linger in grabbing range. I am not suggesting that you never commit to a power shot that engages a bit of over extention, I am just suggesting you should be aware of what you are doing.

My purpose in mentioning this here in *Stop 2* is strictly concerning limb grabbing and being grabbed, not an essay on efficient power striking. Just grabs. Subsequent *Training Missions* will cover hand striking, kicking, stick and knife strikes, even striking with a pistol and long gun, and trying to hit that balance, recovery and maximum power.

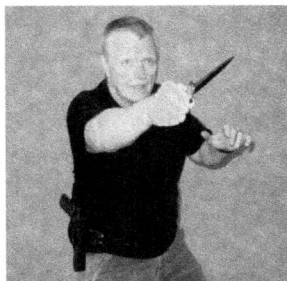

A thrust. Straight line.   *A hook. Curved line.*   *A hit and quick retract, be it a thrust or a hook.*

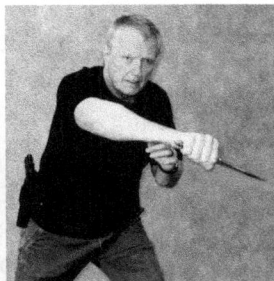

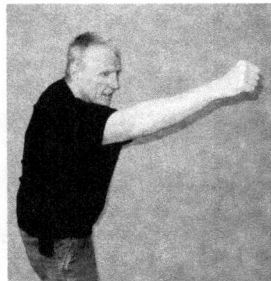

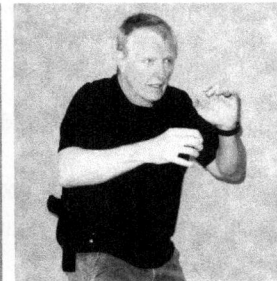

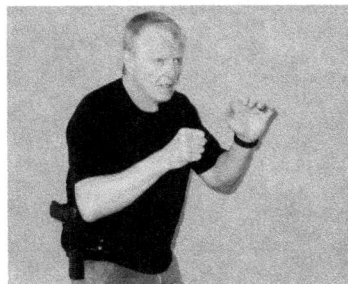

A committed lunge, be it a thrust or a hook. It may well be extended too far and may cause exposed arms and body lean imbalance. Missed targets can cause this imbalance and over-extended limbs.

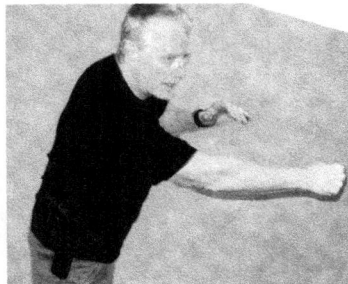

There is much to present and review in this subject, through the hand, stick, knife and gun levels as we progress in these courses. But for now, a theoretic point is a hit and retract imperative can get your limb away from a grab, when standing.

A hit and retract motion is essentially, a natural, "yank back" release from a grab

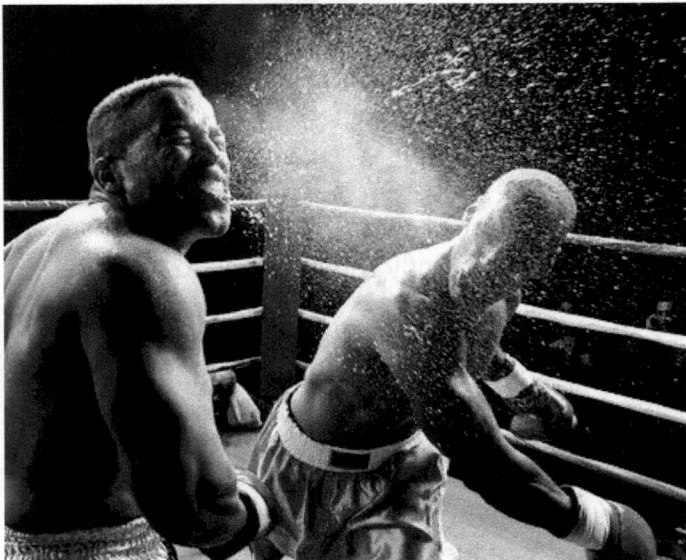

Here is a fully committed, hook punch, "fading-off" way to the side, with q torso lean and still, VERY successful!

attempt or a successful grab. A hit and retract is a bult-in, natural counter attempt versus a grab attempt.

I am not suggesting that a committed, unbalanced lunging strike is always a bad thing. They can be powerful. Fighting history is replete with such successful "over-strikes" and unbalanced seconds.

A question that comes up in seminars when I raise this issue is "but, we are always told to "punch *THROUGH* the person?" I reply with - "define through. How through is through?" This will discussed in great detail in *Training Mission Five* and its bare knuckle punching section. We are sticking with the grab-only subject here in this progression.

A study of knockout punches in MA, boxing, Thai etc., reveal a lot of oddball, off-balance positions, yet still very successful. Performers have to "chase" moving targets. As I wrote in *Training Mission One*, a so-called "fighting stance" is really about balance and power in motion and you will become unbalanced in unarmed and mixed weapon fights and with all sports too, and you should try to regain your balance as quickly as possible. Often the solution is footwork and hit and retract strikes.

     1: *Footwork* to keep and/or regain balance and,
     2: *Hit and retract* strikes to get your limbs and weapons away from grabs.

Exposed? Over-extending strikes, be it a stick, a knife hand, or a firearm, or over-extending your stance, is a risk, as in holding your hands out to far, too long, or holding your weapons out too far, for too long, makes them susceptible to a grab.

His Exposure? Worry about this for yourself but also consider your enemy. Are his forearms, wrists, or hands in reach? Are his weapons like a stick, a knife hand, a pistol, or a long gun in reach? Grabbable?

CHAPTER 5: FOOTWORK DRILL #2 – IN AND OUT

Either the left or right foot remains on the center axis while the other foot travels in and out. This keeps the fighter in closer. He moves out a bit, then back in. Right foot in and out, evading a hand, stick, or knife attack. The left foot remains in the center. The lead right foot moves from about 2 o'clock to about 5 o'clock and then back to 2 o'clock again. Rather then shuffle away and shuffle back, this keeps you closer. Switch sides.

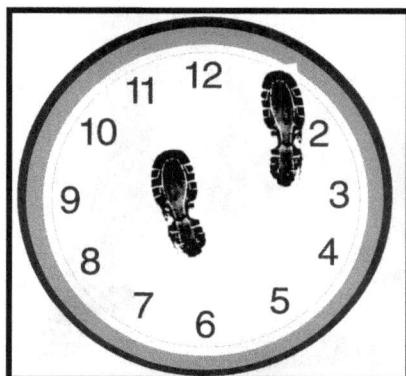

1: Right foot lead start.

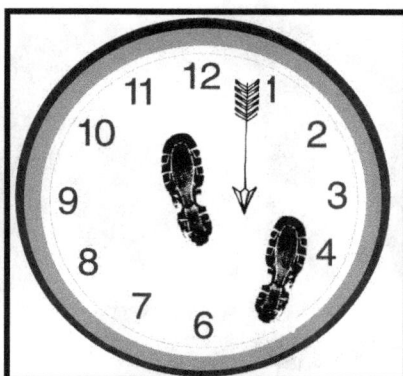

2: Step back to 5-ish.

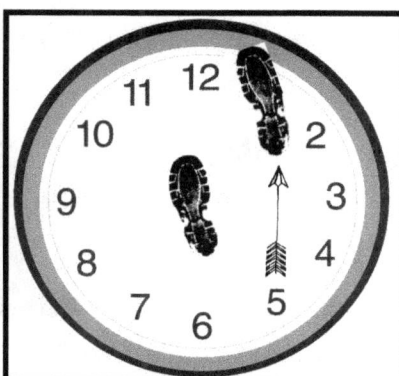

3: Step forward to 2-ish.

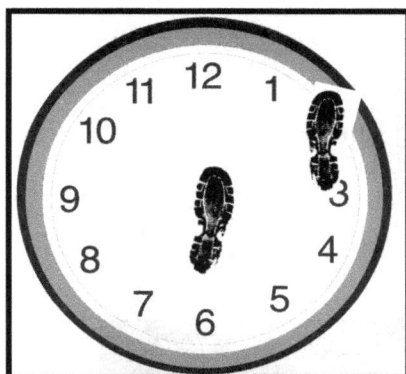

1: Left foot lead start.

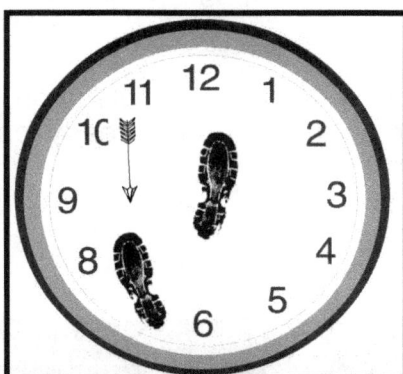

2: Step back to 8-ish.

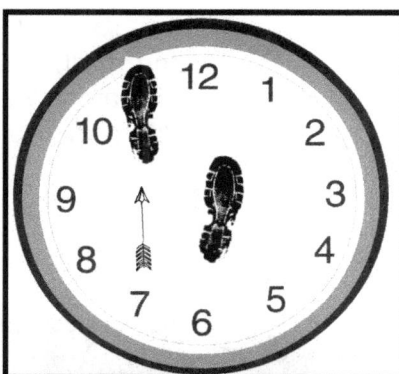

3: Step forward to 10-ish.

Here is a sample of a right foot in-and-out step. The left foot remains. You can step out and right back in. You do not lose ground because the left foot remains. Obviously do the same with the left foot.

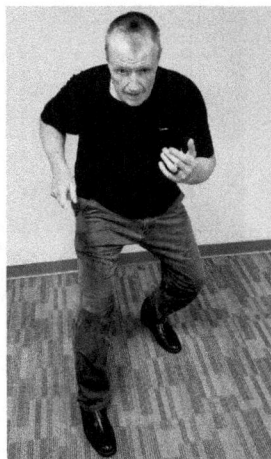

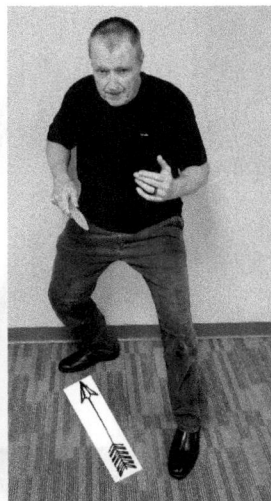

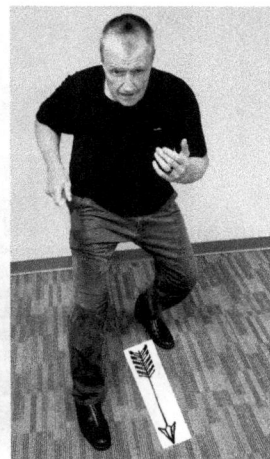

One foot up front, then back, then up front again. In and out.

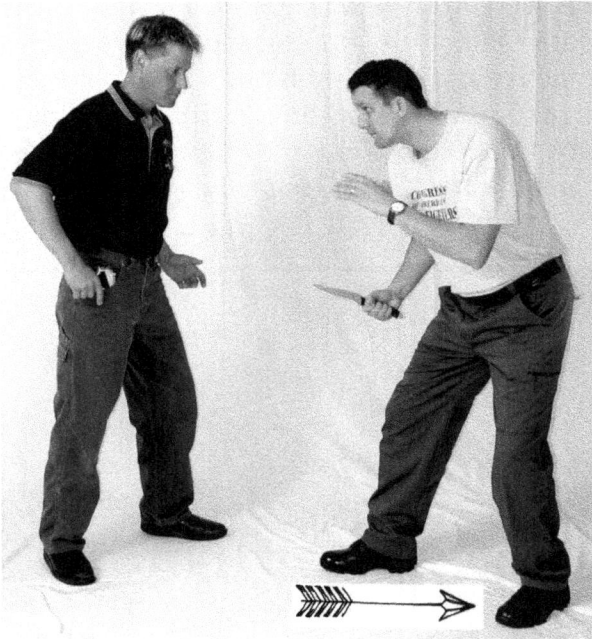

The in and out step, forward or back, right or left foot is done, and should be practiced:

- Unarmed.
- With a drawn pistol, knife, or a stick/baton.
- With a dismounted and/or up and ready long gun.

Suggested reading...

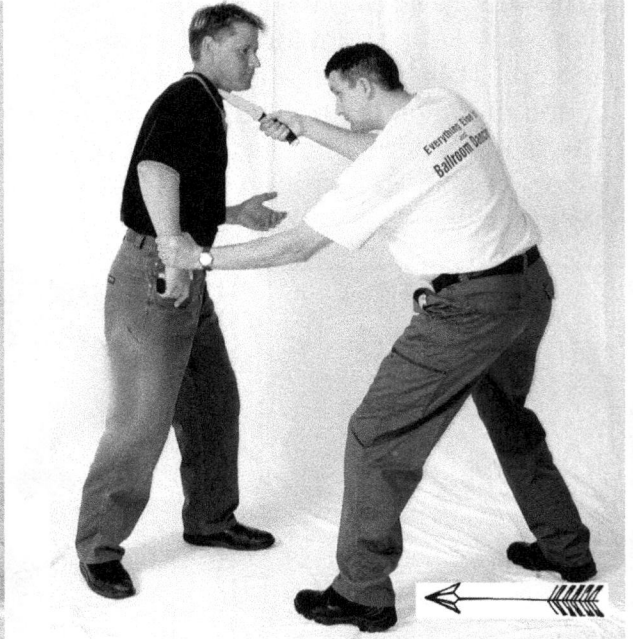

CHAPTER 6: THE STALKING CONTINUES WITH THE MAD RUSH DRILLS

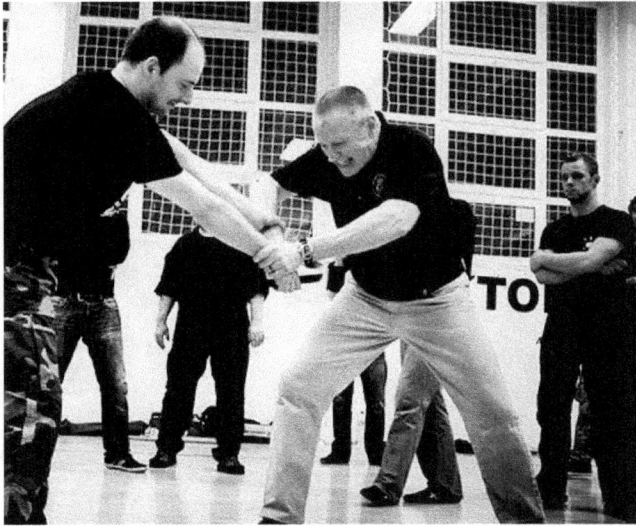

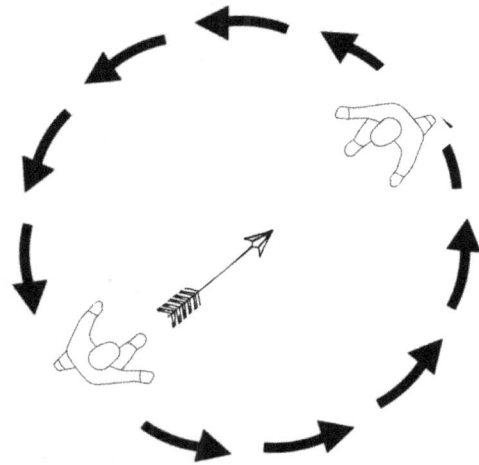

The Stalking Drill continues from *Training Mission One*. Remember, it begins with the idea that when the suspicious person starts to move around and/or position you you must react. You stay away, with some available distance. In the drill, we start with circling. He moves to the right, you move to the left, and vice versa. Full circles, half-circle, Quarters. Back and forth.

For the purposes of *Stop 2* and hereafter, we introduce the Mad Rush inward charge attacks. As in *Stop 1*, the attacker/trainer, circles and then suddenly charges the trainee with *Stop 2* only problems. (It is good idea to start off most all combat scenarios with common, stalking circles, then Mad Rush attacks.)

Of course, not all stalks and mad rushes result in head on, *Stop 2* (or *Stop 2* thru *Stop 5*) collisions and the defined grabs. Some rushes are passed off to the right or left, with various connections to the lower and upper arm. In actuality, the main directions, options versus the Mad Rush, as practiced in upcoming, deeper *Stop 3* though *Stop 5* are:

Mad Rush direction 1: Attacker shoved off to the right.
Mad Rush direction 2: Attacker remains on the face-to-face, center line.
Mad Rush direction 3: Attacker shoved off to the left.

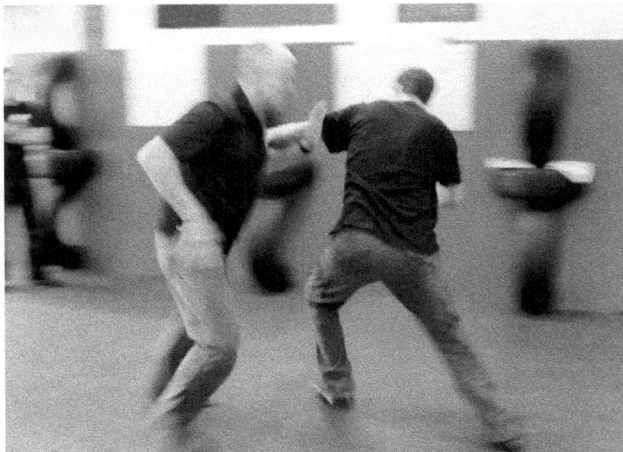

Of course, not all stalks and Mad Rushes result in head on, *Stop 2* (or *Stop 2* thru *Stop 6*) collisions and the defined grabs of *Stop 2*. Some rushes are passed off to the right or left. This passing-off, as done in many sports, should be practiced and we will officially cover in *Stop 4*. But in this subject matter, we are experimenting with rush and grabs.

For the purposes of *Stop 2* study only, to develop these skills within these parameters, the trainer can charge in and only:

- intertwine fingers.

- grab at hands.

- grab at wrists.

- grab at sheathed, holstered knives, sticks, pistols and long guns.

- tries to draw a stick and trainee interferes.

- trainee grabs a drawn stick in some manner.

- trainer tries to draw a knife and trainee interferes.

- trainer holds a knife, trainee grabs the limb in some manner.

- trainer tries to draw a pistol and trainee interferes.

- trainer holds a pistol, trainee grabs it in some manner.

- trainer holds a bayonetted long gun, and the trainee grabs it in some manner.

- don't forget running some exercises where the Mad Rush trainer is shoved off to the right or left.

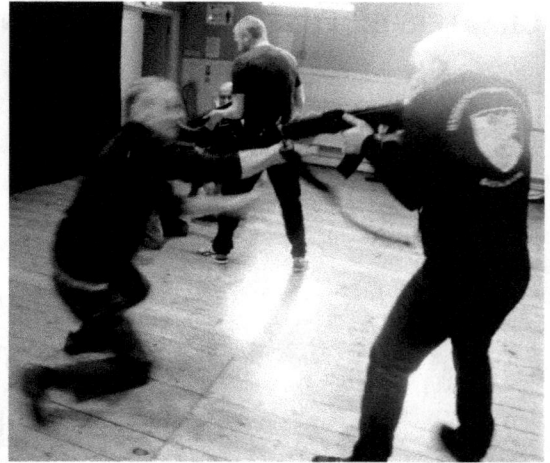

The solutions will be presented in the individual, following chapters. This subject matter is the universal backbone of all *Force Necessary Level 2* and *Stop 2* material. As your progress through this book, try this drill. When you finish the work of this book, the final exams will include this drill. Get good at it.

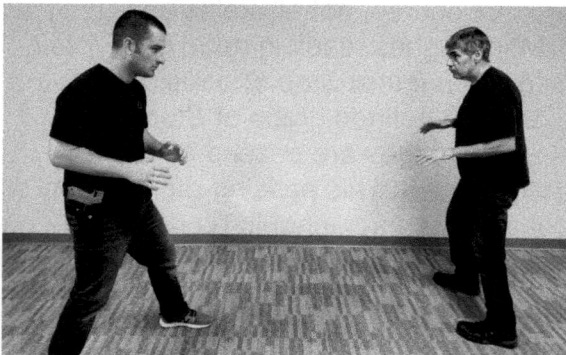

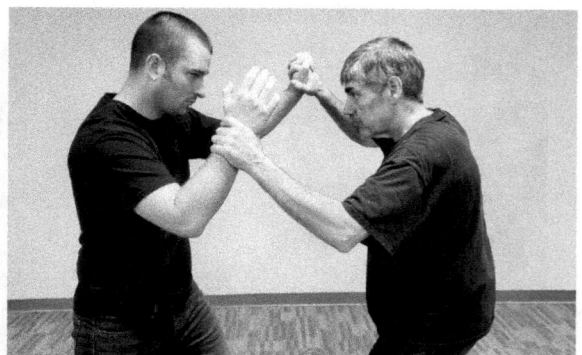

For the purposes of our Stop 2 study, the Stalk and Mad Rush drill will be about rushing into the hands grabs, with, without and against weapons.

CHAPTER 7: LOW-LINE TANGLER KICKS IN ALL STOP 2 PROBLEMS

When stuck *In the Clutches Of*, or *In the Death Grips Of*, one option is to set up (or perhaps even finish?) the problem is with lower-line kicks. One way to introduce the possibilities and drill the steps is through the Statue Drill that I so often use. The trainer stands, legs apart, with the trainer and trainee in the single or double grip situation and you practice kicking and targeting. The trainer and trainee can hold the assortment of mixed weapons.

With a single grip comes the probability that only one leg is within range. With a

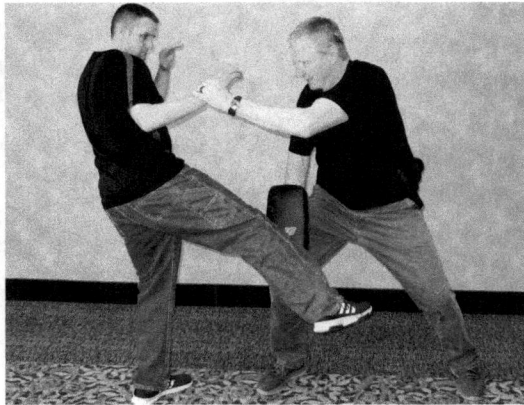

With a single hand grip comes the probability that only one leg is within range. Work against each lead leg.

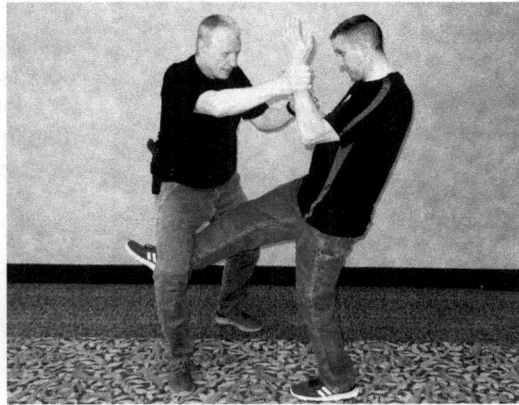

With a double hand grip comes the probability that in closer, both legs are rather "neutral'"and within range.

double hand grip comes the probability that both legs are within range.

Which kicks?
Use only those appropriate for the distance. Experiments prove that the following kicks are achievable in *Stop 2.* In the *Force Necessary: Hand* course Level 1 and here in Level 2 we cover the frontal snapping kicks and stomp kicks. The next few levels will get these other two kicks officially and fully covered, but you can certainly still do them in this *Stop 2* category.
- low round kicks.
- stomp kicks.
- front snapping kicks (shoes to shins, shins to groin).
- knees to knee and maybe thigh and groin.

Kicking
This might be just one kick or if possible, several kicks in *Stop 2* situation. The kick should be delivered as fast and as powerful as possible as all good kicks should be in a fight. If the trainer is holding a pistol, perhaps there is no time to kick! As the kicks are officially introduced in the hand, stick, knife and gun courses, we will reveal the details and individual drills as we progress.

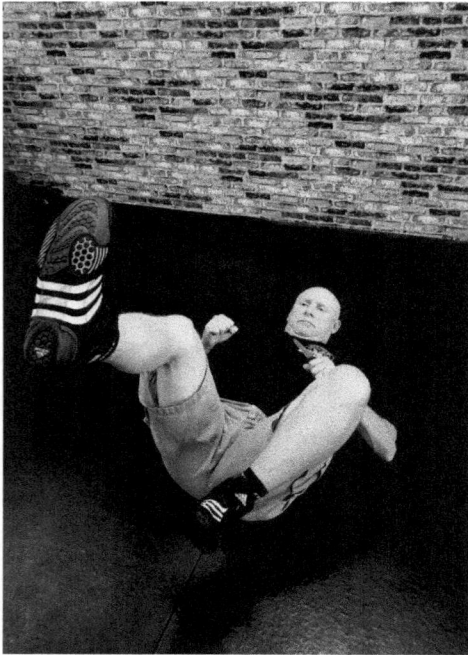

With, without and against weapons, the ground "stomp/thrust" kicks are useful. To the right is a push-pull takedown. More on this in the "Hand" course.

Suggested viewing...

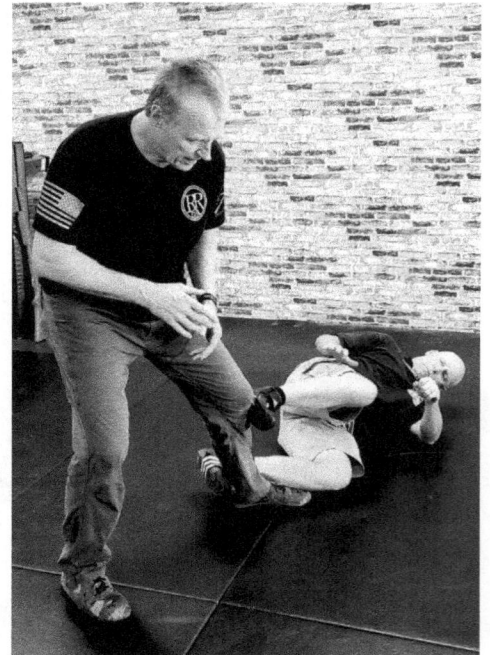

W. HOCK HOCHHEIM'S HAND, STICK, KNIFE, GUN

STOP 6
COLLISION COURSE

KICKS & COUNTERS TO KICKS
STOP 1 THROUGH STOP 6 ARENAS,
WITH OR WITHOUT WEAPONS,
AND AGAINST WEAPONS

APPROX. 2 HOURS

CHAPTER 8: LIMITED USE OF THE HEAD BUTT – A SERIOUS WARNING

Before we deep-dive into the hand, stick, "In the Clutches of" and "The Death Grip," - the knife or pistol formats and *Stop 2,* problem-solving, I would like for you to think about the head butt. Many people see the *Clutches* and *Death Grip* positions and think they can smash the crown of their head, (or even their *face* (Yes!) into the face of the opponent.) But, the other guy"s head moves and that perfect set-up is often not in place or position.

Your brain is jello in a bowl. It vibrates and splashes inside your skull and most people seek the brain splash that causes near knock-outs or knock-outs. When the "Jello" moves sudden and fast, it causes accelerated or decelerated injuries. These injuries can be obvious or be quite micro, accelerated or decelerated. That means if you suddenly bust out with a head butt, or receive a head butt, *your* brain still splashes.

Through the years I have seen a great many simulated head butts in training and they look so good. So cool, don't they? And we all know a few folks who like to do them at bars and other fights. They can all work so well. But they can work so well that they can work against you!

One of the biggest head butt proponents in the martial arts world, famous on the market place since the 80s and 90s, famous for "knees, elbows and head butts," has knocked himself out numerous times doing them...for real! Carried out of places by people I know personally. And...now? He is a known drug addict, a known thief, who at times babbles like a homeless street person.

I myself have brain damage, from 14 knock outs. Two boxing. Two kick boxing. Two car wrecks. Twice in baseball as a catcher, and the rest fighting/working as a police officer. I have sworn myself to warn practitioners of the cavalier attitude about head butts. God did not make your head to be an impact weapon. In fact we have been built to protect our heads. I suffer from several maladies as a result, and they can be unique person to person. This is a training book not a personal, medical history book. Ask me in person and I will tell you.

The latest research reveals that a full knock out is not necessary to add up your "knucklehead score." Now they claim that even little subtle head contacts add up. Have you noticed the UFC fighters that have quit? The UFC fighters that now limit their sparring workouts and harder contact training? Have you noticed whats going on in USA football?

Anatomy of a Head Butt

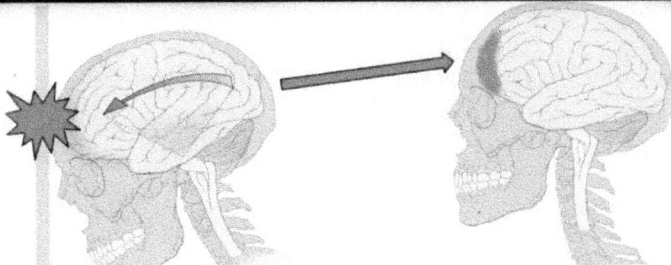

The brain is made up of soft tissue and is protected by blood and spinal fluid. When the skull is jolted too fast in any direction, or is impacted by something, the brain shifts and hits against the skull.

While I am compelled to make this anti-head butt warning, I am also compelled to say that the head butt might be a last-ditch, last resort tool to get out of trouble. If so, let it be the last, not the first option, You could be in a fight for your life and knock yourself out doing a stupid head butt. But I think we can all imagine a physical situation where all we have left is one. Steel yourself and do it as an option. But if there is ANYTHING else you can do? Please do that.

In the 2020 UFC fight, Conor McGregor broke Donald Cerrone's face with his shoulder, popularizing the move for the untrained world to see. Many people do have an option to shoulder smash a face rather than head butt a head in some situations.

There are even "slow-motion" head butts, like the "crown-crush" and other squashing and manipulating that *pushes*, not rams, your hard old skull slowly into the captured, anchored face of an opponent. You need your hands for a crown crush. Your hands will be busy in the stick, knife and gun courses, limiting the anchoring catch and hold.

Head butts have and can work. Really well. But often, I repeat, too well and also work against you. Watch out for the brain-moving impacts.

WHAT IS CONCUSSION?

Concussion occurs when the brain injured following a blow to the head or face

Concussion may occur without an apparent period of

unconsciousness. The signs and symptoms of concussion include any of the following:

• Loss of consciousness

• Loss of memory

• Confusion and disorientation

• Double or blurred vision

• Giddiness or unsteadiness

• Vomiting and headache

HOW CONCUSSIONS HURT

The human brain sits inside the skull with some room to move, surrounded by fluid-filled membranes. So when you take a knock to the head, your skull and brain don't move in tandem.

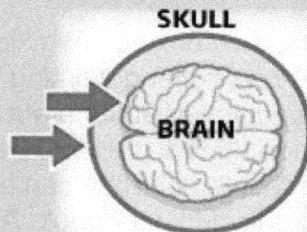

SKULL

BRAIN

A moving head stops suddenly

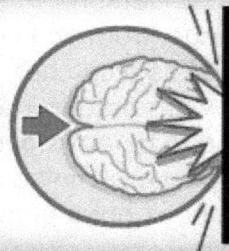

The brain compresses into the skull

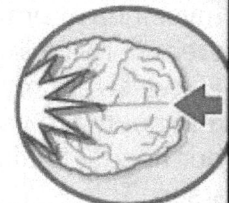

It can even compress again as it rebounds

Traumatic head injuries

A concussion occurs when a blow to the head results in the brain slamming against the skull.

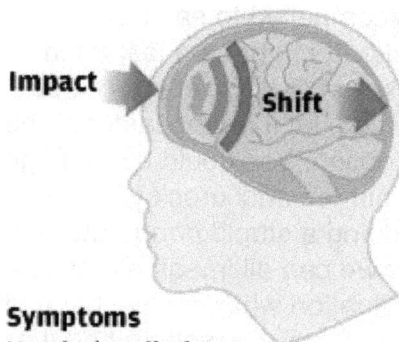

Impact

Shift

Symptoms

Headache, dizziness, confusion, nausea, difficulty hearing and seeing, lack of concentration

Concussion

Brain collides with skull, which can cause bruising, torn tissues and swelling.

Second impact syndrome

When a player who is not fully recovered from a concussion suffers a second blow to the head, it can be fatal.

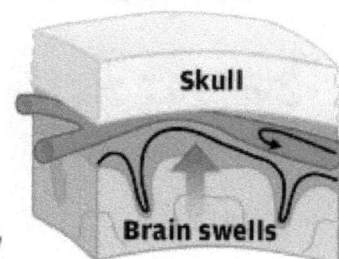

Skull

Brain swells

Blood flow

Massive swelling of brain

Cuts off flow of fresh blood to brain

SOURCE: American Academy of Neurology, U.S. Centers for Disease Control and Prevention, KRT

State Journal

There is much talk about "dirty boxing" and insider fighting and sneaky Thai tricks to get in unnoticed, illegal head butts. When these happen, they are repositories for us to see how effective they are within that situation. There are even videos on the Internet of fighters head butting and knocking both fighters out cold. Such is the consistant risk.

Legal Abstract from Combat Sports Law, January, 2020

"It has long been established that fighting sports such as boxing and mixed martial arts can lead to head injury. Prior work from this group on the Professional Fighters Brain Health Study found that exposure to repetitive head impacts is associated with lower brain volumes and decreased processing speed in fighters.

Current and previously licensed professional fighters were recruited, divided into active and retired cohorts, and matched with a control group that had no prior experience in sports with likely head trauma. This study examined the relationship between age of first exposure (AFE) to fighting sports and brain structure (MRI regional volume), cognitive performance (CNS Vital Signs, iComet C3), and clinical neuropsychiatric symptoms (PHQ-9, Barratt Impulsiveness Scale).

Brain MRI data showed significant correlations between earlier AFE and smaller bilateral hippocampal and posterior corpus callosum volumes for both retired and active fighters. Earlier AFE in active fighters was correlated with decreased processing speed and decreased psychomotor speed. Retired fighters showed a correlation between earlier AFE and higher measures of depression and impulsivity.

Overall, the results help to inform clinicians, governing bodies, parents, and athletes of the risks associated with beginning to compete in fighting sports at a young age."

One of tons of examples: "On April 9, 2017, Japanese wrestler Katsuyori Shibata head butted Kazuchika Okada during their match at Sakura Genesis 2017; the head butt was so hard that it caused the deliverer, Shibata to start bleeding from the forehead. After the match, Shibata collapsed backstage, from where he was taken to the hospital and diagnosed with a subdural hematoma, which is a traumatic brain injury."

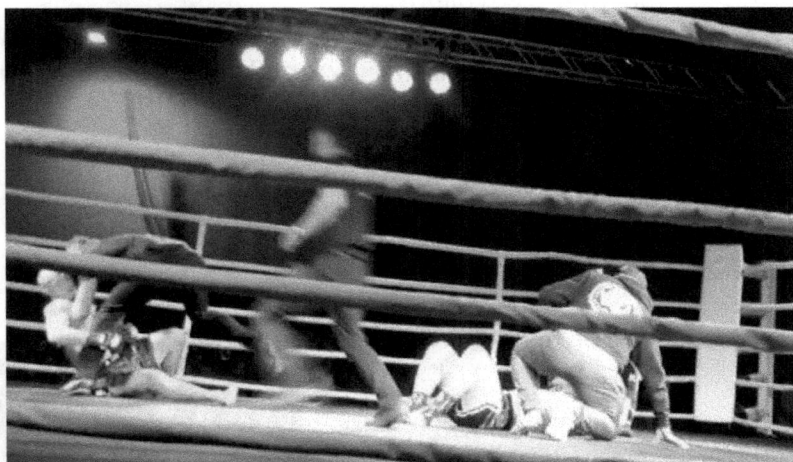

One of many head butt mishaps. Both kick boxers knocked out.

Outside of sports, I see many self-defense programs that emphasize head butts from painfully simple programs on up to the integration of add-on dirty, boxing methods into self defense fighting. In the moves you see a variety of light to hard, head-on-face, head-on-head strikes. I've seen courses where students also smack their faces into focus mitts as part of a simulation drill. Is this supposed to be a face-to face collision?

Of course, the skull, forehead and occular strikes are simulated! Instructors, practitioners remain too cavalier, quiet and/or ignorant about the actual, potential, short-term and long-term consequences of face, head and brain smashing. Short-term, you stun or knock yourself out in the middle of a fight for your life. Longer-term, you may have brain damage.

People usually laugh when I say, "God did not make your head to be an impact weapon."

I still use the term "limited use" of the head butt. I understand there might be times, positions and situations where that is all you have. If so, you must. Again, steel yourself for the prospect of self-stunning, which such steeling is at least rumored to help fortify yourself against unconsciousness. **Made4Fighters.com** reports: *"A study with high school football players found that for every one-pound increase in neck strength, the odds of concussion decreased by 5 percent. Take these findings with a grain of salt, because this study hasn't been replicated with boxers. However, it couldn't hurt to make sure your neck is in good health. You can do exercises with resistance bands to strengthen your neck at home or see a physiotherapist for specific recommendations. If you're new to neck exercises, it's best to consult a licensed professional before trying anything on your own."*

We will explore some of these limited uses and alternatives from pushing to crushing to striking, in *Training Mission 8* as the strike list develops in the *Force Necessary: Hand* course. I mention the subject here because it often seems irresistible to head butt when "In the Clutches Of" and "In the Death Grips Of." It's fun to mimic, and it might be mimicked too much, too cavalierly.

Suffice to say, you should try to avoid being hit by a hostile head butt when "inside," when too close. **Of course, they work.** When you do them, they work so well, they may work against you.

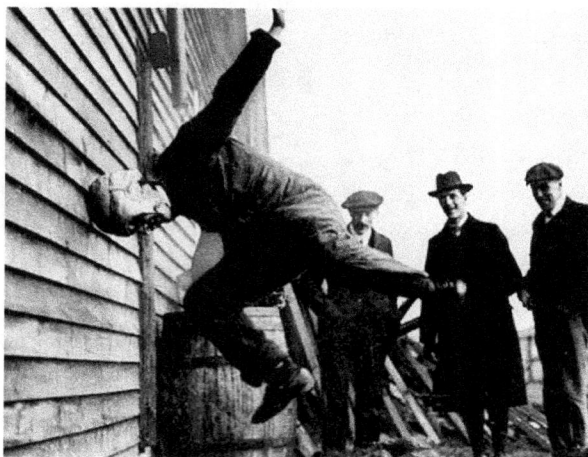

1912 Football helmet testing.

CHAPTER 9: TACTICAL BREATHING THROUGH LIFE, STRIKING AND KICKING

All medical and psychological experts agree that there is one common thread used to counter some of the anguish of anger, pain, and fear. Breathing! And that is a foundational solution. Then we will cover the idea that breath control when striking, as such, is also tactical.

The foundation, good breathing
Yes, simple breath control. No matter who the experts are, from the toughest, scarred, tattooed war vet to the armchair PhD or robe-wrapped yogi guru, or the collared Catholic, all agree that deep and slower breathing can really help control and stabilize the body under stress. You don't have to seek out a monk in China, pray to a god, or contemplate your navel in front of incense or a pink candle. This universal, raw method truly bridges the gap between the police, the military, the martial artist, and the citizen.

In today's mental health industry, *Stress Management* is a major challenge as well as a very prosperous business. Meditation is different. It is hard to meditate when someone is punching your face. For that industry, the majority of problems are marital, jobs, rush hour traffic, raising children, and the like. "Civilian-life problems."

Dr. Beth Greenberg says, "Stress. Unless you live on a heavenly cloud, you deal with it every day. Can you count the number of times you've heard or said, 'I'm completely stressed out!' in the past week? It's probably become routine. And routine, in fact, is what it is. Research has shown that over 70 percent of all doctors' visits are stress-related problems, and in a city the size of Boston, an average citizen has 60 fight-or-flight responses to stress every day!"

"Sixty!" What? That's hard to swallow but there is some stress in most folk's lives. We all have sudden and slow-burning stress problems that involve distorting our bodily chemistry. We all have "before, during, and after" stress problems. But a training and treatment doctrine that includes routine violence and combat is far more complex than for a citizen in Massachusetts or London, England.

Citizens in "everyday life," and soldiers and police have different kinds of stress because in their everyday lives, this "during stress" may be incoming missiles or a butcher knife plummeting down at ones face. Even in most planned and prepared combat, you turn a corner? And boom! You are in sudden combat inside the planned combat. Murphy's Law, etc.

What do all these people feel in their bodies when they get anxious or threatened? Here is, once again just for the record, just for the novice, the classic list. "Rapid heartbeat, shallow, rapid breathing. Tense muscles. Physiological changes take place in the body. The brain warns the central nervous system. The adrenal glands produce hormones (adrenaline and noradrenaline). The heart beats faster. Breathing becomes more rapid. Fast breathing. The person's body is getting ready to do one of two (or more) simple things, confrontation or departure."

Back to this very critical term of "fast breathing," because breathing is the key subject to this report. A normal breathing rate for an adult at rest is 8 to 16 breaths a minute. Most people are not really conscious about their breath count or the way they breathe, but generally there are two types of breathing patterns.

1. Shallow, rapid thoracic (chest) short breathing.

2. Deep or diaphragmatic (abdominal) breathing.

The stressed body needs oxygen, and we need to pump oxygen to the performing muscles. Slow-twitch fibers affect muscle endurance provided enough oxygen is delivered to them. Fast-twitch fibers, which affect muscle strength, develop peak tension quickly and fatigue easily. That is one reason why slower nasal breathing, not fast mouth breathing often works better. Nasal breathing runs by the vagal nerve, which sends calming messages to the brain. Breathing through the mouth bypasses a large portion of the nasal cavity process of warming, moisturizing, and eliminating particles from the air before it reaches the respiratory system. Breathing through the mouth also further triggers the fight or flight response! Sort of a double-whammy, if you will.

Numerous police and military people call this wrestling with breath under stress a "Combat Breathing Event." A singular event? Combat breathing to me should cover an overall bigger "event," as in the "before stress, during stress and while-it's-happening stress categories."

I do like the overall term "Tactical Breathing" used by many, for the before, during, and after. Three parts to it. Three "events." This allows us defined measures for each phase. Combat Breathing should be a sub-category under Tactical Breathing. (Remember, good training programs are all about doctrine, doctrine. Doctrine! Words. The proper skeleton allows for the proper fleshing out.)

Tactical Breathing (three parts)
1. Before the event – preparation breathing before the event
2. During – the combat breathing, hardest to remember to do because you, after all, are distracted.
3. After – breathing after the event to recover

Because Combat Breathing means breathing *WHILE* in combat. For many real performance experts, combat breathing is just in the "act of doing." Doing what needs doing with what you have on hand to do it with. Human kinetic sciences say that good breathing techniques bring the mind and body together to produce some amazing feats on the sport field. Feats well beyond the subject of simple calming and relaxing. Power!

During the fight! Athletes must learn to apply the *laws of pneumatics*, the science of pressurized air, in this case, as a power source by absorbing and transmitting energy in a variety of sports' situations. Most commonly, we know about the exhale when you say, for example, push up in a bench press. Exhale, if you can (as sometimes you can't) when you punch or strike. Firearm shooters and combat shooters (snipers or otherwise) constantly worry about breathing during their trigger pull, but in the chaos of combat, you have to strike or shoot when you have to shoot. Breathing pace often be damned.

So, deep breathing. The only problem is ... remembering to do it inside the fight! It seems that fast breathing is a dirty trick in the biology of survival, doesn't it? It is so easy to forget to breath when the knife is dropping onto your face. But still you must try.

What about breathing before the anticipated fight? Remember, not all fights are ambushes. Here is a trick I learned decades ago from police instructors in the 70s, and one I continue teaching to emergency response folks. I would suggest connecting this type of breathing every time you turned on your police car, ambulance, fire truck sirens or answer any "hot call." Hot calls equal calming breaths. When you hear the siren? Start the proper breathing right then.

Another trick I noticed was no matter what great shape I was in as a younger man, how far and fast I could run in miles, yet often when I dashed up a flight of stairs at the police department or elsewhere, I would still become winded. I could run about a 6 or 7 minute mile, but a sudden, short dash up the stairs would bother me and my breath!

"What good does all this running do when I can't dash up a flight of stairs?" I'd ask myself, at the top of the stairs.

But it is a classic "zero-to-60" situation. I swore then that I would slow/deep breathe every time I climbed any stairwell anywhere. A habit. Every time I looked at a stair step I made it a personal habit. This turned into a major survival tip as we chase and even fight on stairs frequently. Climb any stairs anywhere? Deep breathe. (And, of course, you could run stairs as a workout, another testimony to practicing exactly what you need to do, reducing the abstract).

Responding to emergencies, climbing stairs or crossing the street, the point is to pick a good time to breath like this and make that practice an engrained habit.

Also, for many years I ran a local martial arts class. Often I would have to spar/kick box every student in the class. This was demanding; however, I discovered within myself a certain, calm zone of performance where I could think, coach, and kick box everyone rather tirelessly! I "recorded" a calm spot in my physiology. This zone. Whatever you call it. I could often find this very spot under police stress and confrontations, too. In a way some might call this a biofeedback method (yet another subject I'd like you to research).

Extended and serious exercise usually starts demanding fast lung work, and we find ourselves falling into shallow, mouth-breathing mode. The better shape we are in, the more we push back the problems. Wind sprints are another way to introduce your body to and get in touch with your physiology while it grapples with rising and falling heart rates.

Know where you are and how you feel and think about breathing while wind sprinting. Long-term breath control? Exercise. I repeat and re-shape the above exercise for it is a most important point.

The better shape we're in, the more we push back that falling-apart, disaster crash. Get up and get out and do something. It helps in so many more ways that simple slow breathing cannot alone. If you are having a heart attack while fighting off a criminal or a Jihadist, slow breathing ain't gonna' help you much. Develop both heart and lung capacity. And strength.

Once in "combat," you have a lot going on, and your body wants to immediately breathe a certain way. You make it breathe your way. The best way you can. Good instincts. Good training. Good coaching. Good mental tricks. Good luck. A car going zero-to-60 in seconds becomes difficult to control.

Technically, tactical breathing goes like this. Breathe in through the nose for four or more counts. Deep into the lower lung and the upper "belly" should expand, unlike a shallow breath. Hold for four or more counts; exhale through the mouth for four or more counts. So simple, so respected. So proven, from Lamaze to Basra. It works. For the record, U.S. Military training manuals describe this advice and process:

After the event? Get your act together! Breathe! Get rid of the hand quivers. Assess. Drink some fluids too if you can. You might have an adrenalin dump to filter through.

"Combat, Tactical" Breathing Steps

This technique, known as combat or tactical breathing, is an excellent way to reduce your stress and calm down. This breathing strategy has been used by first responders, the military, and athletes to focus, gain control, and manage stress. In addition, it appears to help control worry and nervousness. Relax yourself by taking three to five breaths as described.

- Breathe in counting 1, 2, 3, 4
- Stop and hold your breath counting 1, 2, 3, 4
- Exhale counting 1, 2, 3, 4
- Repeat

Pneumatics while striking and kicking
Pneumatics (From Greek: πνεύμα pneuma, meaning breath of life) is a branch of engineering that makes use of gas or pressurized air and properly releasing it for power and energy. And our concern here is about air. The air we suck and shove out of out lungs.

For most people, they relate this process with exercising. Like lifting weights. When starting out, they ask - "Why when lifting weights when do you exhale?" The usual expert answer sounds like - "the general prescription for breathing during exercise is inhalation during the eccentric portion of said exercise, and exhalation during the concentric phase. To give an example using the barbell bench press, inhale before lowering the bar to the chest, and exhale when you are pushing the weight away from you."

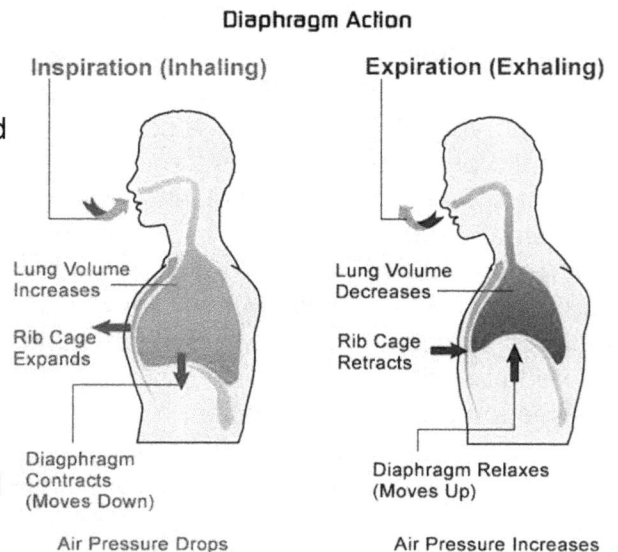

Diaphragm Action

Inspiration (Inhaling) — Lung Volume Increases — Rib Cage Expands — Diagphragm Contracts (Moves Down) — Air Pressure Drops

Expiration (Exhaling) — Lung Volume Decreases — Rib Cage Retracts — Diaphragm Relaxes (Moves Up) — Air Pressure Increases

Still, why do it? Experts use the word "bracing," and explain, "Breathing is cyclical pressure changes in the thoracic cavity allowing for gas exchange in the lungs. Whereas, bracing is the co-contraction of the abdominal musculature that completely encases the abdominal cavity to provide active stability to the trunk and spine."Regular breathing is relaxed and not "bracing." For bracing to occur optimally we must stiffen the trunk and spine." People playing most sports are inherently familiar with the feeling. You can certainly research all this and the definitions and medical jargon is all there for you, if you are interested.

How does this play in the martial world? It might be easy to compare bench press ideas with a punching ideas and you have grasped the concept. But here is a bit deeper look at this by a modern pioneer in martial arts, kettlebells and fitness Pavel Tsatsouline.

"Vinogradov explained the strength increase from straining with excitation of intero-, mechano- and chemoreceptors in the lungs and the abdominal cavity that increase strength via reflex action. The pneumo-muscular reflex has a profound effect on your strength. This neurological phenomenon can be compared to the amplifier of your stereo whereas your brain is the CD player and your muscles are the speakers. Special sensors in your abdominal and thoracic cavities register the internal pressure and adjust your muscular tension like the volume control knob. The higher this pressure, the greater your strength and visa versa.

The Valsalva maneuver is not the only way to up your strength by increasing the IAP. Vorobyev determined that both holding ones breath and groaning increase strength. Screaming is not bad either. According to Ikai & Steinhaus, subjects who shouted during exertion got a respectable 12.2 percent strength boost!" - Pavel Tsatsouline

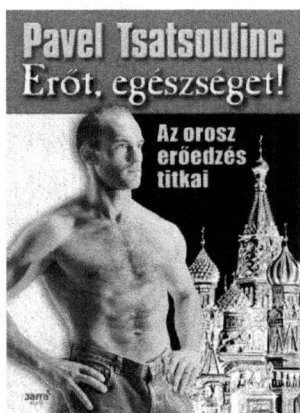

I can attest to "bracing yourself versus incoming body blows. A tightening of the torso with an exhale is important. As I was taught and tested in martial arts. one does not want to be hit while there's a lot of air in the guts, in and around the solar plexus.

On breathing and shooting
I am under my own strict, personal orders not to mention range marksmanship as I declared in *Training Mission One*. But, as a step-aside, on the overall subject of breathing, I will say that breathing is important for range, shooting bullseyes (and being a sniper or taking sniper style shots).

The NRA instructors will say - "Breathing while firing the shot hurts accuracy because it increases the movement of the aligned sights on the target (wobble area). The best time to control the breathing cycle is during what's called the 'respiratory pause.' This is when you're done exhaling, but it isn't something you should have to think about. Don't force air out, because forcing air out makes you contract your chest muscles… which is the last thing you want. During the respiratory pause, your chest muscles are relaxed, and you can stop breathing longer without feeling uncomfortable…"

What of these timed, competition events when shooters are running all over the range and rapidly shooting multiple targets? Are they following the shooters, breathing textbook? To some extent, I think they are, when they can.

Anyway, back on track…off the range, which *is* our bailiwick, we have to remember that most of us will not be taking these lots-of-time, controlled breathing "scoring/sniper" shots in real life. We will be in a fast moving, confusing situations. But each of us should be capable of making/taking that "hail Mary" shot. It has happened, it will happen, and if at all possible? Then breathe right!

Breathe!
Instructors and coaches should make sure their practitioners are breathing while working out. I've had a number of class people who, when engaged in a set or scenario, hold their breath the entire time. I am sure I am not alone. But the practitioners are distracted with the tasks at hand, and are not inhaling and exhaling. This distraction of course, is the same problem in the before, during and after of a real fight.

The American Institute of Stress explains…
"How stimulating your vagus nerve will help you…The vagus nerve (sometimes called the pneumogastric nerve) runs from your neck through to your diaphragm and is the 10th cranial nerve. Broadly speaking, it interfaces with the autonomic control of the heart, lungs and digestive tract.

So why is it important? When you exhale for longer than you inhale, our old friend the vagus nerve tells the body to rely more on your parasympathetic nervous system and less on your sympathetic nervous system.

What does that mean? Parasympathetic control your ability to rest and relax, whereas sympathetic control your in-built 'fight or flight' reflex. By stimulating your vagus nerve, you're specifically telling your body to relax you and not to send you into a panic. This is one reason why breathing techniques are so effective." - AIS

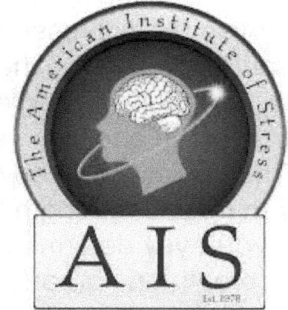

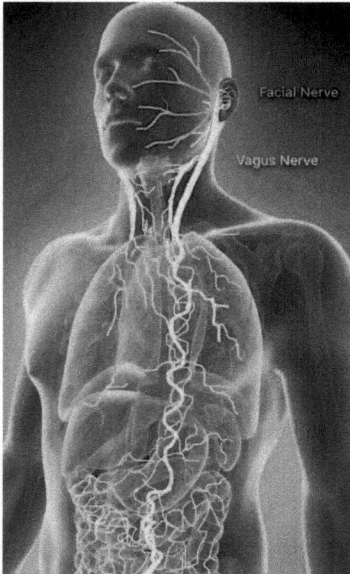

Facial Nerve

Vagus Nerve

In Summary

Tactical Breathing is three parts, the before, the during, and the post of fighting with hands, sticks, knives and guns. While there are some similarities to a meditative style of breathing, "tactical" breathing is not for the yoga mat. It is almost impossible to forget to breath properly in a meditation class. (well, okay, not for daydreaming me, but...). It's hard to remember when you are chasing a car at 100 miles per hour or fighting someone while sliding down a steep, muddy hill in the rain. (That happened to me so I thought I would mention it.)

The methods you use may be very personal discoveries. Generic in concept. Personal in execution. In the end, my friend? I want you to breathe the best breath of all, that sigh of relief when it's all really over and you are still in one "piece" and in one "peace."

Suggested reading...

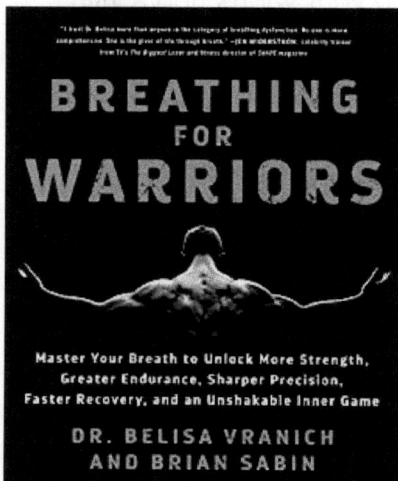

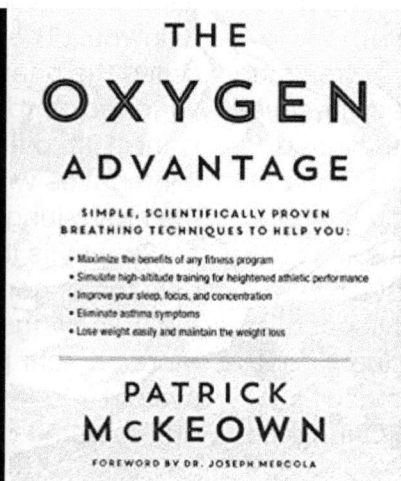

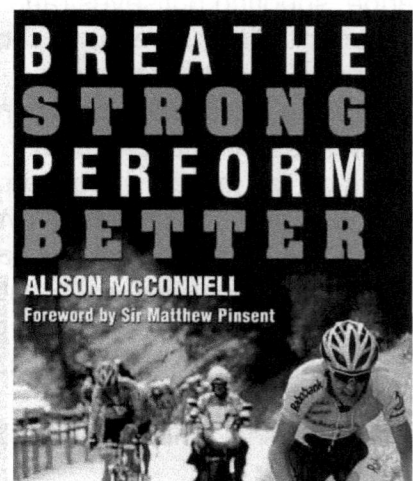

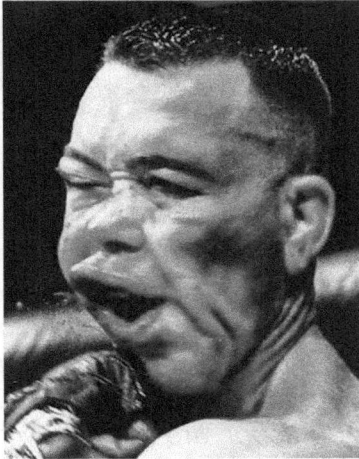

Colby Covington receives the broken jaw.

Loose lips may sink ships, but loose jaws lead to pain and medical operations. Or... How can we remember to close our mouths in the crimes and wars of life?

As the *Stop 6* collision series and the *Force Necessary* series continues here in *TM Two*, at this level we officially move in closer, start hitting hard and also being hit hard, and I feel this is a good time to formally introduce this subject. Breathing in fighting, (mixed with jaw position.)

One of my early detective cases in the 80s was to unravel a country-western, bar fight. About six guys were involved. Some were arrested on the scene by patrol. In patrol I/we sorted out the scene and rarely saw the aftermath. But investigators have to become aftermath experts. I caught the case because there were serious bodily injuries, otherwise it would just be another, unassigned, ignored, knucklehead fight passing through the system. Participants would bond out on simple misdemeanors and the disorderly conduct and bruises would fade away. But, sometimes there were serious bodily injuries. I hated to get these cases through time because they were always complicated and messy to – oh, what's the pop word today – oh yeah... "unpack." You know, who started it? Who hit who? It's a messy suitcase.

I set up an appointment for a statement with a mumbling knucklehead on the phone and he showed up at the station. I quickly saw why he was mumbling. His jaw was wired shut! He took a simple hook punch and crackola! Worse, the doctor had to knock out a tooth so he could suck squashed food through a straw. I thought the tooth removal was extreme, but I guess that's what they did decades ago. Make space for the straw. *Adios* premolar. He said he had to carry wire cutters in his pocket in case he vomited. And could like... drown in his own vomit. Talk about an emergency. He said he would be wired for almost two months.

Jaw wiring sounds and looks so bad I was surprised years later to see how many people have their jaws wired to loose weight (and how the modern docs avoid the old tooth removal idea). This diet is extreme, and people still need to have wire cutters very handy. A very common prognosis is 6 weeks wired up, depending on the fracture.

This was not my first or last jaw-broke arrest or some-such case, but I think it was my first "aftermath" interview with a broken jaw person. Through the years I worked numerous, "simple" punches in the face that turned into serious injuries cases, AKA felonies. I have many of these stories but for this chapter I am fixated on broken jaws.

"But eating is only part of the problem. There's also a strange claustrophobia that comes with having your jaw wired shut. Try closing your mouth and clenching your teeth together lightly. Now imagine that you can't move from that position – not even a little bit, not even for a second – for the next six weeks."- MMA champ Cub Swanson

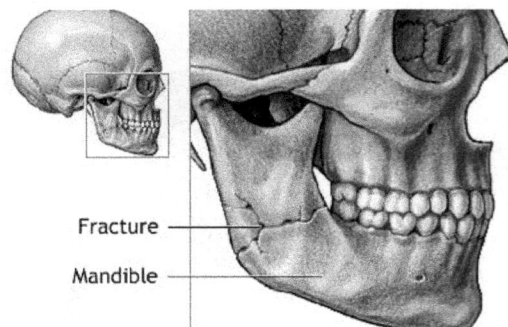

Fracture

Mandible

WebMD states that men are about 3 times more likely than women to sustain a broken jaw. The American Bar Association reports broken jaws come from:

Assault = 50 percent
Slip and Fall = 15 percent
Sport Related = 15 percent
Auto Accident= 10 percent
Other Activities = 10 percent

About 50 percent come from criminal assaults. I believe these US stats are also common in other countries from what I can find. United Kingdom emergency medicine studies state, "Mandibular fractures are the second-most common, facial fracture (after nasal fractures), representing up to 55 percent of all facial and skull fractures. They are most common in 16 to 30 year-old males, and are usually caused by direct force (e.g. physical assault) and motor vehicle collisions.

While people can be assaulted on the proverbial "streets," fights happen everywhere. Domestics in houses. Workplaces. Rec places …yes… country western bars, and some 50 percent of all broken jaws come from these types of attacks.

I always look to the laboratory of combat sports for great resource info. But, as in all sports, this is of course, why God made mouthpieces. (I tend to use the decades-old term mouth "piece" and not the modern term mouthguard. The term mouth piece today gets confused with lawyers, musical instrument parts and other stuff.)

Give me one moment of your attention as we run the classic facts. Stay with me now...

"Mouthguards are a low-cost way to protect the teeth, lips, cheeks, and tongues," the docs say. *The American Dental Association recommends wearing custom mouthguards for, are you ready, "the following sports: acrobats, basketball, boxing, field hockey, football, gymnastics, handball, ice hockey, lacrosse, martial arts, racquetball, roller hockey, rugby, shot putting, skateboarding, skiing, skydiving, soccer, squash, surfing, …"* - repeated by dental gear sales forces

Their advice ends in three "etc." dots, so there are even more hobbies that can't bother typing them all? Is sex in there? And we can't forget that even fighters with big gloves and mouthpieces still get broken jaws in the ring.

"There are three types of mouthguards. Stock, and boil-and-bite mouth guards are usually found in most sporting goods stores. Athletic mouth guards can vary in comfort and cost. A custom-made mouth guard fabricated by a dentist or orthodontist is considered by many to be the most protective option. The most effective mouth guard is resilient, tear-resistant and comfortable. It should fit properly, be durable, be easy to clean and should not restrict speech or breathing."

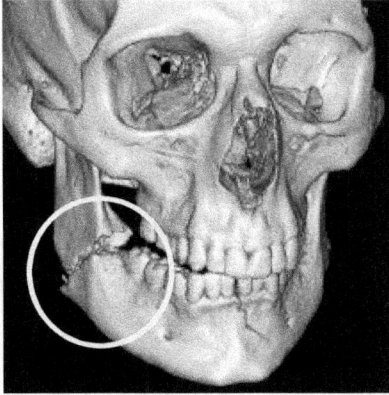

SISU says,

"Mouthguards can also protect others from your teeth. Even if it doesn't hurt you or you don't feel it, you can easily injure another player with your teeth. If another accidentally smacks their elbow on your teeth, it's highly unlikely for your teeth to break skin if you are wearing a mouth-guard."

Remember the stinky mouthpiece you've pulled out from your workout bag? I might add, a mouthpiece or two, usually quite nasty, can be found in all serious workout bags. We need to wash/sterilize them regularly, along with the container - another important health point.

We have officially covered the usually boring, safety and health briefing stuff! We are not playing soccer, but rather punch-ing, palming and elbowing and even kick-ing the lower parts of heads as a matter of routine. And we are being hit there too.

At the US Army military police acad-emy back in the early 70s, some boxer MP cops ran a boxing program off-hours and weekends to augment the official "combatives" at the academy. As a Parker Kenpo Karate guy, I signed right up. One coach handed me a little, new box with a mouthpiece in it and told me it'll save my teeth and would teach me to keep my mouth shut when fighting. I had been

doing all that sparring in Kenpo and no one brought up the subject of mouth pieces. Yet, in the karate tournament so yesteryear, such would be seen.

We have had a long history of confusing messages about mouthguards/mouth pieces and many other aspects of training. But when we are in non-sport combat, de-fending ourselves or others, we can be sur-prised, we'll shoot guns "cold," won't be wearing boxing gloves and we won't be on cushioned mats. It stands to reason, you won't be wearing a mouthguard when at-tacked. But you can practice in one and de-velop good, teeth-gritting, "muscle memory." What can we do about this?

In good theory, rep time wearing your mouthpiece should also reinforce your mis-sion to keep your jaw closed when fighting, which we all know is a key structure for jaw break prevention. In the fight world, the mouthpiece helps us, does teach us, re-quires us, makes us keep our mouths shut. Loose lips do sink ships, but loose jaws lead to medical operations. We would like to create the, dare I say "muscle memory" to keep our mouths shut in bare knuckle fights. But do we wear them all the time? Enough of the time, to create this habit? Do you?

People in the combat-sports-and-de-fense-business don't always train with mouthpieces in. Class after class covering methods in kick boxing, boxing, Thai, Krav, combatives, etc. have people doing tons of drills without their mouthguards in place, creating safer jaw habits. Copious amounts of all kinds of training is worked on and dur-ing so, few even think about their mouth po-sitions, their jaws at all, and least of all shove a piece in for every whole class. Watch any given Thai training film on YouTube, from Thailand and expected super sources and you will spot Thais with-out mouthguards, open jawed, hitting and kicking pads. When they fight they have mouthguards in. When they fight in the alleyway walking home, they have no mouthguards.

I was in a rather popular, international, Thai Boxing association in the 80s and 90s and passed the first 5 levels of 10. There was very, very little actual, interactive Thai boxing in the ring with this famous group, but rather several tons of end-less, mitt/pad work. This is more commonplace in today's world. There was no strict, organiza-tional rule about wearing a mouthguard in training drills. In fact, think about the sound effects you hear in Thai (or other fighting arts, too). With every strike, with every kick comes the

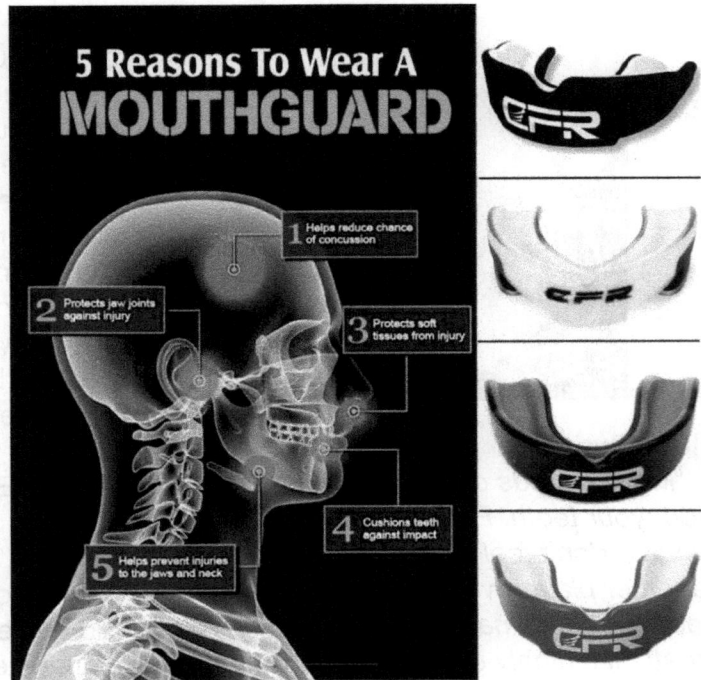

standard "whoosh" or swoosh" from pursed lips. Is the whoosh/swoosh is articulated, not muffled? Such articulation takes a little free mouth and jaw manipulation to produce. No mouthguards evidenced. Tons of class time sans the piece. If you hear a steamy "hissss," you might find a mouthpiece inserted. Instructors need to listen in.

What then about Jeet Kune Do? Wing Chun? Kempo? Combatives? How much time is spent working on a stand-off "duel" like two boxers, and doing entry tricks without an iota of concern, mention, a suggestion about your jaw position. What about stick and knife work?

Even US football players wear mouthguards, buried deep inside the best helmet that technology can produce. In fact I suggest that when you are in the market for a mouth guard you look to the new variety of football options, not the older, kuraty," ones.

With time sparring, you have time and grade wearing a mouthpiece and teaching your jaw to stay shut in a fight, even without a guard. But, it must be noted that breathing well and fully with a mouthguard is a constantly reported problem by many practitioners for all the obvious air, "passageway" reasons, and mouths tend to open. Jaws drop innocently for more air and from fatigue. Dangerous times to be slugged! It stands to reason, you won't be wearing a mouthguard when attacked. But you can practice in one and develop good, teeth-gritting, "muscle memory."

As with the hiss-like sounds, you can still exhale air malevolently with a mouthpiece. When I hit or kick a heavy bag, or work strikes on cable machines, I try to remember to clinch my teeth and hiss, not ignore my jaw and maybe let it drop. Work to make the two parts, one part.

Think about this. Think of you. Think of your friends and classmates. Think about your school, organization. If you're not actually sparring, are you wearing a mouthpiece all of the time? Some of the time? Never? Do you practice for this? Or seemingly…ignore it? Is the idea ignored in your chosen course/school?

Are you? Is your school/course geared for self defense? Or art? Sport? The piece helps keep/train our jaws to be shut, like a prop, and secure when we are attacked in the "outside" world. In real life, we don't have or fight with mouthpieces. They just don't seem to be handy, huh? They are in a smelly little container in a smelly, gym bag somewhere. How does this spell out for you? We have to remember to close our mouths in the military and criminal assaults of our lives.

It's just something for you to think about. It's a topic practitioners should consider, discuss intelligently, and have an opinion on, one way or the other.

And this is my observation for the breathing, mouthguard and broken jaw connection.

(One quick, side story to finish up. I know a Russian bar bouncer in Australia who had a bouncer friend with a successful de-escalation trick. When the friend was having an elevated confrontation with a customer. The friend would put up one finger, reach into his pocket and pull out a mouthguard. He'd insert it. That act alone often quelled many disturbances.)

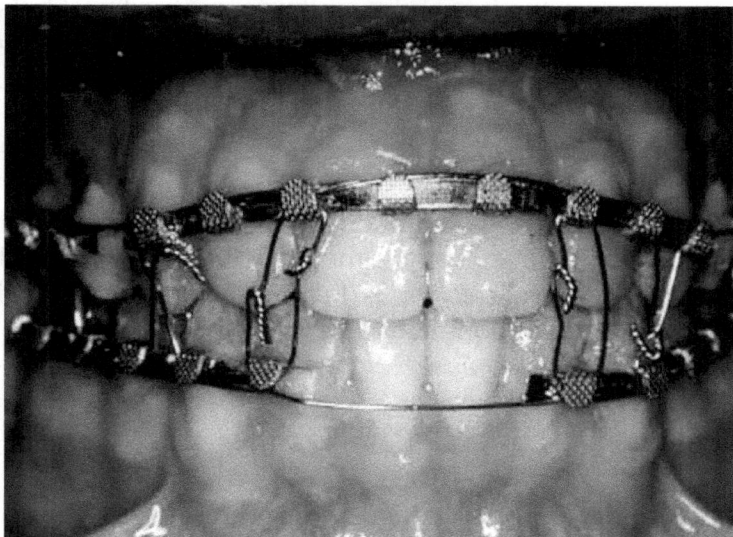

Some first aid tips if you are in civilization:

Call 911 (providing you're not in the jungles of Cambodia.) If the person has:
- Uncontrolled bleeding
- Difficulty breathing
- A possible spine or head injury (do not move the person, await medics.)
- Or if the person is:
    * In shock (faint, pale, rapid shallow breathing)

Otherwise, go to a hospital emergency room.

Prevent Choking
- Allow any blood in the mouth to dribble out or have the person spit it into a handkerchief. Without touching the roots, gently remove any broken or lost teeth from the mouth and place them in cold milk, salt water, or saliva. Take the broken teeth in their solution to the health care provider or emergency room with you.

Immobilize Jaw
Do not attempt to align the jaws. Make a bandage out of a handkerchief, scarf, or necktie, and tie it around the jaw and over the top of the head to keep the jaw from moving. The bandage should be easily removable in case the person starts to vomit.

Control Swelling- apply cold compresses.

Follow Up medical treatment depends on the location and severity of the break. A surgeon may be able to set the bone without surgery, although wires may need to be placed to stabilize the jaw. Surgery may be needed to repair the break. The surgeon will place plates or screws to hold the broken pieces of bone together while they heal.
                    - *WebMD Medical Reference*

CHAPTER 11: THE BASIC RELEASES

Hand, stick, knife, gun in mixed grabs and their releases. A commonality between them all, are the fundamental releasing techniques. These will be used in each Level 2 course chapter showing the unique solutions related to each weapon, such as, what is his other hand carrying or doing while you are grabbed?

Events *before* the grab were covered in *Stop 1*. Events *during* the grab will be covered in this book. Events *after* the grab will be extensively covered in subsequent books, as they are required in *Stop 3* through *Stop 6* and combat scenarios.

This is self defense "101" and must be documented. The escape trick and path depends on the height and nature of the grab. Here, without any support hits or kicks, are the basics. These releasing escapes exist from standing to the ground.

These are just samples. Examples. Standing and for the ground/floor.

    1: Strike once grabbed
            * head and neck, as in face, ears, eyes, nose and throat, carotid, skill base.
            * the grabbing upper arm.
            * the grabbing lower arm.
            * the grabbing hand.

    2: The simple yank-out.
    3: Same-side, step-around.
    4: The slap release.
    5: The joint-lock position release (which are usually half of some circular releases.)
            - full circles, half circles, 3/4 circles, elbow roll-over.

    6: The knee to the low arm grab.
    7: The under-the-arm, shoulder squats.
    8: The arm bite.
    9: The many finger attacks.
    10: Learn the many weapon-specific releases later in this book

Major Release 1: Strike
The opponent has grabbed you to begin to do something bad. Usually you can legally, morally and ethically, instantly strike them, once grabbed in a criminal fashion. Hand, stick, knife, even gun strikes are developed in the correlating Force Necessary courses. He may be grabbing you to strike! More on this later. If your strike the grabber's hand? The bones on the back of a hand are fragile and punching them can disrupt his grip.

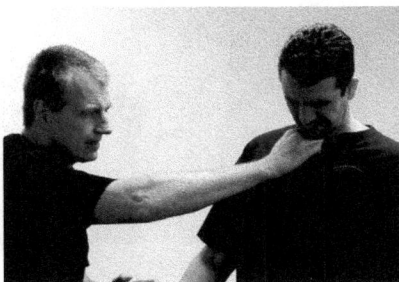

Hit the face, throat or neck.   *Hit the upper or lower arm.*   *Knuckle hit the back of the hand.*

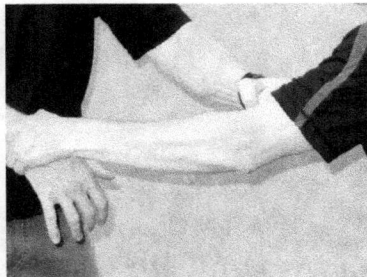

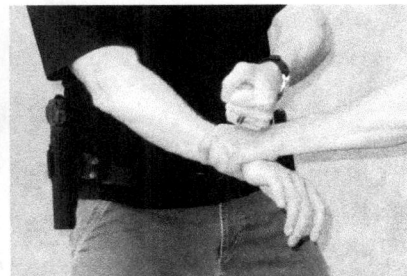

Major Release 2: The simple yank out
Fundamentally, this escape is to powerfully pull-yank free of the opponent's grip. Up, down, right or left, as with the 4 corners of the combat clock. Other than just yanking out, when in doubt vs. a strong grip, a trick is to grab your grabbed hand with your free hand and yank-pull out with both your hands. Your body should move with it, if need be.

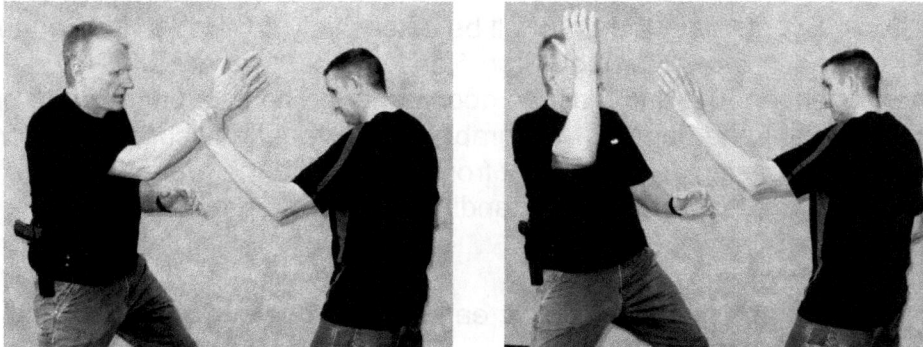

The classic, single hand grip, yank out. Travel toward the opening in his hand.

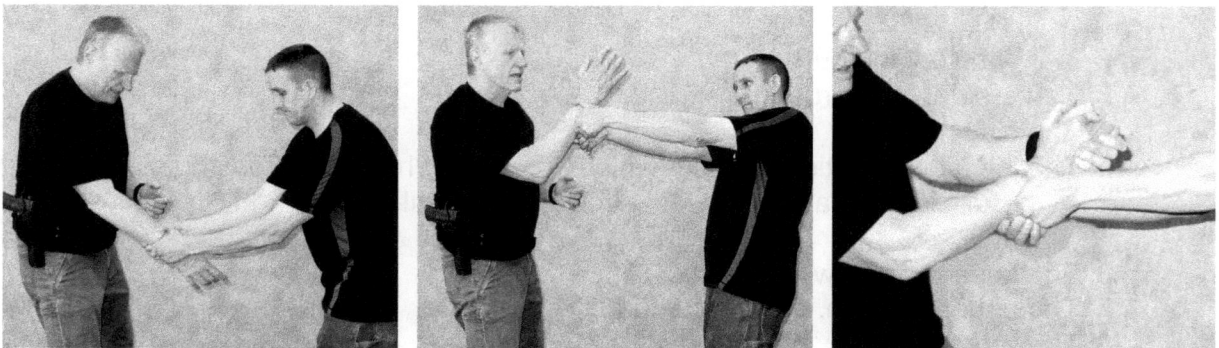

The classic major release - a curl up the middle,

and the two handed, supported "shovel" curl, yank up/out.

Major Release 3: Same-side, step-around
Providing the grabber doesn't "dance" with you, you can sometimes, full-body, turn to the outside and, with a yank, also get free from certain common grips. Sometimes called, "getting elbow to elbow" as seen in frame 3.

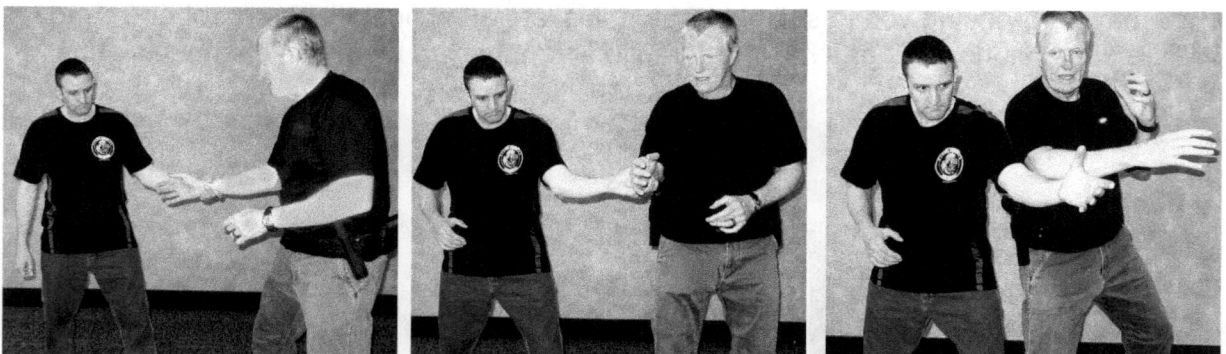

The classic step around, can break a grip (if he doesn't move with you).

Major Release 4: The simple hit-away/push-away, shove release

If you can't or won't, for whatever situational reason, strike the grabber in the face, neck, or throat, you might push the forearm or perhaps the biceps of the grabbing limb.

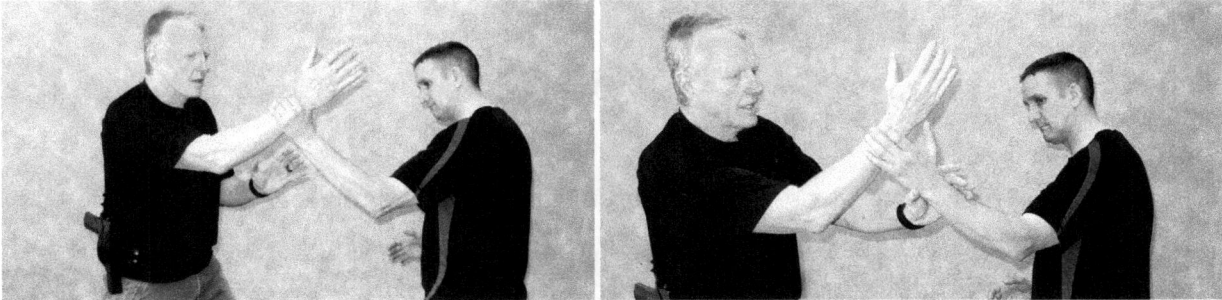

Palm push/shove away the grabbing limb.

Major Release 5: The circular releases

A clockwise circle, or a counter-clockwise circle can often get a release. Experiment to learn which direction is best for what grip. His wrist is in an awkward, weak position.

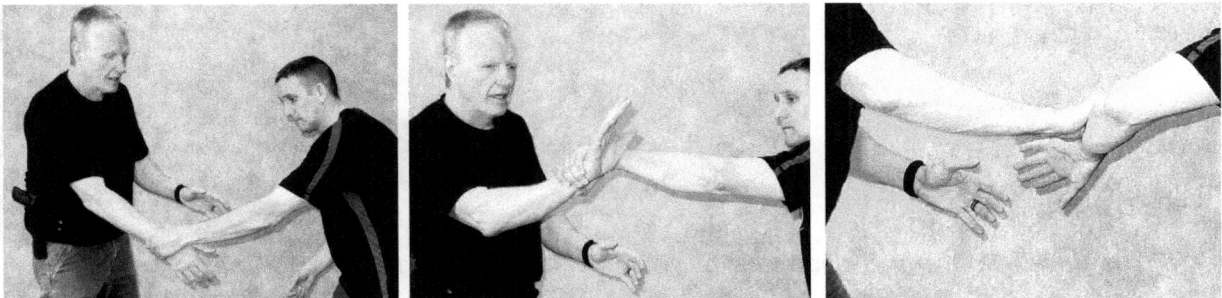

Clockwise or counter-clock-wise circular releases.

Major Release 5 continues: The joint lock releases

Another circle, but often a 1/2 or 3/4 circle. At times during a clockwise circle, or a counter-clockwise circle, halfway through, the wrist is already in a weakened position, such as a center lock, and one can thrust up or down, or sideways and get a release. Experiment to learn which is best for what grip. They work against the wrist. Wrist locks are extensively covered in the *FN: Hand* chapter ahead. This is yet another "center lock," weak wrist position.

      - 1/2 circle and crank down sample.
      - 3/4 circle, circle going palm up, then straight across sample.

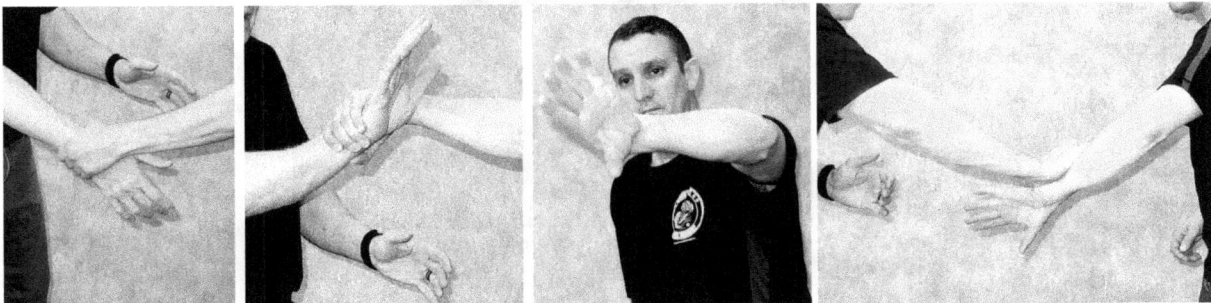

See 1/2 circle and crank down sample. Another weak wrist position. Once atop, shove straight down.

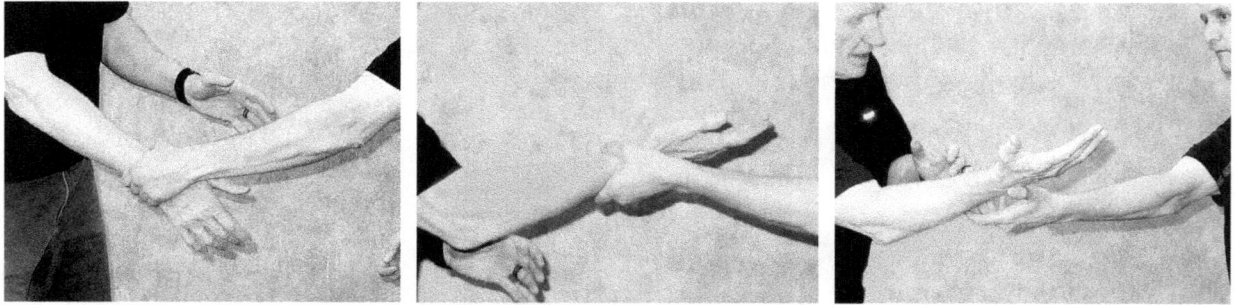

See 3/4 circle, circle going palm up, then straight across and out sample.

Major Release 5 continues: The elbow roll over

The elbow roll over is really another joint lock release, but is so important that it should stand alone. It also attacks the wrist in a center-lock position. As I like to shout, "Elbow up, elbow over (his forearm) elbow down." Against a strong grip, drop your whole body down as you drop the elbow down. Flap your wings and you "fly" away.

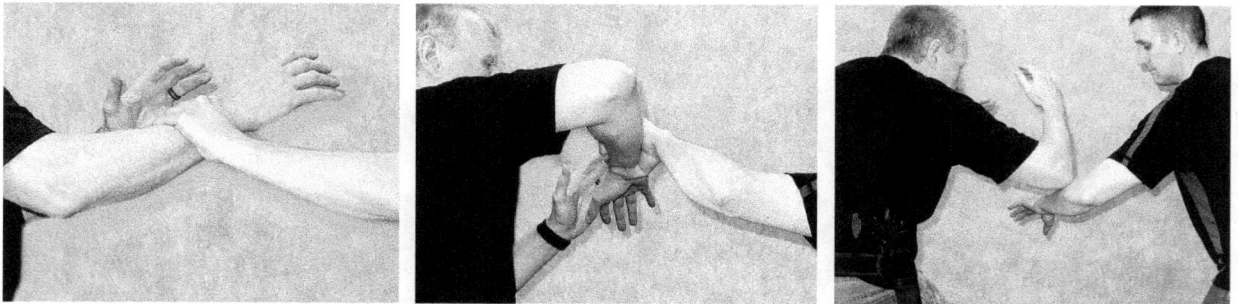

Elbow up, elbow over and elbow (and body) down. This includes bringing your captured hand up.

Major Release 6: The knee shove/strike

If the grip-grab is low and you can't seem to get another release, maybe a knee strike, push-pull might work.

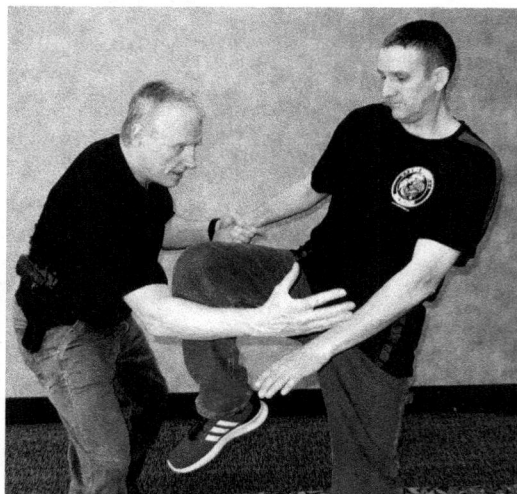

The knee shove/strike, push-pull.

Major Release 7: Shoulder squat

I also first saw this in Filipino martial arts and saw it again in military combatives. A grab struggle ensues. No manipulations are working against his super tight grip. Squat a bit, duck under his arm, with enough shoulder as to save yourself from a guillotine choke. Pull the grab down, thrust your torso up for a release.

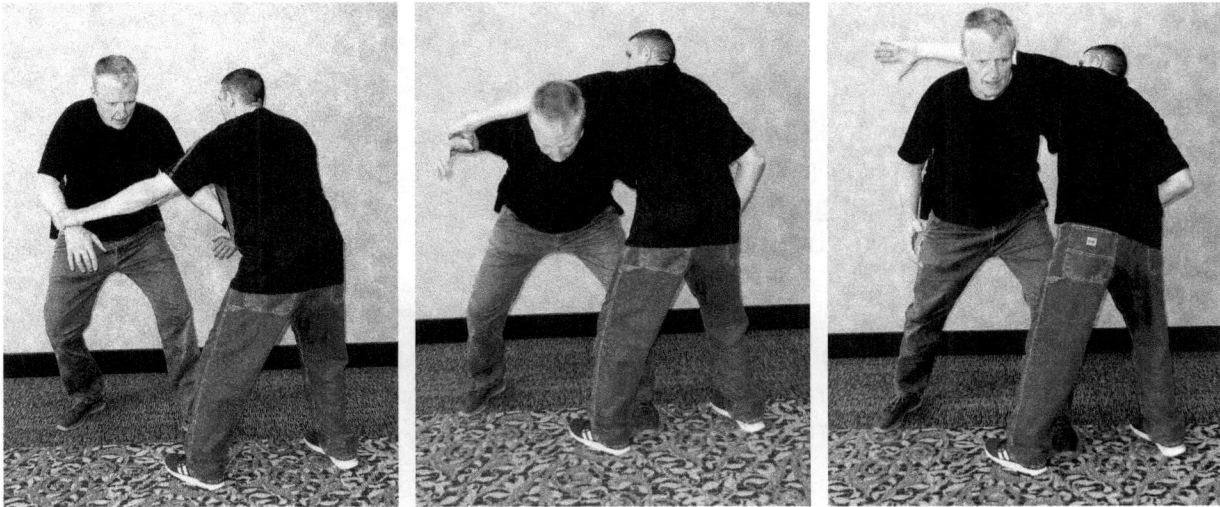

Don't let this turn into a guillotine head lock. Get your shoulder into the armpit. Be fast and furious.

Major Release 8: The arm bite

We cannot forget the arm bite as a possible grip release, should clothing allow for it. If you are fighting for your life, in that can-do instant? Bite! You'll be alive later and can be treated for any infections.

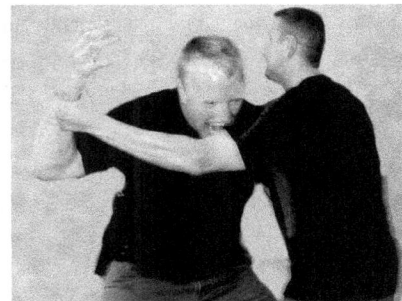

Major Release 9: The many finger attacks

Counter-grabbing fingers, wrenching them, breaking them, are also solutions. These will be covered extensively in this book in the *Force Necessary: Hand* chapter.

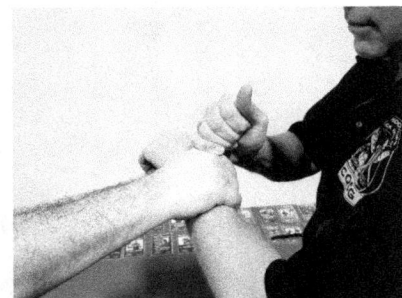

Major Release 10: Escapes from rear and side grabs

Old school fighting systems covered this subject but many modern systems don't. We will, as this can really happen. Remember don't turn into his center for his punch!
Run the numbers of the rear grabs:

1: Mirror hand (same-side) rear grabs.
  - two hands from the rear.
  - right to right grab from the rear.
  - left to left grab from the rear.

2: Two handed rear grabs of one limb.
  - both hands grab the right arm.
  - both hands grab the left arm.

3: Side and somewhat side grabs.
  - right to right.
  - left to right.
  - both hands grab right.
  - both hands grab left.

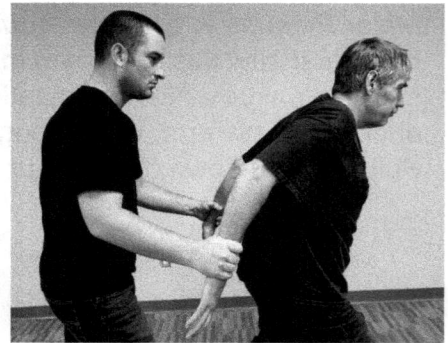
Two-hand grab from behind.

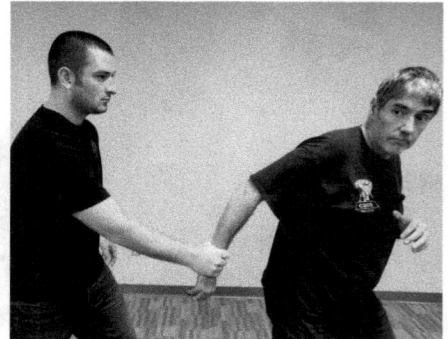
Right grabs right from behind.

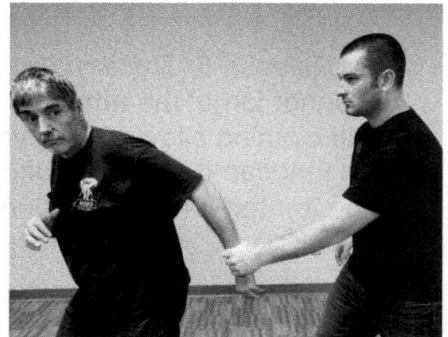
Left grabs from behind.

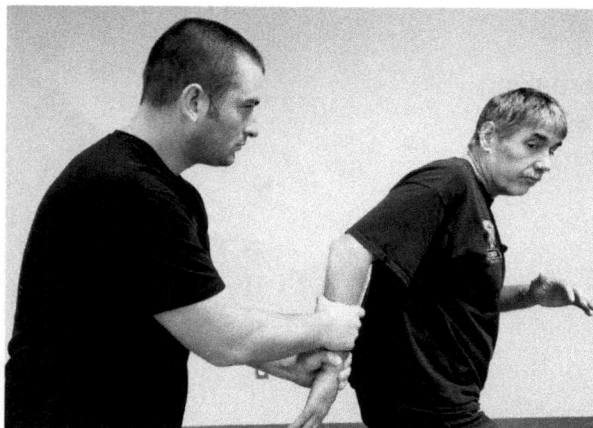
Two-hands grab right from behind.

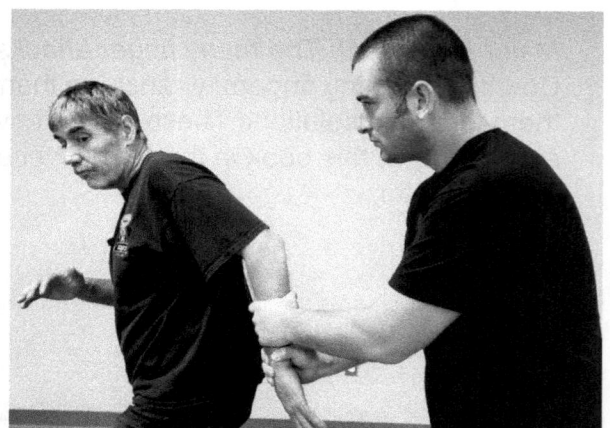
Two-hands grab left from behind.

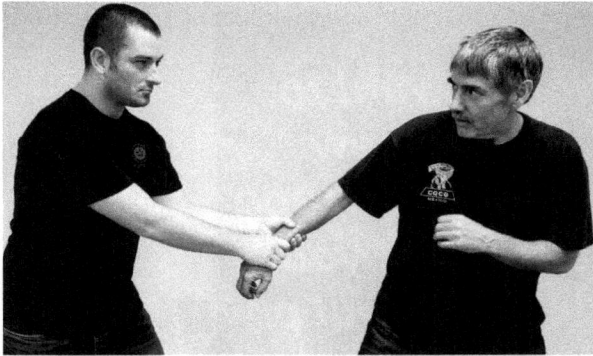

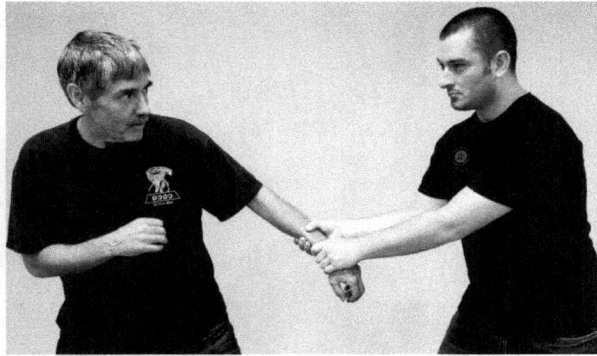

You might be grabbed with one or two hands from the right or left side.

Some possible solutions to rear and side grabs...

   * Kick the grabber
     Can you by feel or glance know
     how/where the grabber stands? Kick
     the knee, groin, etc.
     Do more damage and/or escape.
        * back kicks to the rear.
        * side kicks to the side.

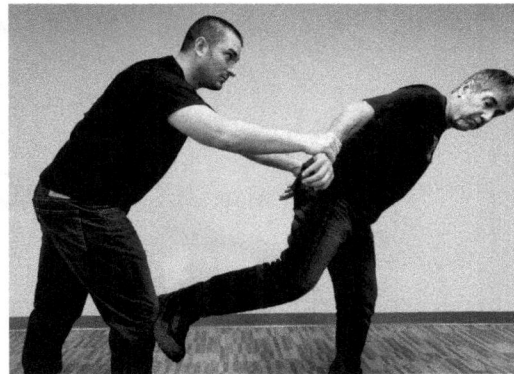

Kick the grabber.

   * Power turn
     This is an important move, but prepare to
     be struck. If you feel a two hand grab?
     Then his hands are too busy. The best
     direction is situational, based on your
     experiments. Turn to his "outside."

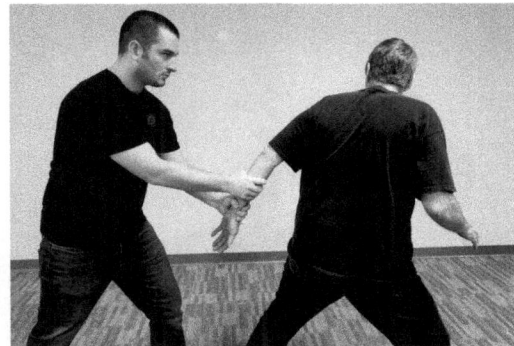

   * Upon turning, then many of the frontal
     hand releases can work, such as slap
     releases and circular releases.

   * Power turn with punches/strikes to the
     gripping limb or torso? Head? Neck?

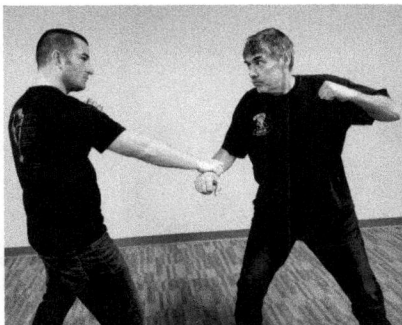

*Power turns which can include
hand releases and kicks and strikes.*

Power turn and strikes.

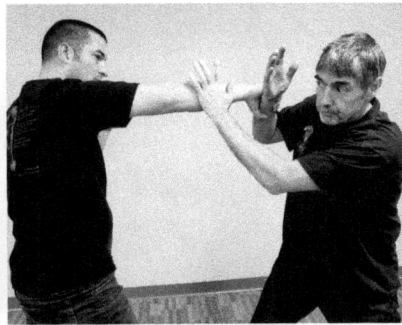

Power turn and slap releases.

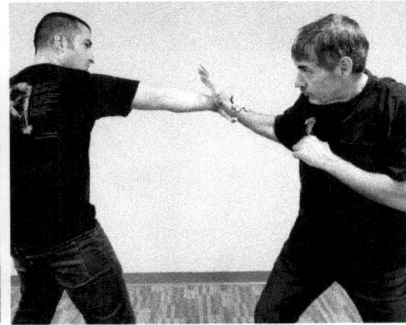

Power turn and circular release.

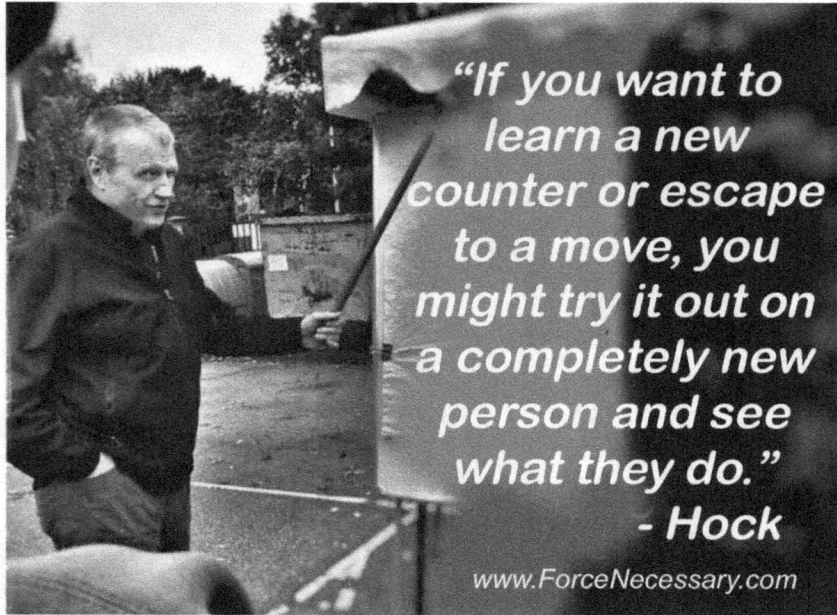

"If you want to learn a new counter or escape to a move, you might try it out on a completely new person and see what they do."
- Hock

www.ForceNecessary.com

Suggested reading...

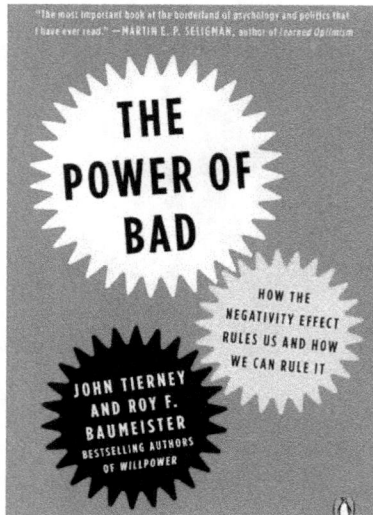

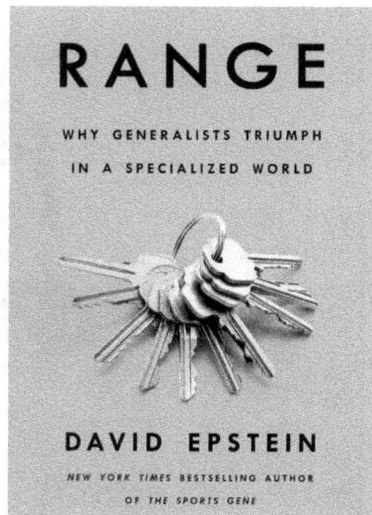

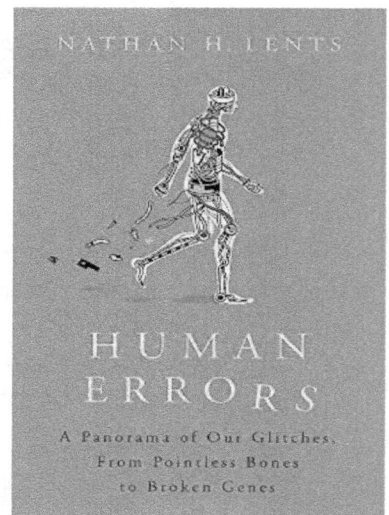

CHAPTER 12: THE "HAND DROP," FEELING THE SUDDEN DRAW

This is a universal concern to hand, stick, knife and gun. You have collided into a *Stop 2* Tangler! A one-handed or a two-handed grip. When entangled you should be aware that he might release himself from your grip, or let go of you, and move his hand to a carry site to draw a small or expandable stick, a knife or even a gun. Official studies, such as the one by the US FBI crime reports suggest that a large percentage of people we fight are armed, usually with a knife or a pistol (and not so much a stick.)

Why is he suddenly letting go of your limb? Why is his hand dropping to a common weapon carry site on his body? Or, why is he letting go or getting free and reaching somewhere off of his body?

We have already spent a copious amount of time in *Training Mission One*, worried about the hand pathways to reach and draw a weapon. These same pathways exist when you are tangled up, with the exception that the beginning of the process begins with the *Stop 2* entanglement. We are closer in. We have less time to respond to that draw.

With that release, with that reach, you may have to charge in and interrupt a weapon quick draw, even before pulling your own weapon. This interruption can be done many grappling ways.

Quick point of review and interest - some 9 out of 10 people are right-handed.

In *Stop 1* we covered the three weapon carry sites. For review, here they are again:
- primary carry sites (belt, belt line of pants, pockets, etc.) think "quick draws."
- secondary carry sites (boot knife, boot gun, neck knife, etc.) think "back-up."
- tertiary carry sites (off the body) think "lunge and reach."

The belt, or belt line, a common primary carry site
It is rather well known that in the gun world, criminals usually do not wear hosters. So, even though we are using a belt for this explanation, imagine a weapon that is tucked into the criminal's pants, with a belt. These are good *Combat Clock* training references.

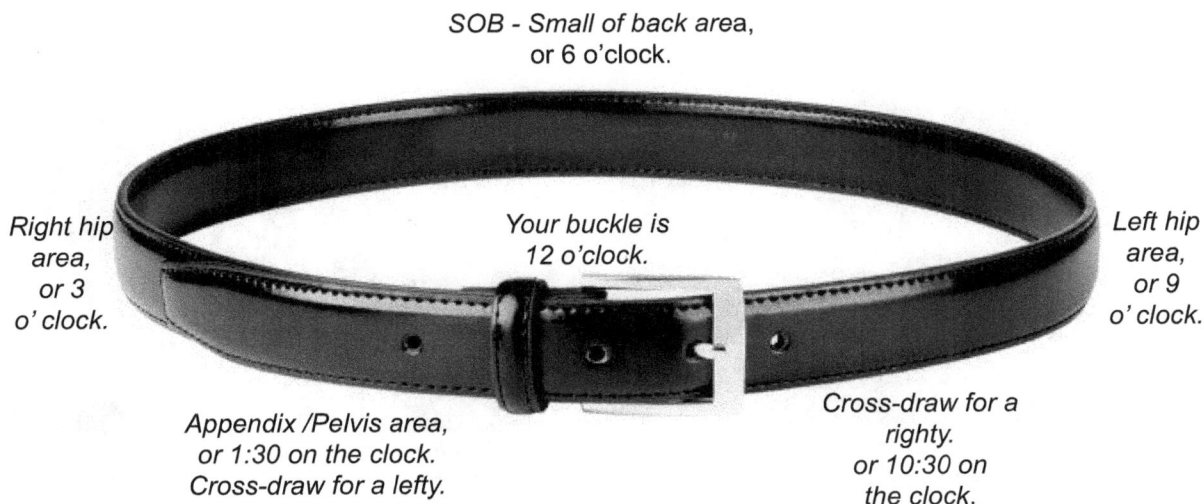

SOB - Small of back area,
or 6 o'clock.

Right hip area, or 3 o'clock.

Your buckle is 12 o'clock.

Left hip area, or 9 o'clock.

Appendix /Pelvis area, or 1:30 on the clock.
Cross-draw for a lefty.

Cross-draw for a righty. or 10:30 on the clock.

The shoulder holster and other on-the body, carry sites
Not many criminals have belt holsters but there may be some that delight in having a shoulder holster as seen in movies and TV. We would see these once in a while used in armed robberies. This requires a cross draw. The cross draw from a shoulder holster is a high 10:30 and a cross draw from the belt is a low 10:30, based on the "belt clock." Do the math. Right hand crosses over the torso to the left. Left hand crosses over the torso to the right. Nine out of 10 people are right-handed. It is not a good sight for you to see a hand cross the torso to the armpit or belt line.

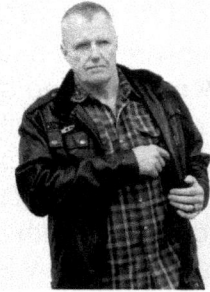

The shoulder holster is another quick draw carry site.

Trouble signs for his coming draw.
You are tangled up. He either holds you or you hold him. You feel the release and his hand drops down? Why? Must be to pull a weapon from a common carry site.

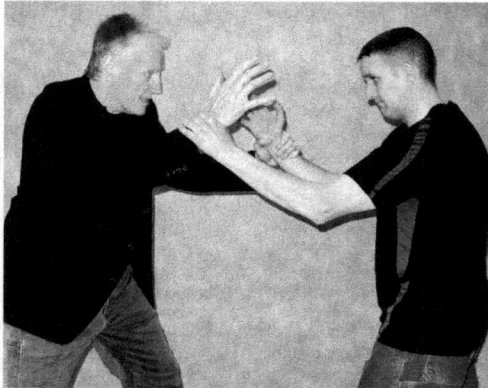

Two hand tangle. Which is his or your weapon hand?

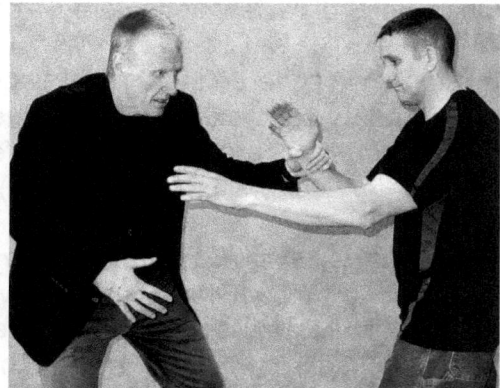

You feel the release...

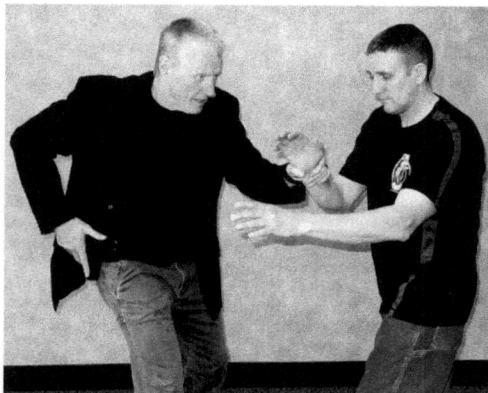

...and his free-hand drops to a carry site and he maybe takes a step back.

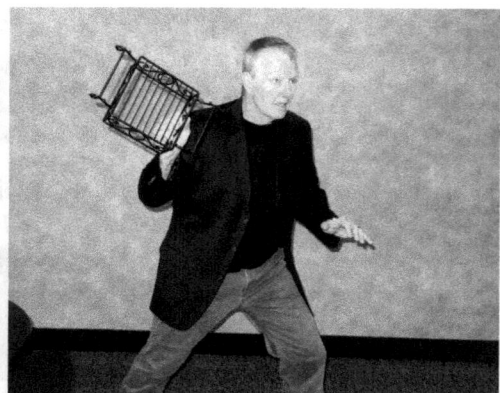

His freed hand may reach for some nearby item as a makeshift weapon.

Quick weapon-draw solutions
We will tackle these problems inside the particular hand, stick, knife and gun courses, but generically for them all, here are some overview solutions.

* Get entangled? Quick kick to the shins, knees, groin which may short circuit his idea to draw. Fight on.

* In a vacuum? Punch. (As Bruce Lee would say.) If he releases, don't leave your hand in the air. As soon as it's free hit his face, and/or throat.

* If he is reaching off his body for a lamp, a hidden weapon, whatever? Instantly, fight on.

* Riding the hand down, so to speak. If he releases, don't leave your hand in the air. Ride the escaped hand down his hand path to draw a weapon and interrupt his quick draw with unarmed combatives. A common solution is the rear arm bar hammerlock because the arm is usually bent in his quick draw process. More on this "ride" in the upcoming, gun chapter.

* If possible? Release and/or draw your weapon and instantly use it. But the reality is, as we see this in practice with simulated weapons, you are behind the "eight ball," as they say, action beating reaction, and the best choice may well be to interrupt his draw first and then you draw.

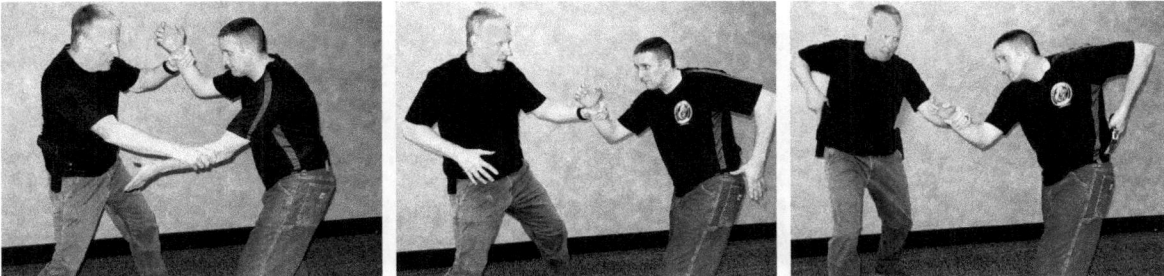

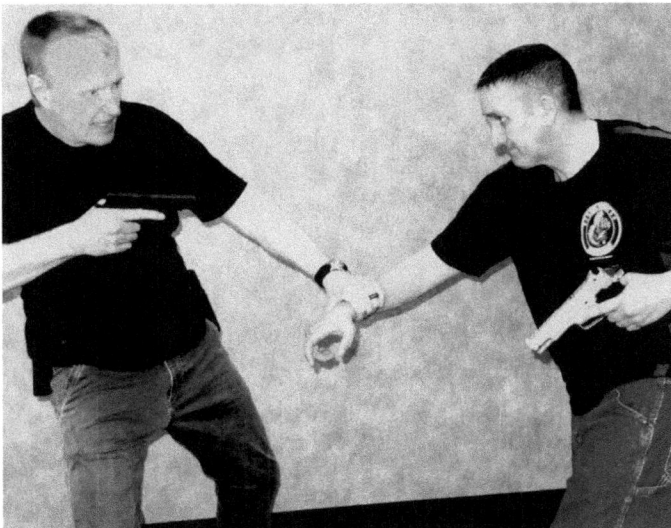

Remember, action beats reaction. He goes for his gun, you see that and then go for your gun, you are behind the curve, behind the timeline, and he may well draw and shoot you first.

It might be better to interrupt his draw with strikes, grappling, even a knee or groin kick, and then pull your pistol.

If he is pulling a folding knife or expandable baton he has to open it, giving you time to react.

More solutions to follow in the gun chapter.

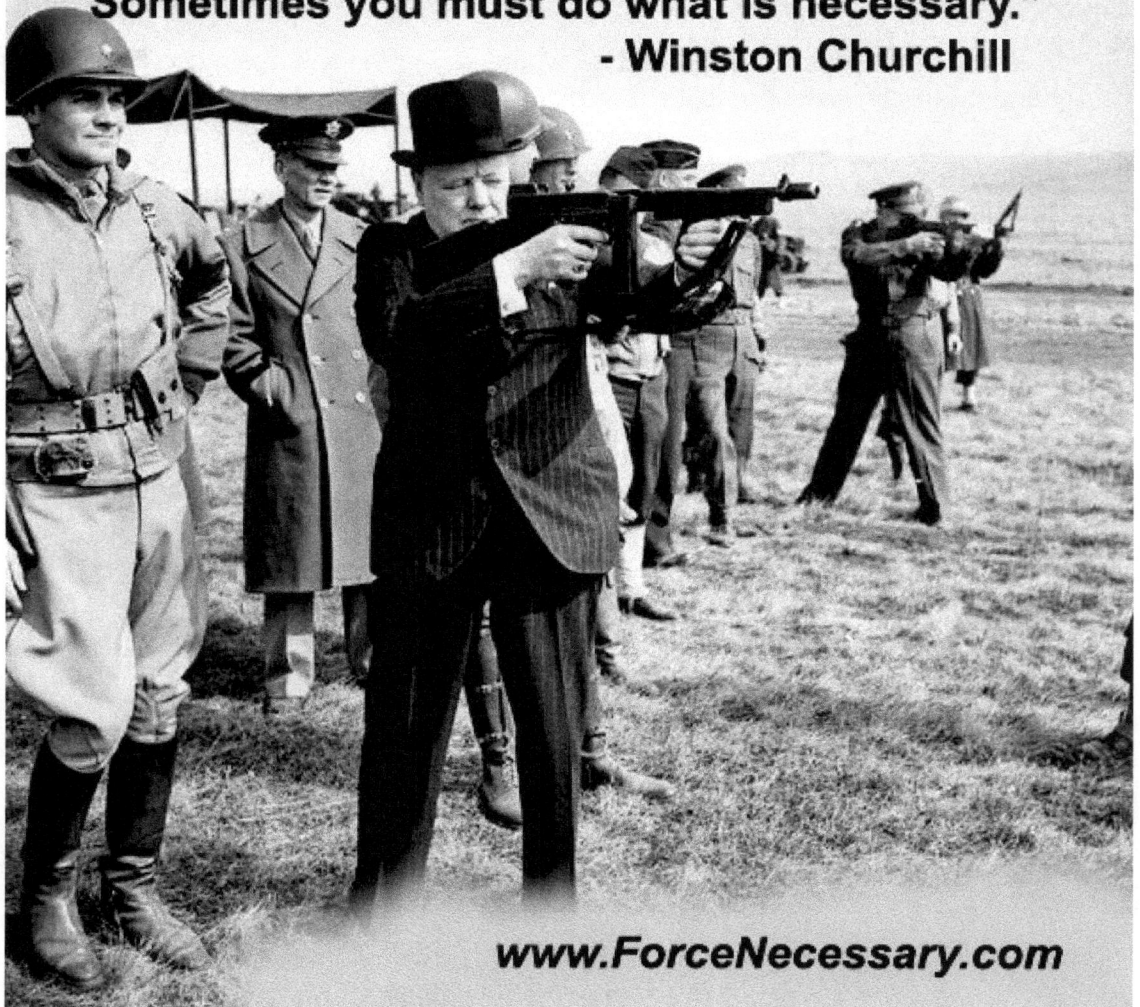

"Sometimes doing your best is not good enough. Sometimes you must do what is necessary."
- Winston Churchill

www.ForceNecessary.com

CHAPTER 13: COMMON, WEAPON RETENTION PROBLEMS

It's a hand, stick, knife, gun world. Throughout this book and further *Stop 6* and *Training Mission* studies, we have to remember that the fight may start unarmed. This is why unarmed combatives is so important. And, we know not all fights start with this *Stop 2* "hand" entanglement, but some do, and some may move in and out of *Stop 2* after the fight starts. You and your enemies may be armed. Weapons may be drawn. He may use one or two hands to snatch. He may well try one of these or more tricks to disarm you.

> 1: strike you in an ambush, or from a son-man conversation.
> 2: grab you somewhere. Throat? Arms? Bear hug? Not just the hands and wrists.
> 3: grab and strike together.
> 4: hide and jump at you.
> 5: sneak up on you.

He may try all of these things before he attempts a weapon steal from you. *Stop 2* is the beginning of hands-on, and that means hands on weapons too.

Weapon retention covers these five elements:
> 1: Protect your weapon at the carry site.
> 2: Protect your weapon during the draw process.
> 3: Protect your weapon during the full presentation.
> 4: Protect your weapon while you are striking, or blocking and/or firing.
> 5: Weapon recovery after your weapon has been snatched (disarming him back).

Intermixing unarmed combatives as much as possible is a necessity. You do not need to become an MMA champion (although that would be terrific) to problem-solve common unarmed problems, or weapon-related problems. Learn to dodge, block, stun, strike and kick, grapple and so forth. It's all in the *Force Necessary* courses. We will cover stick, knife and gun retention in the respective categories, in upcoming chapters and books. For now, know and think about these commonalities.

Protecting the Belt. Commonalties for Stick, Knife and Gun

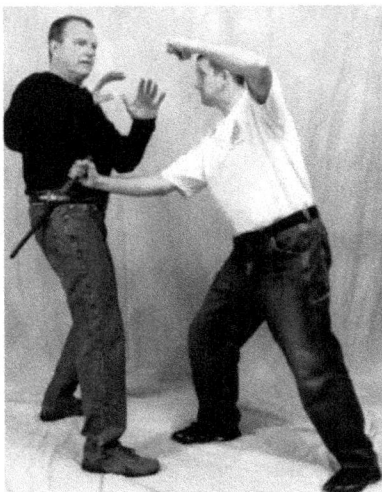

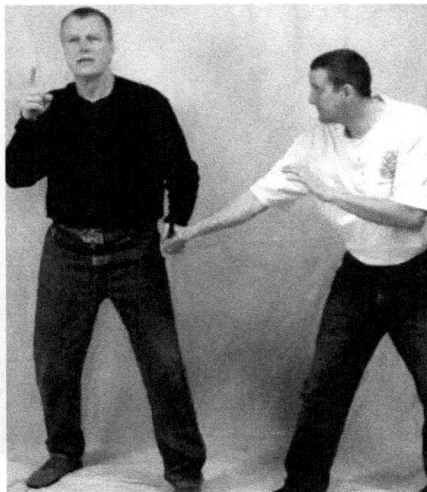

He may strike you.	He may approach you from all sides.	He may use one or two hands.

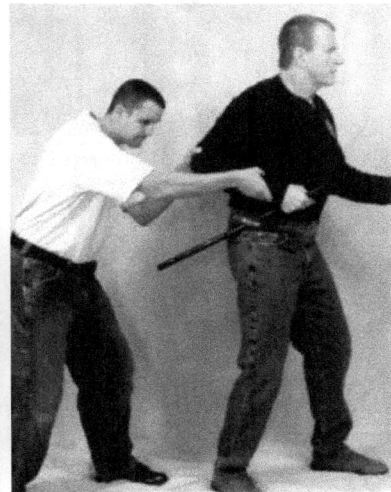

Retention Commonality 1: Slapping, shoving, blocking grab attempts.
Retention Commonality 2: Capturing the enemies grab, for more action.

We will cover retention in great detail in the upcoming chapters.

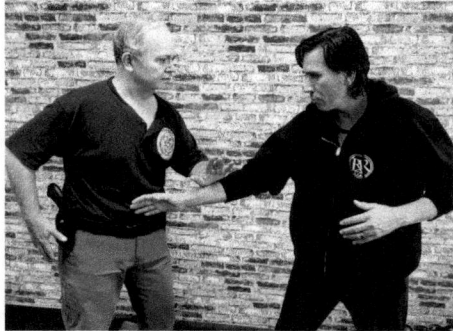

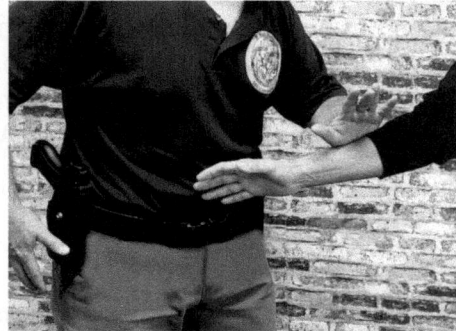

Slapping, shoving, blocking grab attempts.

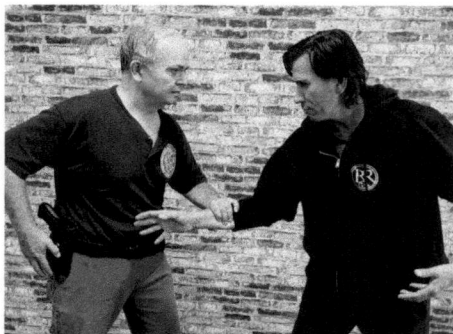

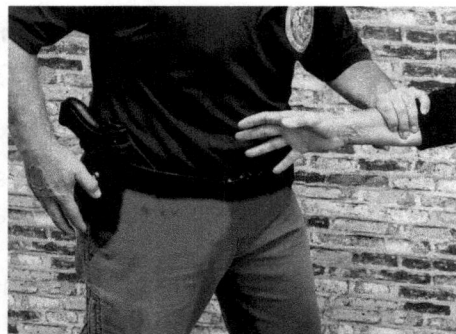

Capturing the enemies grab, for more follow-up action.

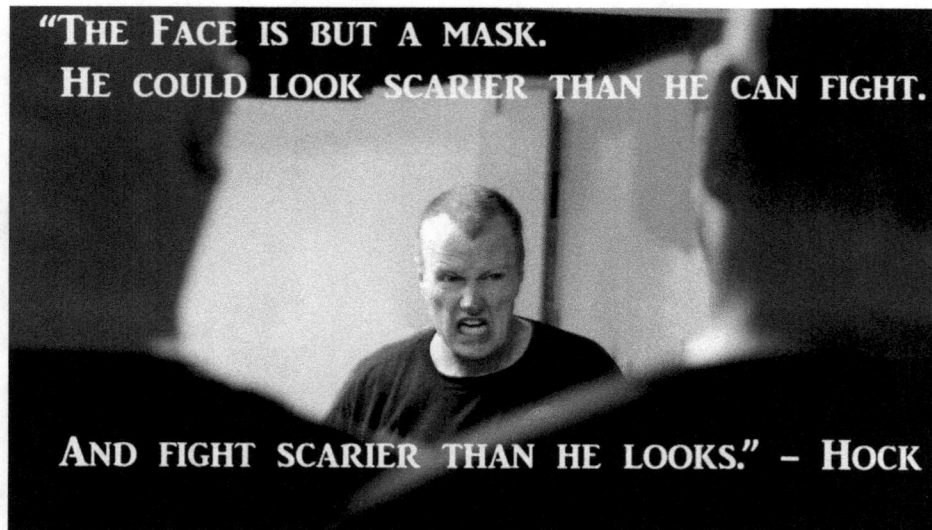

"THE FACE IS BUT A MASK.
HE COULD LOOK SCARIER THAN HE CAN FIGHT.

AND FIGHT SCARIER THAN HE LOOKS." – HOCK

Getting a Grip on Your Grips! Weapon Handling!

A quick reminder from **Training Mission 1** and its relationship to firearms, knife and baton retention. Slick weapon handles in your hands make it harder for you to keep weapons when someone is pulling them from you.

Johnny Cash once wrote about the "kicking and the gouging and the mud and blood and the beer." There's also guts, water, oils, sweat, bad gloves and other substances that can make life very slippery and your hands and tools very slippery. Legend has it that the Gurkhas would dip their kukris in motor oil and then train with slimy grips. And what if your hands are injured and-or are freezing? I always shake my head when I see slick, metal knife handles gun handles and stick handles.

A considerable amount of time, money and research has gone into making working tools like hammers, saws, screw drivers etc., very grippable. Still you will find slick-handled hammers and tools too! But like wise tool-makers, many wise gun and knife makers and sellers have also labored to make your weapons stay put in your hands with textured grips! People like to suggest that textured gloves solve some of these problem, but will you ALWAYS be wearing gloves 24-7?

I am not endorsing anyone or anything here. I am just making a suggestion: forego pretty and slick, and get the most textured grips on your firearms, knives and sticks-batons.

Get a damn handle on your handles!

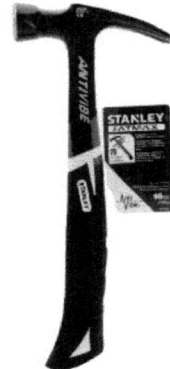

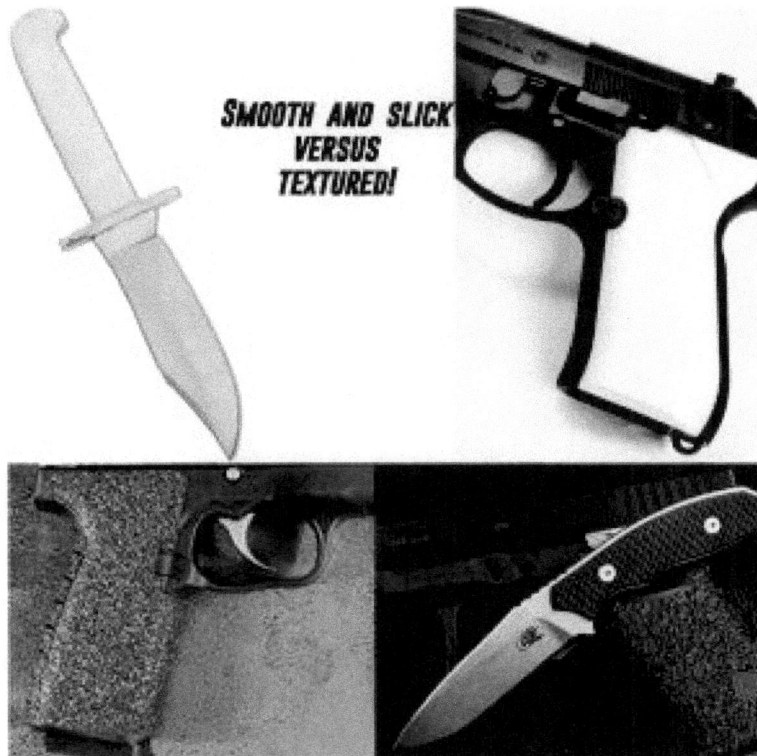

SMOOTH AND SLICK VERSUS TEXTURED!

Chapter 14: Weapon Disarming Overview

The material in *Stop 2* and *Training Mission Two* will center more on weapon retention than disarming. But it is difficult to cover retention without a quick study of some disarming. In this early stage of our common sense, survival, progression study we are still pulling our weapons out under stress and trying to keep them in our hands and use them. Protecting the belt, protecting the draw and protecting the use. The *Stop 2* mission study.

While it is true that grabbing weapons to disarm them is a very "handy, hands-on" subject, and would seem to fit perfectly in this subject matter, and I agonized on this, I believe that the disarming of sticks, knife, pistols and long guns require a lot of support set-ups, striking, kicking and grappling and would be best covered in later *Training Mission* books, just as combat scenarios are highlighted later after some official training.

Of course, any instructor can teach any subject at any time in classes and seminars, I am making great effort to proceed in a official, smart progression as a point of doctrine. Disarming is usually considered a "hand/unarmed combatives" subject, but disarming of weapons can occur while people are holding weapons also. There are nuisances involved with "while-holding" situations.

Some stick, knife and gun disarming will follow in later *Training Mission* books. Stand by. Here is one devastating disarm scenario example I learned in the US Army. "The Military Body Pitch." It is hard to practice, but when you are 18 thru 22 years old, everyone survived! (We did use mats.)

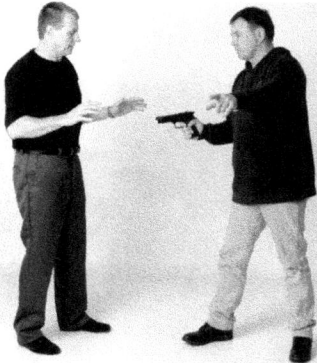

The capture.

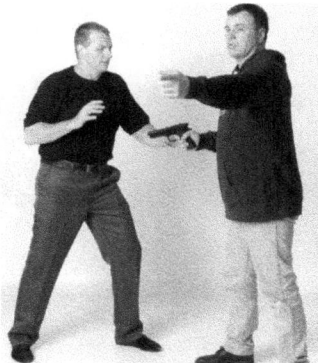

The situational distraction.

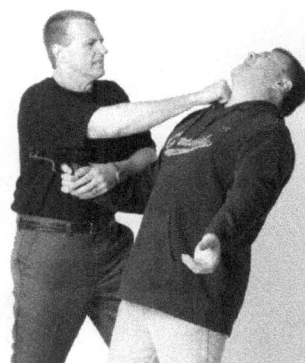

The gun grab and stunning blow.

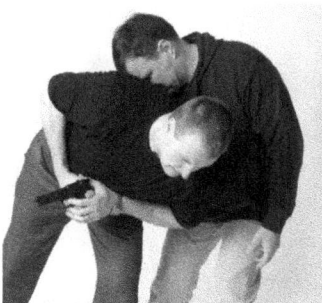

The leap.

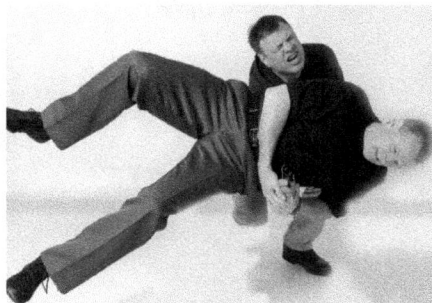

The full body dive, a bit of a forward roll direction to force the attacker down to his front.

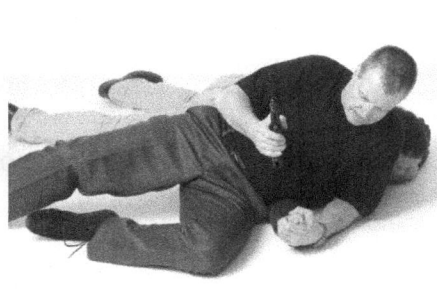

The devastating finish to the shoulder and arm. And take-away.

I am not suggesting to embrace this particular disarm, I just wanted to show you an old school, military example.

I have said that the best way to learn retention is learn how the trained and untrained do disarming. I just don't want to overload these early stages of the progression with this massive amount of weapon disarm training. See future books.

In *Stop 2 weapon retention,* we emphasize:
>1: Protect the belt.
>2: Protect the draw.
>3: Protect the presentation (or firing).
>4: Look at common disarms to defeat them.
>*Note: More on this in the upcoming chapters.*

For an early look at disarming to come, here are some downloads available at www.ForceNecessary.com

CHAPTER 15: GRABBING THE PISTOL. WHAT HAPPENS NEXT?

A hand, stick, knife and gun *Stop 2* grab commonality is grabbing the opponent's pistol in a close quarters fight. You might be armed or not? Here is a quick list of variables to think about and exercise through:

    You could be grabbing a revolver.
    You could be grabbing a semi-automatic.
    You could be unarmed and grabbing an opponent's pistol with one hand.
    You could be unarmed and grabbing an opponent's pistol with two hands.
    You could grab his pistol, move it off of you and pull your pistol.
    You could grab his pistol, move it off of you and pull your baton/stick.
    You could grab his pistol, move it off of you and pull your knife.
    You could grab his pistol and your pistol is already out.
    You could grab his pistol and your knife is already out.
    You could grab his pistol and your baton/stick is already out.

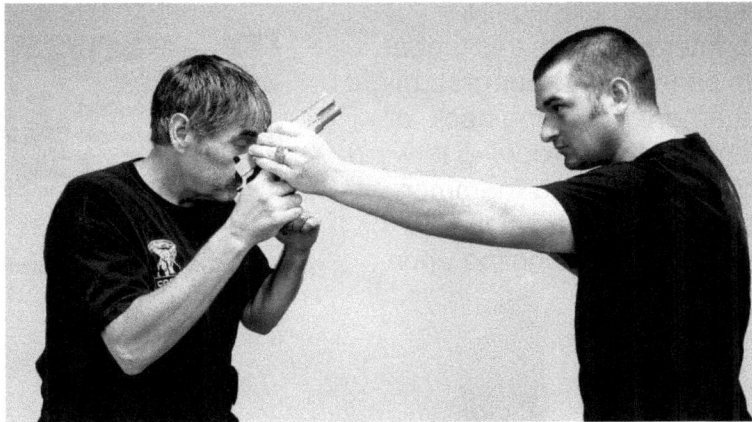

There are a series of common concerns in this situation.
    Concern 1: Still being shot?
    Concern 2: Will his pistol still work once grabbed?
    Concern 3: Will my hand break or burn if the gun goes off?
    Concern 4: And then, what happens next?

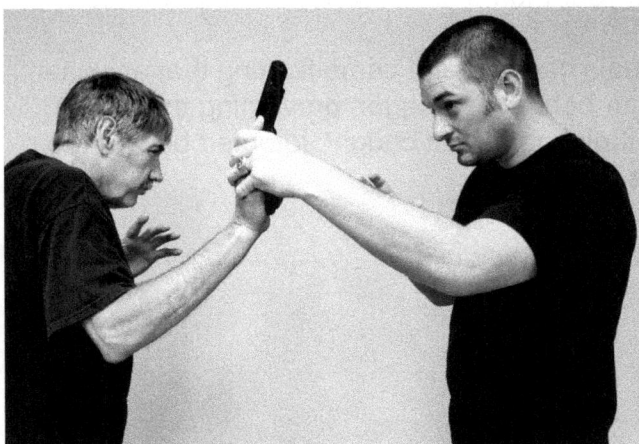

Concern 1: Still being shot?
If you grab the gun, you must point it away from you. This is easier said or read than done. It becomes a quick arm wrestling match that might bring the pistol right back to bear on you. Be prepared to move out of the way too, and be prepared for his natural, common "yank back." You can use invading footwork to chase the gun in. You cannot keep this dance up and must take immediate action.

Concern 2: Will his pistol still work? After a grab?
There is an old military and police expression, "Your pistol grab might render the gun from a 'no shot' to a 'one shot' weapon." We must look to the two basic kinds of handguns, the revolver and the semi-automatic.

Revolvers. In our modern world we see less and less of revolvers, but quite a number of people, myself included, have small revolvers for self defense. Though some say that revolvers are "enjoying a massive resurgence of popularity." Most revolvers have a hammer. The hammer can be cocked back by hand, or drawn back by the trigger pull. The hammer must then fall upon the frame for the bullet to fire.

Hammer

If your grab interferes with this trigger action, the gun cannot fire. Your grab might prevent the hammer from going back, or prevent the hammer from dropping forward.

Some revolvers are called "hammer-less" because you cannot see a visible hammer. This weapon will function upon the trigger pull.

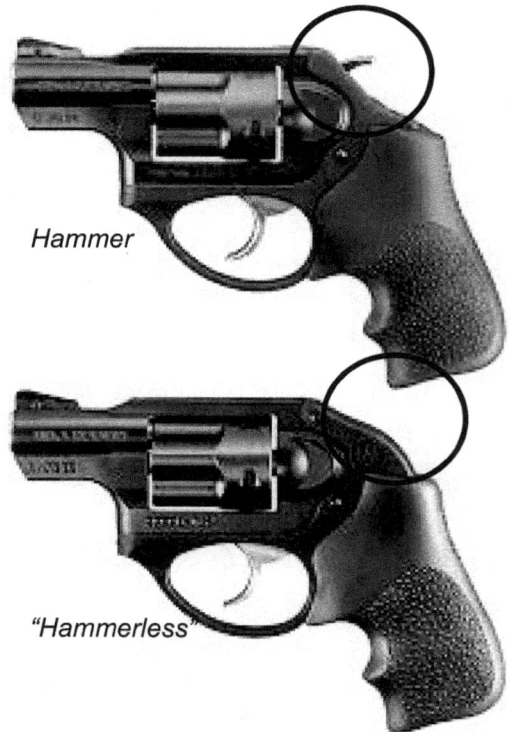

"Hammerless"

I began my police career in the 70s, in a world of "wheel guns," and we trained certain ways to grab a criminal's revolver. One was on the top. With the trigger pull of a double action revolver, the cylinder turns. If the suspect has cocked the hammer, the cylinder has turned. The hammer is not cocked the trigger finger muscle pull, essentially one muscle, turns the cylinder and draws back the hammer.

The police academies suggested to seize the pistol from the top in a "c-clamp, so that your palm and FOUR finger muscles (versus his one finger muscle) stop the cylinder from turning. In a perfect world your thumb or pinky hopefully interferes with the hammer action.

It has actually happened in the annuals of crime and crime fighting that a winner has, and usually by accident, got a finger behind the trigger, preventing the trigger pull. Some survivors of this report that their fingers got caught, jammed behind the trigger during the subsequent struggles.

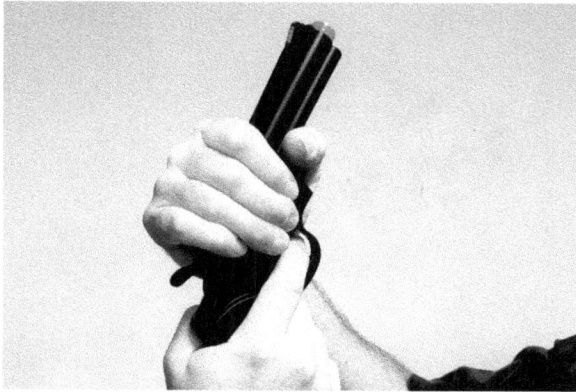

Your c-clamp stops the cylinder turn. All your finger muscles working versus one of his, his trigger finger muscle.

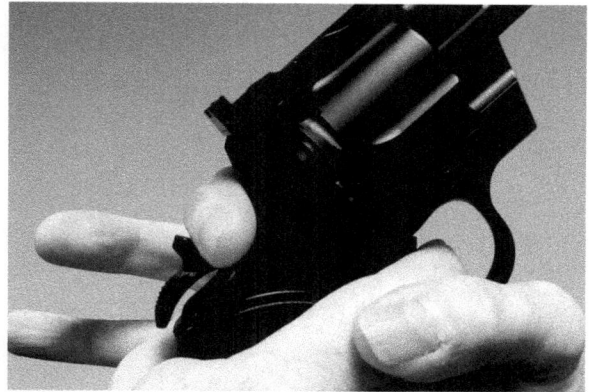

Your finger falls between the hammer and the frame of the gun.

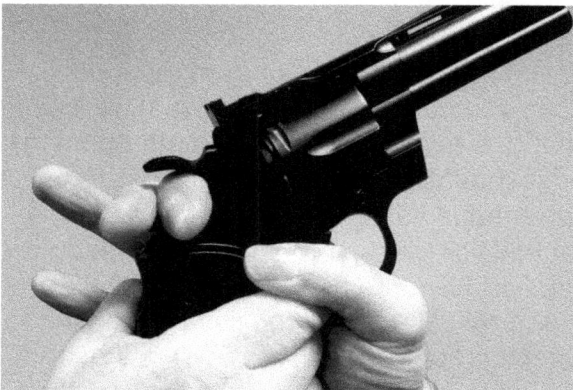

Your finger falls behind the hammer, preventing the hammer from moving back.

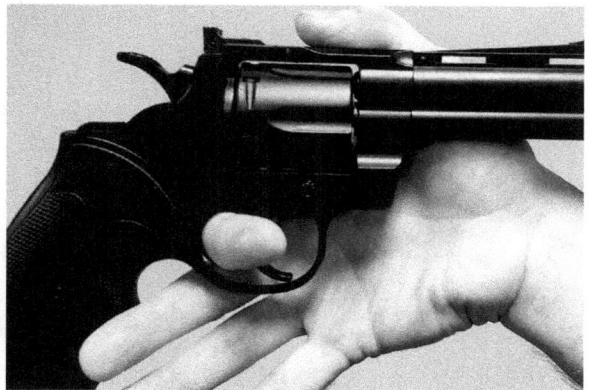

This has happened in struggles, A finger gets behind the trigger!

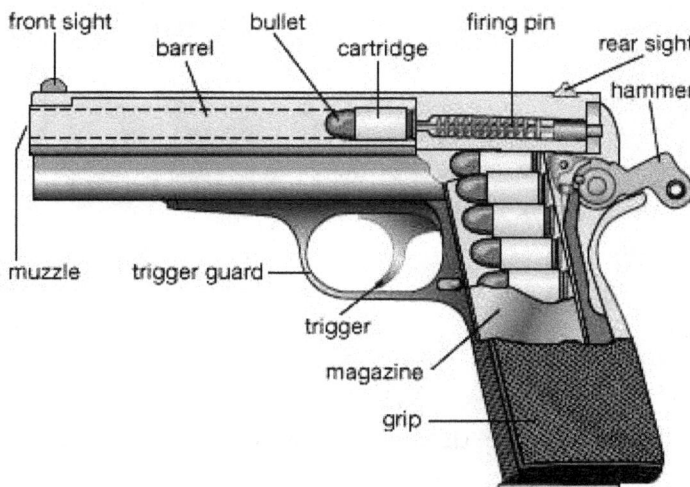

front sight · barrel · bullet · cartridge · firing pin · rear sight · hammer · muzzle · trigger guard · trigger · magazine · grip

An automatic, just for the record here, is like a machine gun. Press the trigger and cause continuous fire. A semi-automatic is not a full "machine gun" automatic. One trigger pull shoots only one bullet.

The slide atop the weapon blows back with the explosion, and it ejects the empty shell out and frees the space for the next bullet to be pushed up by the spring in the magazine. The returning slide pushed that rising round into the chamber. Suffice to say, it stands to reason that the back and forth slide action-function is important.

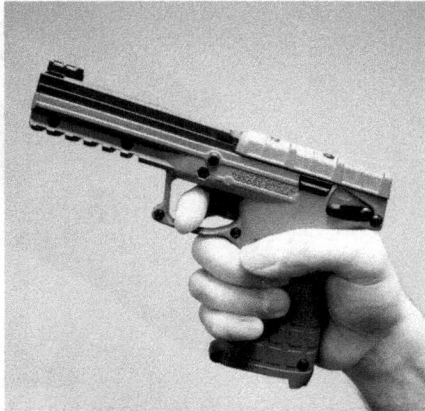
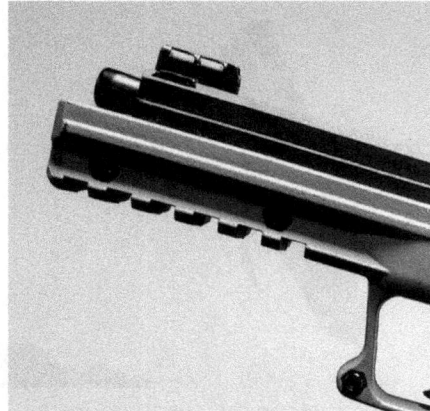

The slide is "flush" with the end. If the slide is pushed back just a slight bit, it may still fire. Back just a bit more and it may not fire.

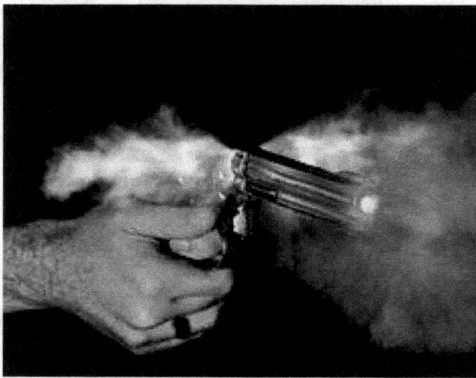

Concern 3: Will my hand break or burn if the gun goes off? Can you hold on to a fired pistol? Will it burn your hand. A revolver (left) has frame openings and will somewhat "explode" out of the sides. It will be an instantaneous flash. If your hand is on the open areas, you will feel something. Lots of people have grabbed and held semi-auto pistols with little to no problems. It will take some consistant shooting to make a barrel too hot to touch when not being fired.

The moral of the story is, if you are fighting for your life? Do not let go of the handgun.

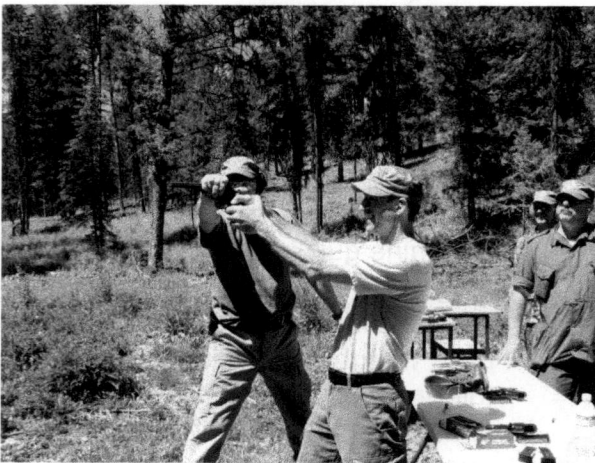
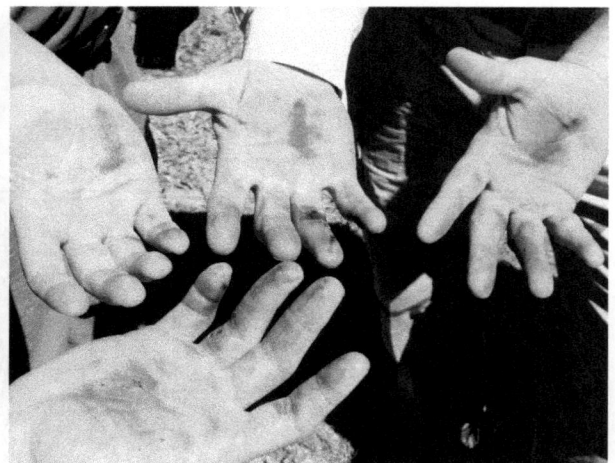

British military war vet and old friend, Alan Cain was assigned to study this problem for the infantry, using a variety of handguns. Revolvers caused some pain but semi-automatics did minimal damage to the hands.

Concern 4: And then, what happens next?
Get a hand on a pistol, deflect the aim from yourself and, as simultaneously as possible, punch the gunman in the head. Sound familiar. This is Israeli Krav 101. But chances are it might not work out as well as it does in class.

Where on the head are you punching?
Will all your one-punches work like magic?
Will he fall?
Will you rip the pistol out of his hand, with your gripping hand be fast enough?
Should you ride the gun down?

Ride the gun down? I mean that you **cannot** let this enemy fall backward with that pistol in his hand. It is too risky. You have to hold on to it if you can't disarm it. Ride it down.

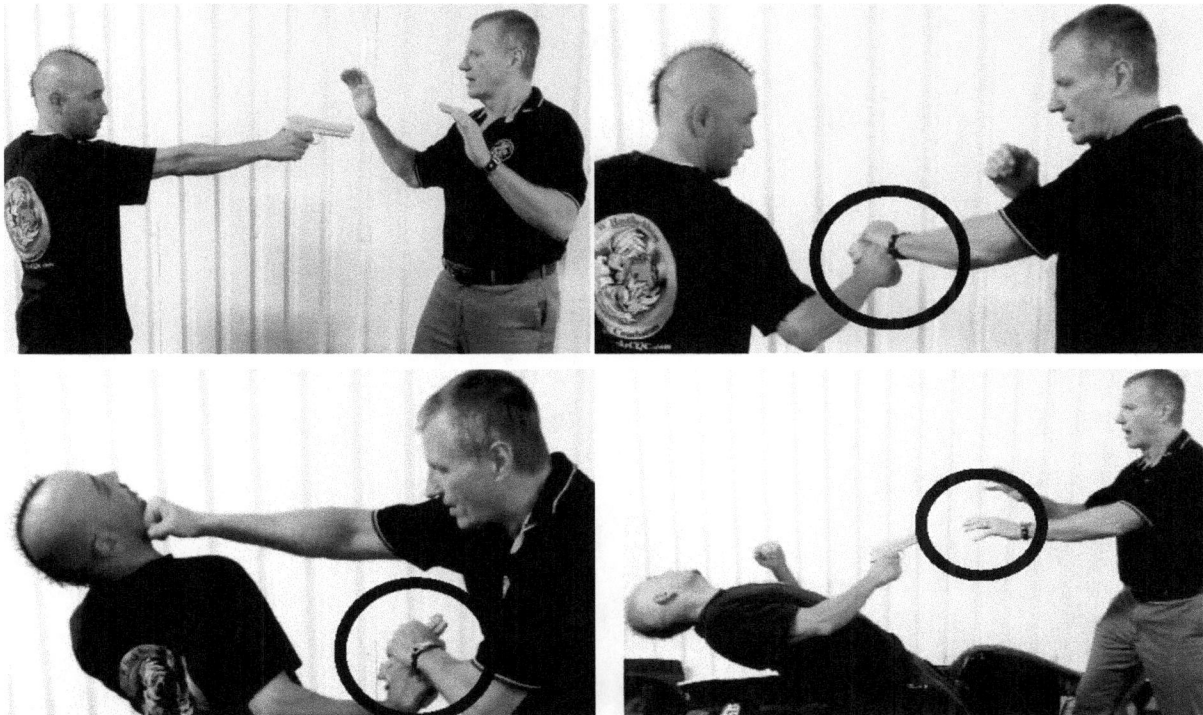

You can't let go of the pistol, or lose the grip.

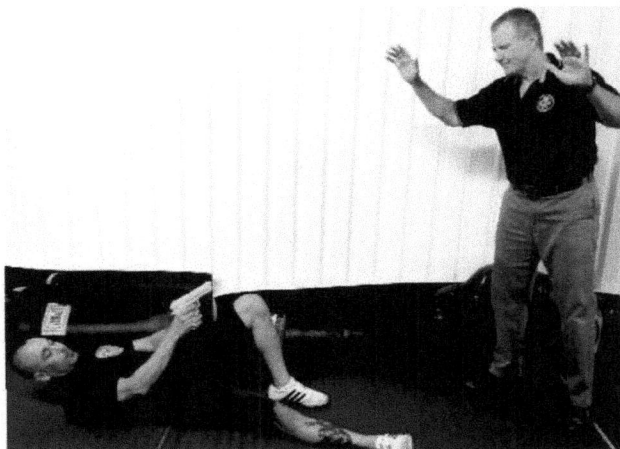

Ride the gun down. Unarmed, or you are armed with a stick, knife or gun in your other hand, remember this problem. He could shoot you on the way down, or shoot you when he hits the ground.

This theme should also appear in your stick, knife and gun course training. You can draw your weapon as you ride his gun down. Or, you might strike him with your drawn stick, knife or gun.

CHAPTER 16: ANGER MANAGEMENT

What are the *Force Necessary* "Three Managements?" Anger management, pain management and fear management, all to be reviewed in commonalities sections of these *Training Mission* books. This book introduces the important topic of anger and anger management.

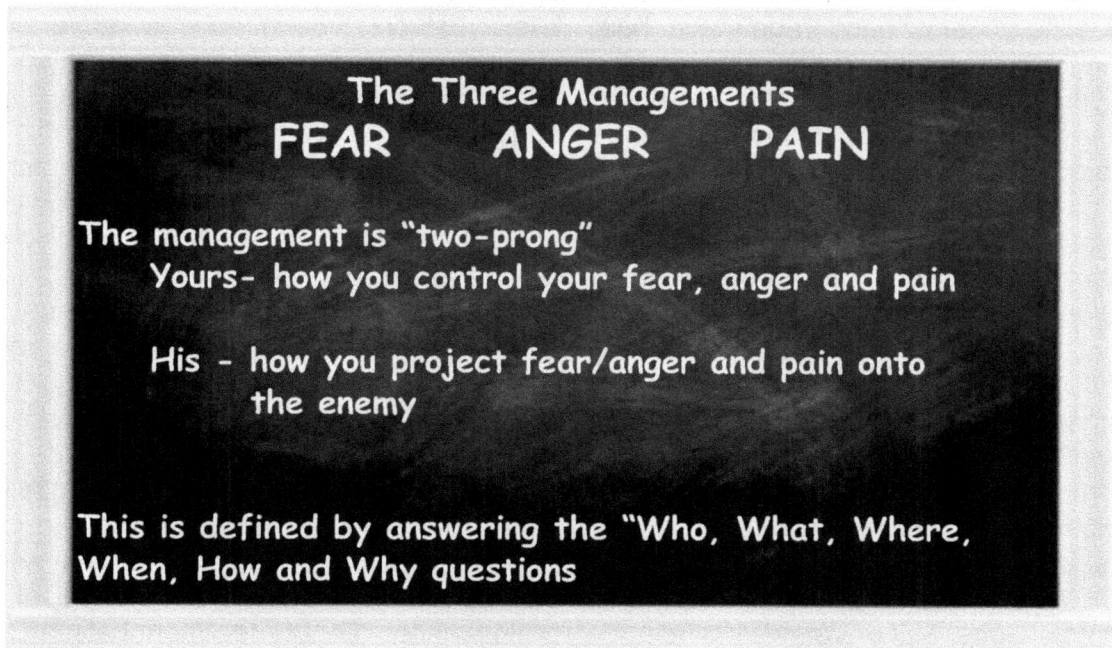

The Three Managements
FEAR   ANGER   PAIN

The management is "two-prong"
    Yours- how you control your fear, anger and pain

    His - how you project fear/anger and pain onto
        the enemy

This is defined by answering the "Who, What, Where, When, How and Why questions

I am not a psychologist. I can only quote psychologists and inspire you to do appropriate research. But I am convinced that anger, pain and fear, their "managements" are three important aspects in all kinds of fighting. I hope this will inspire you to do more research.

One of my favorite people I could call a friend and advisor, who has passed away, was David "Hack" Hackworth, author of *About Face* among other books, and at one time he was the most decorated US Army soldier, a vet from WWII, Korea and Vietnam. He recalled a wartime trench fighting incident where a fellow soldier who happened to be a Samoan, got so angered by the loss of his fellow troops, so enraged, he stood up screaming and charged the enemy blasting away. He did some initial good, but he was cut down. Hack said he'd never minded his troops getting angry, in fact he

depended on it, but not that kind of "crazy angry."

This is an example that anger to the level of losing total control of your rationality, even your skills and becoming the Hulk - may certainly be detrimental to your physical and legal survival.

I think everyone from time to time has anger issues. If you read my police memoirs books, *Don't Even Think About It* and *Dead Right There*, you will find several times that I foolishly "lost it." I added them in as educational warnings for new (and old?) police.

In today's YouTube world, cops are consistently caught "losing it." The motives are varied, the obvious and unobvious.

"Anger management is a process of learning to recognize signs that you're becoming angry, and taking action to calm down and deal with the situation in a positive way. Anger management doesn't try to keep you from feeling anger or encourage you to hold it in. Anger is a normal, healthy emotion when you know how to express it appropriately. Anger management is about learning how to do this. You may learn anger management skills on your own, using books or other resources. But for many people, taking an anger management class or seeing a mental health counselor is the most effective approach." – *Standard Psychology*

1. anger is the cause of many fights.
2. it is interwoven with adrenaline and adrenaline issues.
3. "controlled" anger can also be used as a source of strength. Amy Morin, LCSW and medically reviewed by Steven Gans, MD of Verywell Mind, remind us that "your anger might give you the courage you need to take a stand or make a change."

In terms of this quick mention about crime, war and violence, anger is broken down into the classic three "fight" categories, before the fight, during the fight and after the fight. Trying to recognize and control yourself when anger brews is the realm of professional counselors, your culture and lifestyle.

Controlling anger to a positive performance level is the goal. Use it. Don't lose it. Don't abuse it. I know. Easier said than done. There are some options if you are not completely ambushed and overwhelmed. When time is available, some people use humor when under threat. Some even smile. Learn to calm yourself physically. Learn to use physical relaxation techniques like "centering yourself," a term not easily explained on paper. Take slow, deep breaths and concentrate on your breathing. The tactical breathing, as discussed in a prior chapter. Tighten and release small muscle groups. Repeat a word, phrase, vision or ideal that reminds you to stay in control and remain confident. These are just some methods known to work, *when time is available*.

I always like to investigate the duality of things. Yours and his. What about his anger? In some pre-fight situations, you might be able to control the anger in your opponent by how you act and what you do or don't say. This effectively is trying to manage his anger, not just your own.

This subject contains several college degree's worth of material, not stuff for a seminar or two, or a martial class specialty. But, in the survival, self defense business, keep a Wolf Man or Wolf Woman alive inside you in a cage. Feed it once in a while. Rattle its cage. You may need to set it loose.

Numerous psychologists warn that anger can rob you of 80 percent of your logical brain function. Dr, Diane Wagenhals, an anger management specialist, tells us it takes about 20 minutes to calm down and "get a grip." Wow, 20 minutes! Counting to 10 does not help? Do we have to count instead to 1,200?

The goal of anger management is to reduce both your emotional feelings and the physiological arousal that anger causes. You can't get rid of, or avoid, the things or the people that enrage you, nor can you change them, but you can learn to control your reactions.

The following comes from a public health pamphlet from the *American Psychological Association*. Since you may never see this pamphlet, as a public service, here are some key elements of their anger management message.

"Are You Too Angry?

There are psychological tests that measure the intensity of angry feelings, how prone to anger you are, and how well you handle it. But chances are good that if you do have a problem with anger, you already know it. If you find yourself acting in ways that seem out of control and frightening, you might need help finding better ways to deal with this emotion.

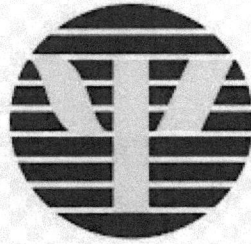

AMERICAN
PSYCHOLOGICAL
ASSOCIATION

Why Are Some People More Angry Than Others?

According to Jerry Deffenbacher, PhD, a psychologist who specializes in anger management, some people really are more "hotheaded" than others; they get angry more easily and more intensely than the average person does. There are also those who don't show their anger in loud spectacular ways but are chronically irritable and grumpy. Easily angered people don't always curse and throw things; sometimes they withdraw socially, sulk, or get physically ill.

People who are easily angered generally have what some psychologists call a low tolerance for frustration, meaning simply that they feel that they should not have to be subjected to frustration, inconvenience, or annoyance. They can't take things in stride, and they're particularly infuriated if the situation seems somehow unjust: for example, being corrected for a minor mistake.

What makes these people this way?

A number of things. One cause may be genetic or physiological: There is evidence that some children are born irritable, touchy, and easily angered, and that these signs are present from a very early age. Another may be sociocultural. Anger is often regarded as negative; we're taught that it's all right to express anxiety, depression, or other emotions but not to express anger. As a result, we don't learn how to handle it or channel it constructively.

Research has also found that family background plays a role. Typically, people who are easily angered come from families that are disruptive, chaotic, and not skilled at emotional communications.

There are numerous books in the marketplace on this subject. Do not rely on martial instructors and martial artists to teach these topics to you unless they are multi-qualified to do so. Martial folks such as myself and others can only skim the surface, only offer very brief overviews and steer you to the real experts.

Some suggested reading...

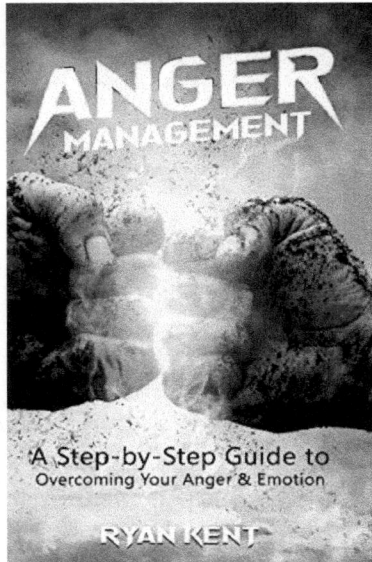

ANGER MANAGEMENT
A Step-by-Step Guide to Overcoming Your Anger & Emotion
RYAN KENT

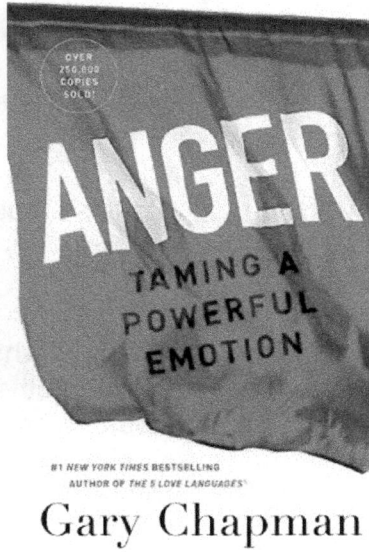

OVER 250,000 COPIES SOLD!
ANGER
TAMING A POWERFUL EMOTION
#1 NEW YORK TIMES BESTSELLING AUTHOR OF THE 5 LOVE LANGUAGES®
Gary Chapman

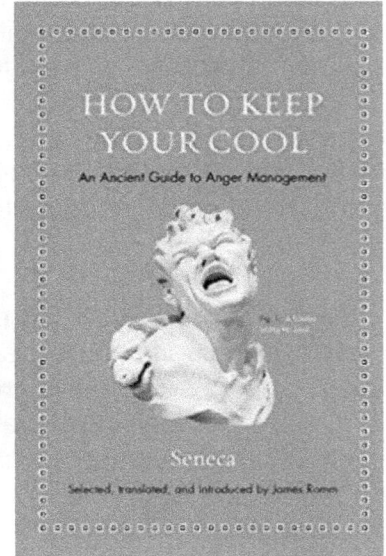

HOW TO KEEP YOUR COOL
An Ancient Guide to Anger Management
Seneca
Selected, translated, and introduced by James Romm

CHAPTER 17: FIGHTING COLD!

No, fighting cold is not about being mugged in Alaska or just a concern for the 10th Mountain Division. "Shooting cold" is a term thrown around here and there by smart people in the gun training business, but also relates the ambush in the hand, stick and knife world too. It should be a major concern for all, because generically, it's really about the ambush, surprise attack. And you must respond - cold.

Usually you hear the term with snipers or hunters. Folks who have to suddenly shoot a long gun from a distance. And from a clean barrel. Once in a while you will hear of a "one-shot" competition.

> **"Participants will be allotted a single shot, cold-bore (unfired rifle) @ 1000 yards. (30 Caliber & under) Time & hit determines the winner."**

They have those things because, they are challenging. The sin weighs heavy with that icy-cold rifle, but what of the shooter? There's also an important concept of "cold bore shooters." I guess you could remove the word "bore." Cold shooters. I think in terms of training and then real life crime and war ambushes, there might be a nickname, "Frigid Bore Shooting," or "frigid shooting." Here's what I mean.

Chilly? Cold? Frigid?

After all, who wants to fight cold or shoot cold in competitions for scores, trophies, money and bragging rights? Who doesn't want to take a few warmup shots? I know I often like to do a few dry-fires before live-fires. I use to participate in some police shooting competitions and they were often complicated paths, chores and obstacles involved. You had to be briefed on your routes and goals, and this would include a "walk-thru," or a "dry-run," or even a live-fire run before the official

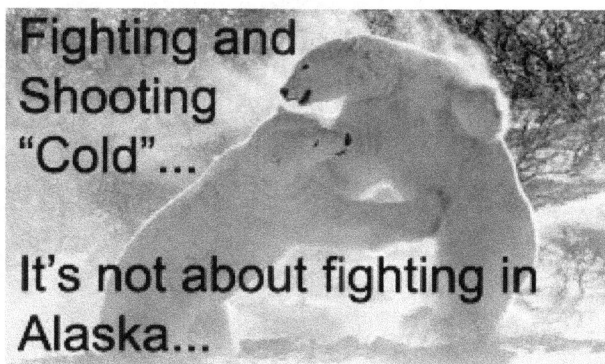

run. Same with police training courses and qualifications. It could be safety issue.
Chilly? Cold? Frigid?

After all, who wants to fight cold or shoot cold in competitions for scores, trophies, money and bragging rights? Who doesn't want to take a few warmup shots? I know I often like to do a few dry-fires before live-fires. I use to participate in some police shooting competitions and they were often complicated paths, chores and obstacles involved. You had to be briefed on your routes and goals, and this would include a "walk-thru," or a "dry-run," or even a live-fire run before the official run. Same with police training courses and qualifications. It could be a safety issue.

So just how cold is it, though? Completely frigid? Cold? Or chilly? They call it "cold shooting," or reverse the phrase, "shooting cold," and it kind of is, in a way. Sadly, oddly, some of the best shooters I know, don't do as spectacular in their first set, as they wish, and this is one reason why they keep score of this process over time. And often they do about as good as I can when we all start, and I do not shoot as much as they do, nor do I labor and belabor and ponder the art, science, love and dedication to trigger pressure and bulls-eye, pistol, target shooting as they do.

They admit, fighting and shooting cold is challenging for most. And, it frustrates some. Then they very quickly get much, much better after a "warm-up," quickly surpassing ol' mediocre me. (And yes, yes, we all know some special gun gods and rockstars with so much time and grade they do awesome right out of the gate. Pew-pew! More on that later).

Some regular, range shooters I know and hear about will always keep score of their first set, their "cold shooting" when they first step up to the firing line and shoot a set. But was it a true cold-virgin experience of the day?

Was it completely virgin? They want to keep track of how well they do after they:
- set the time and date, pack their gear at home,
- drive to the range,
- get out of the cars,
- get some gear from the "back" of the car,
- maybe sip some coffee, talk about guns,
- chat with the "range masters," and course instructors, or a classroom?
- If at a class? Listen to the instructor's intro, lecture,
- carry their gear to the spot, stand, table, shelf,
- shuffle up to the target and paste up a new one,
- wander back to the shooting line and,
- shoot…"cold."

So a cold shooter on gun day is not on a "frozen-solid-ambush" when they shoot at a range. Neither are folks starting a gym workout or a hand, stick, knife class. The mind and body are cooking just a little to prepare to train.

A hunter has worked on the trip, sometimes insanely so, before departure, going over equipment and plans in his or her trip.

I became interested by this idea of shooting and fighting cold. What does mean in the bigger picture? How does it relate to self-defense, in crime and in war? You know, all the "who, what, where, when how and why" questions I like to kick around.

Subliminal preparation? Years ago it was common knowledge in the fitness field that if you packed for the gym and drove to the gym about the same times, your body/brain knew the routine as we are such creatures of habit.

You drive, park, walk the lot, climb the stairs. All the while your body/brain is saying, "Okay, okay, we're coming. We're getting ready." Once in the gym, is this moment a true zero? Or, maybe 10? 10 to 60? Last month I parked on my gym parking lot and saw another guy, a bit older than me, park too. He got out of his car, got a gym bag and stopped. He took his ball cap off, looked to the sky and said a prayer. I spied his lips moving. Then he donned his cap and made for the gym doors. He really pre-prepped for a work-out! What did he say in prayer, I wonder?

"Dear Lord, let me crush everything?"

"Dear Lord, don't let me die of a heart attack this morning?"

What would your prep prayer be? Have one? Need one?

Routines. Preparation. Getting ready. Not always short term. We have all gone to a shooting class, or a martial tournament that we anticipated and our inner engine was revved up more than just the morning before. Even the night before. Even longer than that. I once took a shooting course, to prepare for the tougher shooting course the following weekend.

How powerful can mental preparation be? Surely you have heard of, or read the studies about how positive this mental approach can be. It is important.

I recall even back in 1972, in Ed Parker Kenpo Karate, teachers and students gossiping about another martial arts system and how the system sequestered students in dark rooms, assigned them to imagine the moves over and over in their heads as a basis of performance. 1972! None of us could fathom this being successful. Yet, quite a number of studies say this works! It somehow works for some. So, does the simple act of going to the range to shoot on gun day, mentally prepare you for the target/bulls eye process? I think so. A bit. It is one step back from dry-firing if you think about it.

Just getting dressed for work, be it a guard, or police, lawyer, truck driver, or an accountant starts churning up, the work mind, whether you realize it or not.

Frigid? How about being asleep?
It's especially cold-cold when you consider the old attempts at testing the responses of police when *THEY WERE ASLEEP!* Yes. They would bed down a series of state troopers in a sleep clinic environment and tell them that they would be harshly awakened at some point and they would have to wake up, grab a nearby gun and shoot a target near the foot of their bed. The results were not so good. Often bad in fact. Another similar sleep-study let tested police wake up on their own and they had to remember this assigned chore of immediately shooting. They were groggy-slow to remember the assigned chore, but most did grab and shoot…and also not too well, but they did remember. Where does this information fit in the "chilly, cold and frigid" charts of our considerations?

It starts in the mind.
When you actual started doing physical stuff on your jogging route, or at the gym or at the "dojo," or the shooting range, you are not really, fully working out "cold." The same is true with getting your uniform on for work, or slinging your vest on in the military. You are not cold-cold (unless of course, much time passes between the prep and action and you "chill out," which is a whole other set of study we talk about in other essays). And the same mental prep is true of the drive to the shooting range, the lugging of gear, the chat with the range master.

The inner gears are working. This type of first round scoring, cold shooting is not as frigid as you think. Not like a zero-to-60 ambush frigid. (Think for a moment about all the mental and physical prep before SWAT arrives on a scene.)

Life is either...
My old catch phrase is – "life is either an interview or an ambush" that people hear each week that I teach. I hope they never tire of it. The greatest armies in the world have been defeated by ambush. The simple element of surprise. The greatest fighters too. I get a kick out the internet comments when location cameras around the world catch a criminal jumping a victim in the most "ambushy" types of locales.

It does come back to the element of surprise and the ambush, doesn't it. There is always a wise-guy, arm-chair-est that comments "that person was not alert!" and the sage advice, "you must always stay alert." As if he, she, or we all, walk around with enough cortisol scorching our veins and heart, to be scanning EVERYWHERE, ALL the time.

We always hear the expression "you don't pick the time and place of your attack, the enemy does," so as everyday walk-around folks, or someone on common police and military patrol, you will probably, suddenly be fighting chilly or cold.

It is certainly a good idea to worry about and consider "cold-fighting" and "cold shooting," in your training, even though we simply cannot really replicate that "zero-to-sixty" frigid to red hot, encounter. I don't think we need a chart the size of a doorway like the new OODA Loop demo diagrams have become, to explain this simple "Boo/Surprise" idea. The element of surprise and reaction to it, can be as simple as a foot fake in football, rugby or soccer.

There are many startle responses to the sudden boo/jump, (one modern textbook counted 30 responses) not just one or two, hands-up, as you might have been sold to believe by martial and gun marketeers. Let's hope you don't fall right down or feint, which are two of the startle responses! You instead, have to deal with the attack.

Immediate Action Drills
Again, the element of surprise has defeated the greatest militaries of the world. I first learned about all this Ambush/Counter-Ambush in the U.S. Army in 1973, and it was a big deal. They trained us in what was called back then, "Immediate Action Drills," things done so many times that you may well jump right into that response groove when ambushed. Hopefully. It is reinforced by many, many repetitions. Here are some of my old Army manual notes (minus the small and large unit suggestions they offer) on the ambush drill idea that relates to citizens and police.

"Immediate action drills are drills designed to provide swift and positive reaction. They are simple courses of action, done immediately. It is not feasible to attempt to design an immediate action drill to cover every possible situation.

It is better to know a few immediate action drills for a limited number of situations that usually occur (in a combat area.)

1. Can be designed, developed, and used by anyone, (any unit).
2. Are designed and developed as needed for the anticipated combat situation.
3. When contact/ambush, is at very close range and maneuvers may be restricted."

This does work often, and then…sometimes not, because you might be too frigid, or too cold to respond well. Just some notes. As I have stated many times before, when students approach you with concerns about "how-fast" and "will-they" react properly to an sudden attack, you can honestly shove them back on the floor and tell them to do more reps, and explain why. "Fortune favors the prepared." Build confidence, yes, but darn it, cold is still cold, and frigid is still worse.

But, back to the shooting guns, cold subject. One of my friends said after reading this when first published back in 2011:

"Hock is right about this. I suck shooting cold, but that is how I am going to shoot, cold, stepping out of the Waffle House and suddenly in trouble, on any given night."

So, it's hard to replicate shooting cold or fighting cold in training, because you are never completely cold-cold when you plan, dress and travel and lug-in and gear-up for training. Maybe they should call a real ambush response "Shooting Frigid?" or "Fighting Frigid" instead of just being cold? Frigid bore shooting?

Am I getting warm, yet?

CHAPTER 18: THE RITUALS OF DEATH (BEFORE THE DEATH, NOT AFTER!)

The rituals of death. Understanding them may save your life. But, when you try to research the term, all you are most likely to uncover are after-death, practices of various worldwide religions and funerals, like tossing a handful of dirt on a coffin to name but one. I guess the trouble with the research quest is the word "ritual" - so quickly associated with religions. Dig a bit deeper (no pun intended) and you'll find a few ceremonial pre-death rituals like when archaeologists discovered that the Incas got their children sacrifices drunk before their deaths on coco leaves and alcohol. Still after much digging, not much is mentioned about before the death.

If you broaden your own definition of "rituals," of death, it starts you thinking. You might recall the many other kinds of political and religious killings, ones before the flame, the shot, the needle, the hanging, the guillotine, the firing squad, the electrocution, etc. We remember some pre-death, rituals with them. Before such events, we have been exposed to ritualistic habits like, "the last meal." The "last cigarette." The blindfold, "any last requests?" "any last statements?" These are also rituals of death, before the act. Why do people bother with them?

Think about the ritualistic procedures in the United States over a prisoner execution. There are many ritualistic steps and protocols. Think about how people gather in to witness the execution.
In the olden days, people gathered for the public hangings, nowadays seating is assigned at the prison death chambers to watch a person die.

I feel as though any of the death row prisoners would much rather be surprised by a shot in the back of the head at some late point rather than go through all that extraneous legal, ritual, nonsense. And, consider this irony, there have been postponements in prison executions because the prisoner was too sick on his

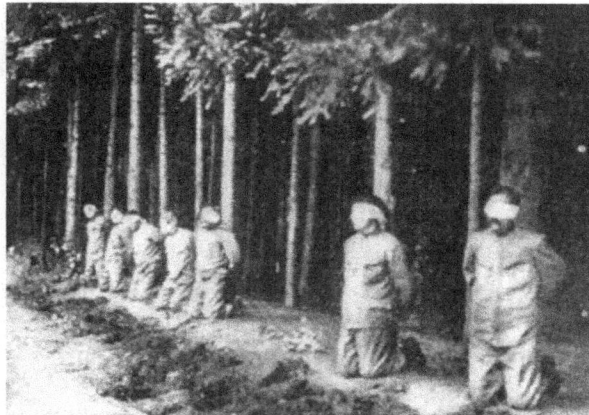

Who, what, where, when, how and why are these doomed prisoners all on their knees? Blindfolded with white cloth? Tied to trees? It's a ritual.

death date. Too sick to die? "Let's clear up that flu before we kill him."

All these numerous rituals alone, suggested to me that most humans have a certain significance attached to death. They hold a regard about death and often do things, also in crime and war to postpone, celebrate, or commemorate death. A ritual, however slight or small, might be created. It often seems to be in our human nature.

I would like to write about a very particular situation when someone is cornered, captured, kidnapped and-or taken hostage. They may be held hostage short-term or long-term, and about to killed. As a police detective most of my adult life, and a graduate of a police, criminal profile course, I came across numerous cases, mine and others, of victims executed, or who received threats of execution in the final act of rape, kidnapping, robbery, assault and so forth. And what about in war? Such as when someone is taken prisoner, or cornered? What did those last few seconds look and feel like? What small ignored, rituals existed or still exist for the killers. If we knew what the killers did, we might better prepare people to read upcoming signs and find ways to counter them.

In recent times now more than in the past, instructors like to present lists of pre-assault cues with all the anger, tip-offs. That list is long (and far from new - as the first one I saw was back in the military police academy in 1973.) What of pre-crime clues? They are different and largely ignored as people tend to dwell on the pre-assault cues. With pre-crime there might be a no-anger greeting, usually presented by smiling con-men criminals setting you up with a minimum tip-offs, or not. Maybe just an overwhelming, sudden ambush?

In this same vein of study, but not like the pre-assault, and pre-crime, are the verbal, physical and situational, last ditch rituals of...pre-death. Situational? The overall situation also counts like a ticking time bomb.

So, I became fascinated, in crime and war's last moments, especially the last few seconds, the last few steps of these killing actions. What exactly went on? And to see if there are any big or small "rituals" even in these instances. They may or may not be spontaneous. The crime may be pre-meditated, but the physical act itself un-planned. What happened? Learning this as a self defense, martialist instructor for civilians, police and military, might warn and prepare people for last resort counters to these problems.

For example, think of all the pistol dis-arms taught. Think of the more rare, long gun disarms. Think of the knife disarms. Think of the strangulation escapes. Lots of..."techniques," as they say. But hardly anyone understands or covers the total "who, what, when, where, how and why" (the Ws&H) the victim wound up in this terrible moment, these terrible, critical last, few seconds. The context. The situation. What last ditch, last resort things could be done to counter the murder attempt?

The techniques? I have told this story for decades as an example of the "classroom disarmer," of a student who learned two pistol disarms techniques earlier in the day at a martial class. He goes home and tells his friend how great the disarms were. The friend says "wow, show me," and he gets a "clicker," replica pistol and stands before the student, face-to-face, gun aimed at the student's head, execution style.

The student and friend stare at each other, (like a Western showdown that actually hardly ever happened). The friend is a live wire, watching anxiously for ANY slight sign, a "tell," (tip-off or clue) that a disarm attempt is coming. The student tries one of the disarms, j...u...s...t barely flinches and...CLICK. He's "shot!." The student tries and tries and can't do either of the disarms. Disillusioned, depressed, he confesses, "I guess they don't really work."

Like the Western showdown, how often does a criminal stand in front of you with 110 percent attention like this... waiting... waiting...

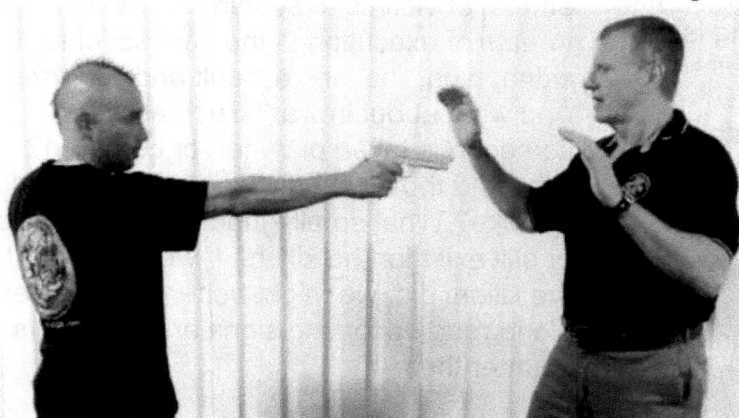

The gun threat training partner is just waiting breathlessly for the ever so slight movement to pull the trigger and thwart the disarm. Would this really happen? Or would the killer just produce the gun and shoot? Or would the criminal be ordered compliance? Or grilling for information?

This evaluation could be very wrong because forgotten is the unusual, multi-faceted crime and war situations people are thrust in. Gun men are often preoccupied running their overall crime scenes and rarely, if ever, are they in this sterile, "face-to-face," "anxiously waiting-for-the-disarm" waiting to pull the trigger, classroom situation.

Ws&H questions for examples...

The Who Question? For the purposes of brevity, let's loosely list a few general "who's-who" to get you thinking about this topic. (Remember I am not a psychologist and you must investigate these typologies yourself.)

* *Psychopath.* Someone who might kill in an instant, without remorse, without ritual.

* *Psychopath who terrorizes.* Someone who might kill and wants to enjoy torturing someone. There might be a ritual in involved.

* *Realistic actor.* Someone who is not a psychopath, but is somewhat "forced" into killing you due to circumstances. He might be resigned to the act.

* *Reluctant actor.* Someone who is not a psychopath, but is really reluctant and really "forced" into killing you due to circumstances. He might be angry or depressed and resigned to the act.

* *Impulse actors.* Various criminal studies state that many criminals have poor impulse control.

We could of course, slice and dice these very generic characterizations forever. But, anyone of these might have tip-off tells of what they will do, verbal or physical.

Perhaps your best predictive luck or chances are with the realistic and reluctant actors. If a true, cold-blooded psychopath decides to kill you, they might well do so in an instant. No rituals. No tells...just boom. Imagine a hostage situation where there is food for seven people and he has eight hostages. Boom, a random death upon discovery of the problem. Now there's food for seven. If a non-psychopath has to kill you, he might say or do something...specifically at the moment...that is "ritualistic."

The What Question? There are numerous examples of what might be said or done in these situations.

* Verbal. A psychopath may say nothing, or in the terrorizing version, enjoy saying extra-frightening things. Their rituals might be very personal and impossible to understand by sane people. A non-psychopath might ask for somewhat ritualistic things like, "Get down on your knees?" or, "Lay face down," or "Turn-around." This is because he doesn't want to fully see or not see your face. It is old military psychology now that you are harder to kill face-to-face for most "normal" people. The reluctant's voice may get mean with a certain resolve and resignation. This could be because he is actually angry at himself and-or the situation.

* Sounds. And this is not just about voice. There is a case in Gaven Debecker's book *The Gift of Fear* when a rapist left the victim's bedroom and turned the volume way up on the living room stereo. The victim realized this increase was to cover the sounds of her murder and screaming. She managed to sneak out of her apartment while the rapist was in the kitchen to get a knife. Translating sounds. What of the sounds of loading or cocking a gun?

Opening a trunk or a van door. Endless, normal sounds can be situationally suspicious.

* Physical. Sudden deep breaths before actions. Serious facial expression changes. Some might easily be read as a resignation that the reluctant has to kill. A terrorizing psychopath might smile with enjoyment. It has been observed in a variety of situations that someone holding a long gun at hip level, resigned to murder, will grimace and lift the weapon to shoulder height. They might elevate the pistol from low to high. They could just shoot from the hip. These are last second "tells."

The Where Question? First off, a rule of survival, never go from "crime scene A" to "crime scene B." If you can fight and resist at crime scene A when you discover a planned transport? Do so. B is usually a prepared place of torture and-or death. A psychopath might kill you anywhere, or at crime scene B.

A non-psychopath might ritualistically march you off to somewhere else, and often for no real reason. It seems to be a ritual of death to do so. The back room refrigerator of a convenience store for just one example. These marches may take you to a place where there are no sight or sound witnesses.

The When Question? The brewing situation should help a victim tell if an execution is forthcoming. Understanding the overall situation can set the clock for predicting your planned demise. Many victim can predict their eventual doom by just seeing the face of a criminal.

The How Question? How will the murder be accomplished? Are you being marched off to a cliff? The meat locker? Does the

criminal or enemy have a stick? Knife, pistol? A long gun? If so, do you know the common striking, stabbing and shooting positions? How close is the killer standing? Where are you standing? Has he approached with an "angry" strutting walk and face? How will your respond?

The Why Question? By keeping close track of your dilemma, can you anticipate why you need to be killed. Whim? Delight? No witnesses? Revenge? Understanding motives. Think of an on-premise, witness to a crime. Think of a crazed spouse, violating a protective order after many violent threats, showing up at a house with a weapon. Why must things end this way? The killer usually needs a motive, whether you understand the reasons, or not. Again, studies show that many criminal have poor impulse control.

Quick summary. I would like for you to think about these Ws&H points. It usually takes about 6 passes of the Ws&H questions to collect satisfactory information. You might get down to the "when" question and you realize you need to reexamine the "who" question again. And we can't forget that crime patterns, in your region, your city or street, can be a copycat ritual. Examine if you will, the many gang shootings in Chicago. How do they unfold?

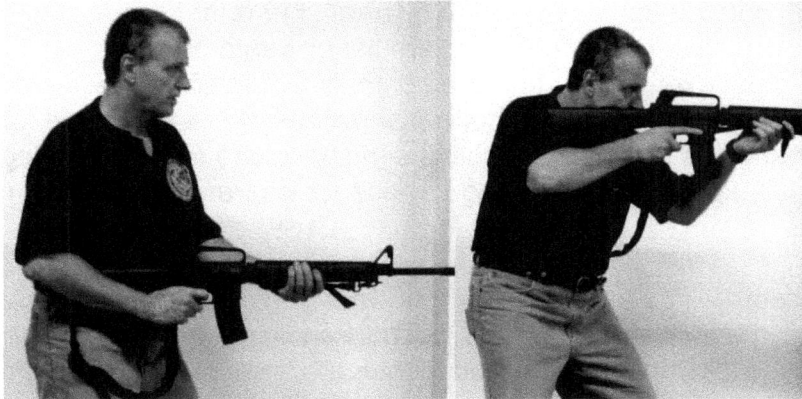

The sudden weapon lift might well be the last ritual step before execution.

What might the rituals of pre-death be?
* You are cornered, captured, kidnapped and-or taken hostage. Short-term or long-term, and about to killed.

* Verbal clues like tones and words.
* Sound clues like weapons preps - racking, chambering.
* Visual clues like facial expressions.
* Crime patterns may be involved.
* Situations that history and common sense lead to executions.
* Brewing, overall situations.
* Has he approached with an angry walk and face?
* Last request questions.
* Suddenly being treated nicely. A "sorry, good-bye ritual."
* Being marched to questionable and isolated places with a lack of help or witnesses.
* Sudden lifting of firearms into common firing positions.
* Sudden lifting of sticks, bats, clubs and tool into striking positions.
* Sudden drawing of weapons.
* ....continue to develop your own lists.

On the rituals of suicide.
I have probably worked more suicides than murders through the years and they might have their own meaningful rituals and death scenes. Some organized scenes were fascinating and not appropriate for this essay theme. But, recognizing the organized suicide scene and any ritual evidence is important to classify and conclude the case, but again, suicide rituals are another subject.

But I must mention that in the police world, we are long cursed with "suicide by cop" situations. There is suicide by civilian or also military. Whether cop, citizen or soldier, these suicidal people get you to shoot them by presenting you with these same ritual of death moves we cover here, like drawing a weapon, lifting a weapon, marching upon you armed, with angry walks and angry faces. Perhaps really over-acted to get your reaction! Recognizing apparent suicidal situations may save you great expense and grief and legal expense later on.

My goal here is not to teach any weapon disarms, but rather to translate events, see clues and tip-offs, or "tells," before counters are life-or-death needed.

Of course you must exercise all unarmed combatives to solve these problems. Standing, kneeling, sitting, grounded on top, bottom and sides. All must include knowledge of weapon operations, yours and his. All positions must include striking, kicking and what might be called "dirty fighting" or "cheating." These topics transcend typical martial arts found everywhere.

The rituals of death. They are not just about what goes in a funeral mass or at the cemetery after you die. It is also about the last things killers often physically say and-or do, just before they try to kill you, and how you must learn them to stay out of the deep end of a cemetery.

*(And I remind you again, I am **not** a psychologist. Keep researching this and make your own lists. I only wish to provoke thought and planning.)*

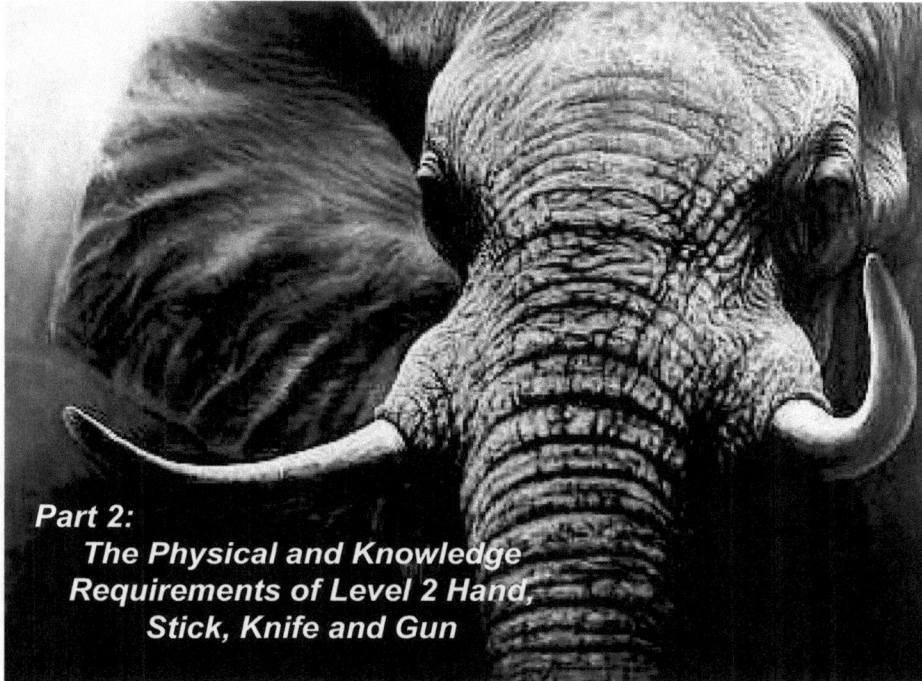

Part 2:
The Physical and Knowledge
Requirements of Level 2 Hand,
Stick, Knife and Gun

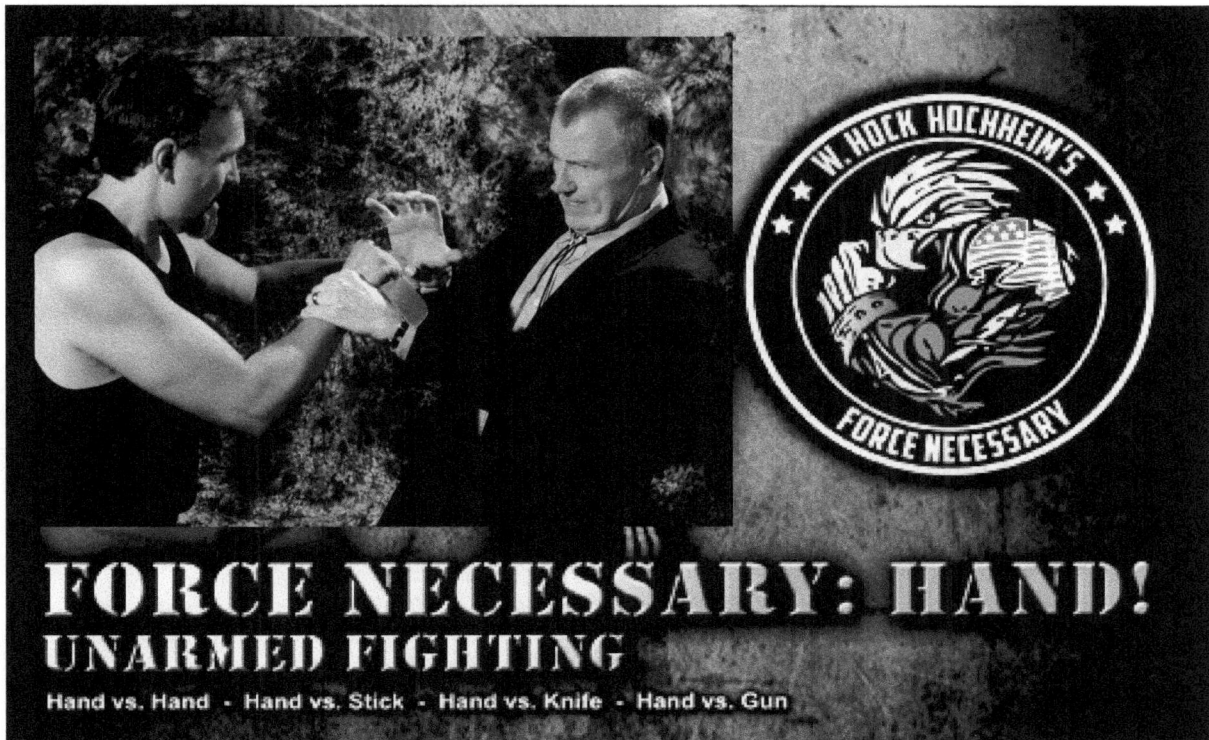

FORCE NECESSARY: HAND!
UNARMED FIGHTING
Hand vs. Hand - Hand vs. Stick - Hand vs. Knife - Hand vs. Gun

CHAPTER 19: FORCE NECESSARY HAND – LEVEL 2

Review Training Mission One

Commonalities

Examine Stop 2 as explored within the Level 2 Hand context.
Examine the "What" question as explored within the Level 2 Hand context.
Examine the Footwork Drill #2 - The In and Out Drill.
Examine and remember the basic, grip releases chapter from Part One.
Review the *Stalker Drill*, adding the *Mad Rush*, and *Tangler,* and work on these within the Level 2 Hand context.
Continue studying your local self defense laws.

Physical Performance Requirements

The *Palm Strikes Module.*
The *Agitating Push Module*, added to *Stalker* and *Mad Rush* Drill.
The *Stomp Kick* Module.
The Level 2/*Stop 2 Grappling.* Study Finger and Wrist Grappling.
  - the "5 Wrists," counters and 1 lock/crank flow.
  - the "10 Fingers" and counters.

Stop 6 Stopping Review: Caught Red-Handed! Common Hands-on Stops.
Ever watch the TV news and see a fight in the Taiwan parliament or someplace like the West Palm Beach City Council meeting. There you will often see people in these hand-on-hand, *Stop 2* situations, like a palm-to-palm stop, of some sort. It is really not an uncommon stop or catch. Fingers entwine. Hands grab hands and wrists.

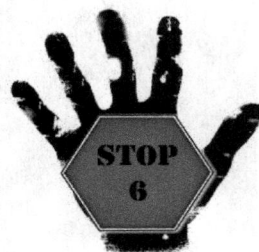

   If you charge someone to grab them, push them, pull them or grapple with them, or even arrest them, you do so with your hands up. They often reflexively respond with their hands and arms up too, which is why this catch is a common occurrence. This *Stop 2* contact could be:
   - fingers in fingers.
   - hands on fingers.
   - hands on hands.
   - hands on wrist areas.
   - hands on stick, knife, gun carry sites.
   - hands on drawn sticks, knives and guns.
   - a combination of the aforementioned.
   - here in *Training Mission Two*, we nickname these contacts as "Tanglers" as your fingers, hands and wrists are tangled up with your opponent's hands, and/or your weapons.

   Remember that while the *Force Necessary: Hand,* unarmed course also covers *Stop 2* problems. The unarmed course is very big and also has its own progression proceeding along inside and outside the parameters of *Stop 2*.

The "Ws and H" Survival Questions continues with the "What" Question Review.
   * *What* belongs and what doesn't belong, at a location?
   * *What* can really happen to you inside your home?
   * *What* can really happen to you in your home area?
   * *What* can really happen to you on your travels away from home?
   * *What* crime did you anticipate? What event?
   * *What* is happening in the actual event? Exactly. Step-by-step?
   * *What* is he doing in the actual event? Exactly.
   * *What* are you going to do? Exactly.
   * *What* weapon will you choose?
   * *What* will you carry?
   * *What* training course will you take?
   * *What* happens next? The big overall, question lecture. Are you arrested?
     Are you sued? Are you home safe? At your house, HQ or your base?
   * *Continue* to develop the what questions.

Review The Footwork Drill #2 - The In and Out
Read that chapter in the front part of the book. You should be able to, while unarmed, work this in and out footwork on the Combat Clock. *(Obviously Drill #1 appears in* Training Mission One.*)*

Level 2 Strike Module: The Open Hand, Palm Strikes

Lecture Point 1: The common strike deliveries, as expressed here in palm strikes
    1: Thrusts or,
    2: Hooks, both delivered by either:
    3: A hit and retract, or,
    4: Committed lunge.
    Note: These are the only 4 ways that *ANY* strike is delivered.

Lecture Point 2: Remember the Force Necessary Combat Clock
We use the Clock for strikes, blocks, footwork, etc.

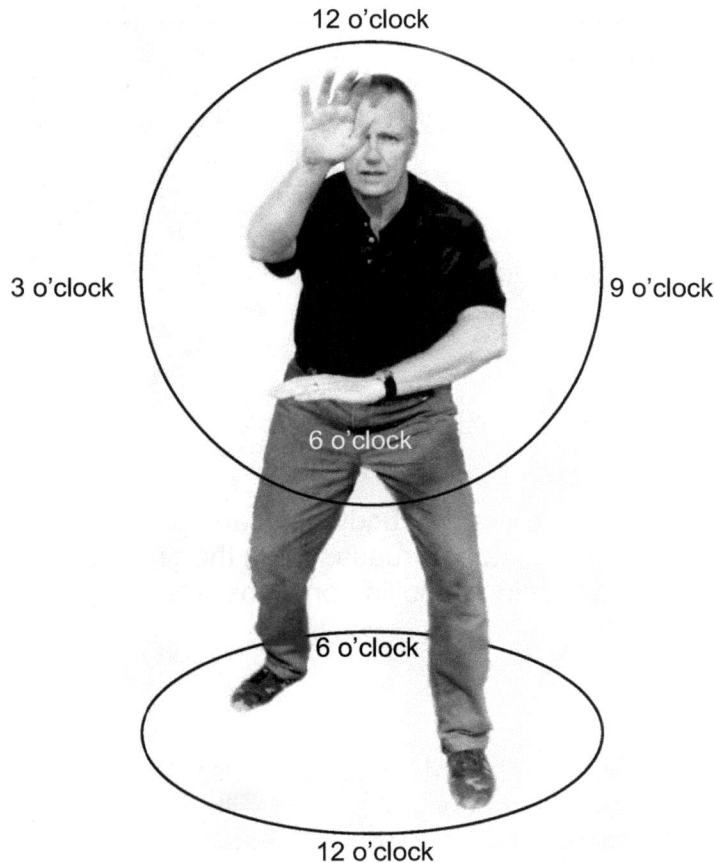

Lecture Point 3: Broken fists
Fearing broken hands that often arise from punching the head, more specifically punching the top half of the head, or the old, "bicycle helmet" area of the head, many combatives programs prefer the open palm strike. Do remember that palms and connecting fingers, wrists, even forearms are not invincible either, are subject to injuries, when striking. Champ Bas Rutten suggests you strike trained fighters with palm strikes and punch the untrained. How they stand before you and how they begin to fight are clues to this status.

Lecture Point 4: Legal stigma
The open hand strike also seems to carry less of this violent, *legal* stigma. For example, some US police agencies do not allow their officers to "ball up their hands into fists," yet have no such restrictive rules on palm strikes.

Lecture Point 5: The overall palm list, variations on a theme
The palm can be used in so many way. Here in a *Stop 2* strike study we will emphasize a few. Topics like blocking, trapping limbs, will appear in *Stop 3, Training Mission Three*. Most strikes via thrust, hooks, lunge and hit and retracts. An overall study and workout list should include:

- thrusting and hooking palms.
- slaps.
- web hand.
- single hand palm strikes.
- double hand palm strikes.
- face mauls.
- hit and shove.
- single hand push.
- double hand push.
- straight arms. (Think US football.)
- trap slaps and pins.
- blocks.
- pushing in general.
- pushing (with pulling) in weapon disarms.

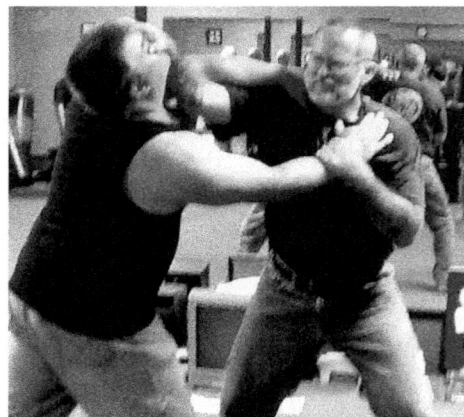

Long time FN instructor "Big Dawg" Kerwood of Mississippi, works on the palm strike.

Lecture Point 6: Targeting
With thrusting and hooking deliveries, any body part can be hit and/or shoved. Favorite targets are the head (overall face, nose squash, chin), the groin, the torso, but the palm can be used for targeting as pushing or pulling on limbs, and involved in weapon disarming.

The Thrusting Heel Palm
These strikes are often called "heel palm" strikes because when thrusting, the heel of the palm is used as a solid, striking surface in alignment with the forearm for power, and it helps prevent the hand from hyper-extending at the wrist.

A 6 o'clock delivery can produce the popular "chin jab," favored by so many. The chin jab may set-up an immediate eye attack, too, as well as a leg sweep takedown and many other options. Many people believe, after the chin strike, one can push the head back even more.

Of note, the old, Marine Raider, heel palm to back side and back of the lower head, neck area, once called the infamous "Gerber" strike, because as they described it, once hit, you will be eating Gerber, baby food for a week. This is an illegal target in sports, for that reason.

For solo command and mastery work and bag and mitt work, we can cover the basic Combat Clock training, exercising the 12, 3, 6 or 9 o'clock corners, and if needed the advanced training, Combat Clock exercising all 12 numbers/angles of the Clock.

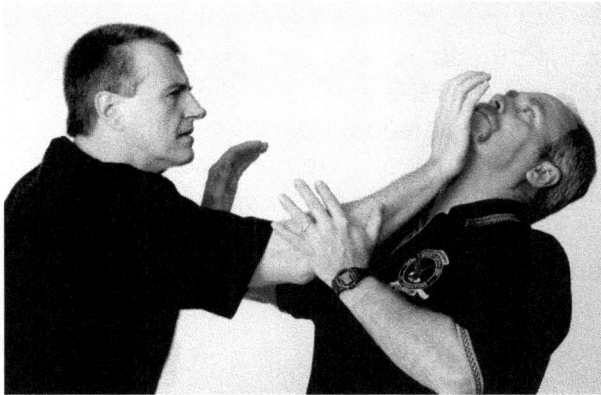

The 6 o'clock, thrusting palm is the classic "chin jab."

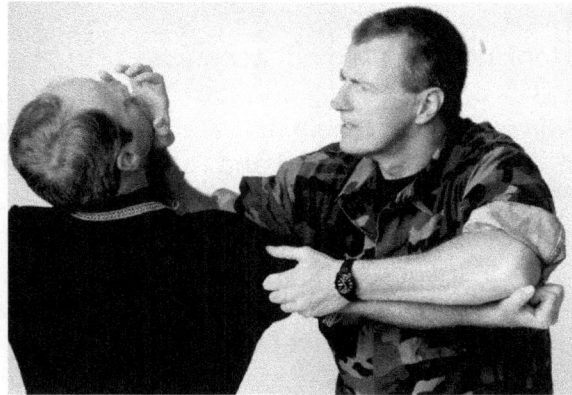

A chin jab may also lead to an incidental, eye attack, an old military tip.

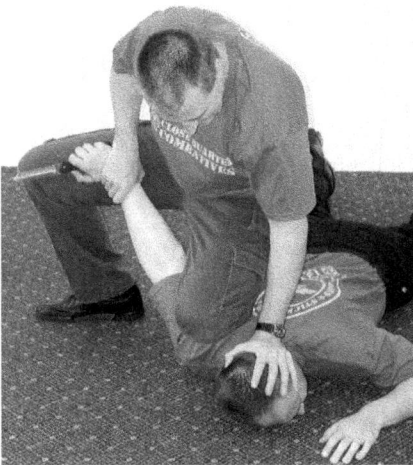

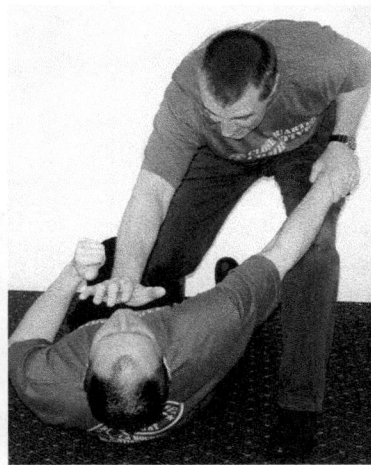

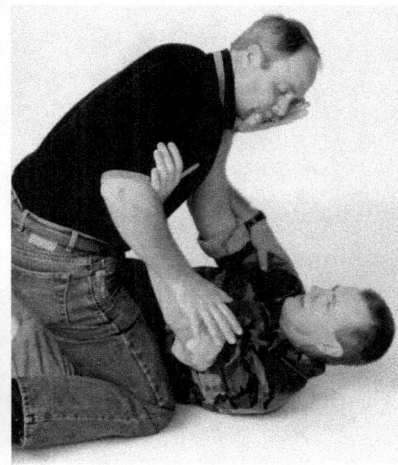

You can hold down or bounce a head off the floor, or a wall, or a car door post, whatever, with a thrusting palm.

Another Thruster - The thrusting web hand
A web hand strike is usually a thrust with an open hand, as in the thumb is way out, usually the upper and lower throat area as the target. You have to watch out not to hyper-extend your thumb, and realize that a windpipe may get seriously damaged.

For solo command and mastery and bag work, we can cover the basic Combat Clock training, the 12, 3, 6 or 9 o'clock corners, tightly delivered, and if needed the advanced Combat Clock on all 12 numbers of the Clock, again tightly delivered because you need that center line access to hit the target.

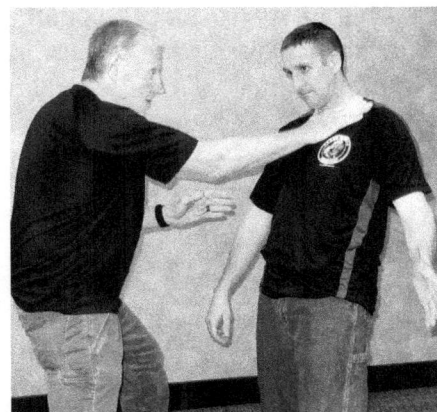

The web hand strike. Take care not to hyper-extend the thumb.

Hooking palms

Hooking palms do not accentuate the heels as the thrusts do, and use a larger impact surface, or slapping surface. Fingers can sometimes rake the eyes and stun the nose. It takes a hooking palm to make single and double ear claps and other devastating shots.

For solo command and mastery work and bag and mitt work, we can cover the basic Combat Clock training, exercising the 12, 3, 6 or 9 o'clock corners, and if needed the advanced training, Combat Clock exercising all 12 numbers of the clock.

Military and fighting experts all suggest hitting the "sports-illegal" area behind the ear, lower skull area with the heel of your hooking, open hand. This can also hook behind the sport-glove-face coverage.

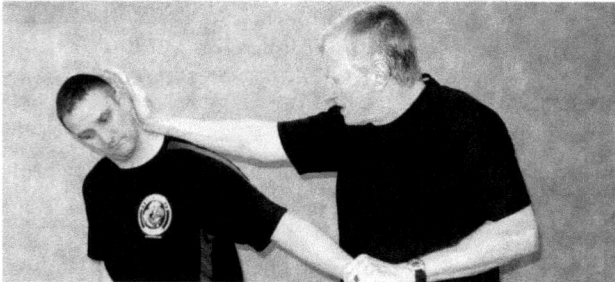

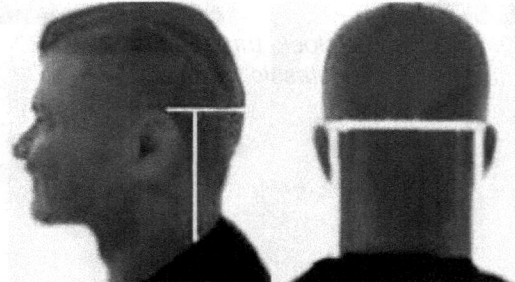

A great target for a hooking heel/palm is the sports-illegal area behind the ear, lower skull.

As presented in *Training Mission One*, when emphasizing the eye strikes, here is a military ear clap series I was taught in the US Army.
- right hand to left ear clap, right thumb into eye.
- left hand to right ear clap, left thumb into eye.
- double ear clap, double eye attack.

Unlike some training suggests, you do not need an oddly, cupped hand to hit the ear. The flat or your palm is a better striking surface upon the ear.

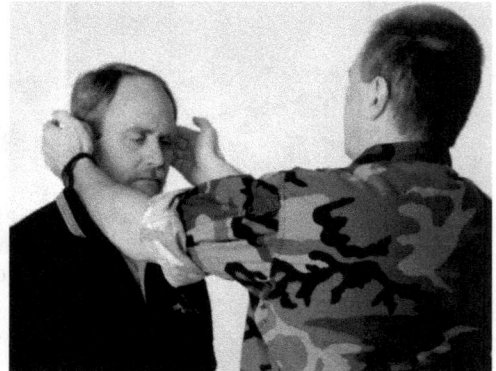

Double palms (or double palm stops/restraints)

There's not a successful American football or rugby player worldwide that doesn't use two, simultaneous or almost simultaneous palm strike/pushes to get past, knock down or position someone. Downward palms/hands, or upward ones are used in many predicaments, not just double ear claps or double palm, chin jabs. Thrusting or hooking.

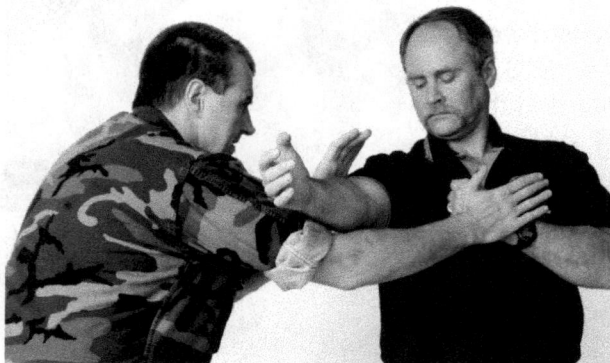

Here are two examples in one photo to the left. My left palm passes/blocks Tom the-Arnold-Barnhart's attack, while my right hooking palm traps, pins his hand to his chest.

Comprehensive blocking and trapping with the forearms-hands will be covered in *Training Mission Three*, in one packaged presentation, as it is a *Stop 3* problem, area, collision.

Marine Raider face maul

The old Raider program, at some stage, had the "face maul", kind of a nose squashing, palm strike to the face that stays there and rips and mauls the face. One or two hands. Get two hands involved if possible, because the head must be caught in some manner to really rip and tear up the face. (Try it in survival, groundfighting.)

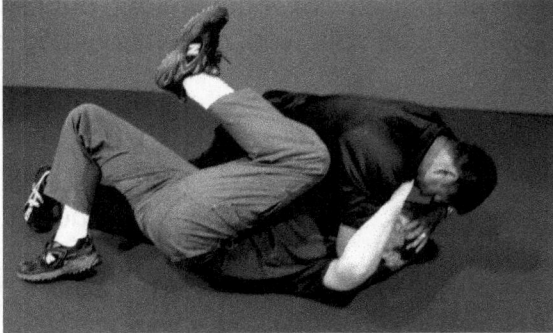

Here Tim Llacuna and Mike Belzer mix it up, to demonstrate a face maul on the ground.

Training the Marine face maul, The face maul is a *major* self defense move. By maul, I mean a ripping, tearing, circular motion that cover the eyes, nose, mouth - the face in general, as passed down to me from the Marine Corp Raiders of yesteryear.

Single hand. Double hand. You can't really train a face maul in class. So, I ask practioners to use their partners shoulder instead of their face. Do a single maul on the shoulder. A double hand maul.

This at very least seriously interrupts his mind and attack, standing or on the ground. Make it a point to do this on the ground. The opponent tries to escape this and one way is to reflexively grab your attacking wrist. Then you must resort again to the releasing methods of *Stop 2*, to free your hands to do more damage.

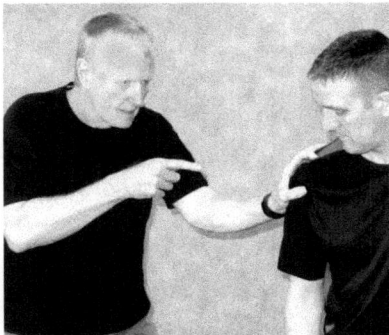

Single hand face maul, as practiced on the shoulder of your friend, such as Rawhide Laun.

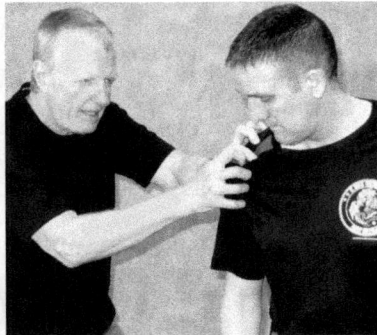

Double hand face maul, as practiced on the shoulder of your friend.

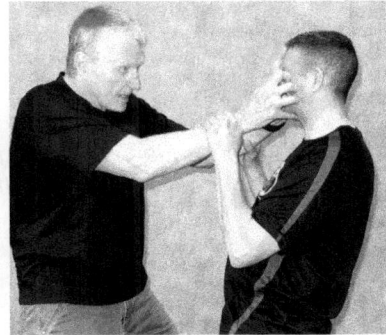

He will no doubt grab you as your maul, and you will need to get a release, as emphasized later in this book.

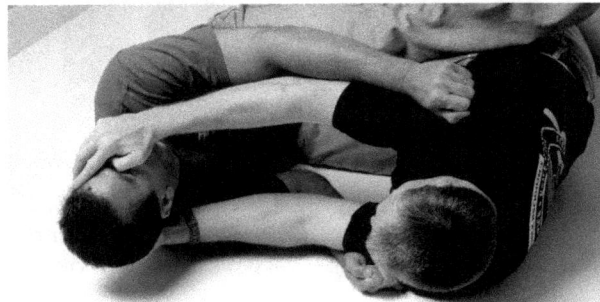

Solo Command and Mastery of the Palm Strike

An instructor should lead practitioners through the solo work in classes and seminars and observe them to make sure they have the overall, correct proper body synergy. Usually the basic 4 Combat Clock is done, with a run-through of 12 on the advanced Clock.

Feel free to change footwork as everyone progresses through the standing versions. When grounded, I remind all not to fly flat when on their backs, legs straight, but rather to move, rock and roll energetically. This category includes solo work on a heavy bag or similar apparatus.

Thrusting right palm on the Clock.
Thrusting left palm on the Clock.
Thrusting both palms on the Clock.

Hooking right palm on the Clock.
Hooting left palm on the Clock.
Hooking both palms on the Clock.

><

- right hand.
- left hand.
- both hands.
- standing.
- kneeling.
- grounded.

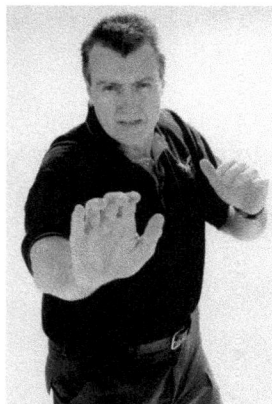
Right 12 o'clock start thrust or hook.

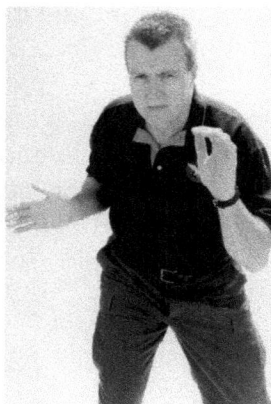
Right 3 o'clock start thrust or hook.

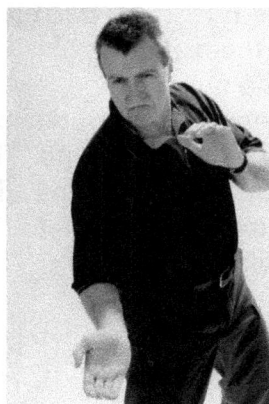
Right 6 o'clock start thrust or hook.

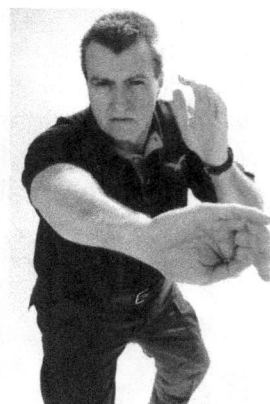
Right 9 o'clock start thrust or hook.

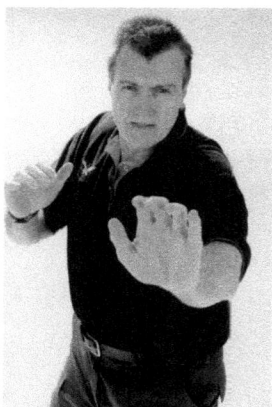
Left 12 o'clock start thrust or hook.

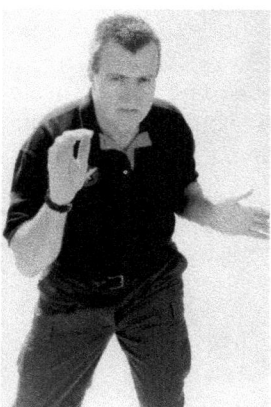
Left 3 o'clock start thrust or hook.

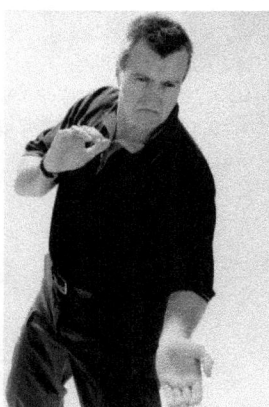
Left 6 o'clock start thrust or hook.

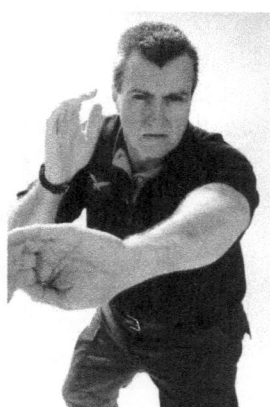
Left 9 o'clock start thrust or hook.

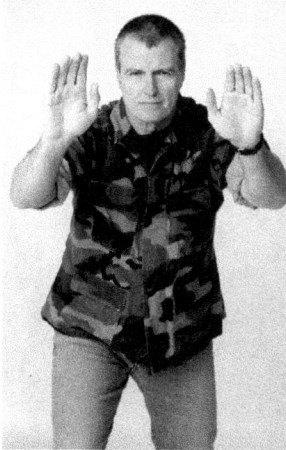

| 12 o'clock or from high on down. | 3 o'clock anything from the right. | 6 o'clock of from low on up. | 9 o'clock anything from the left. |

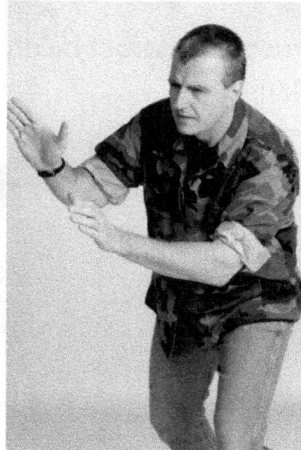

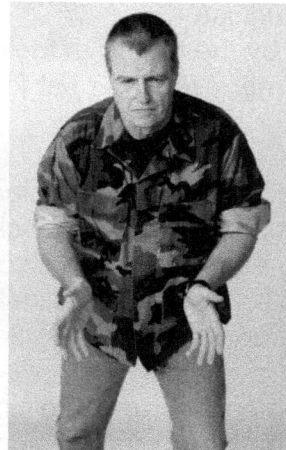

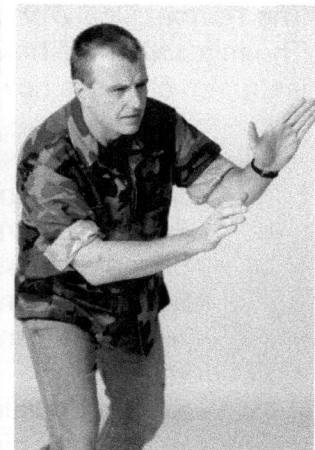

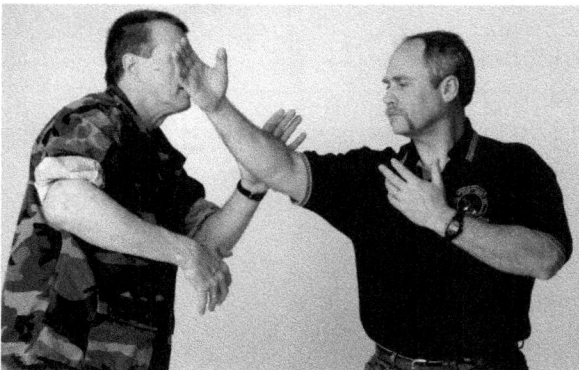

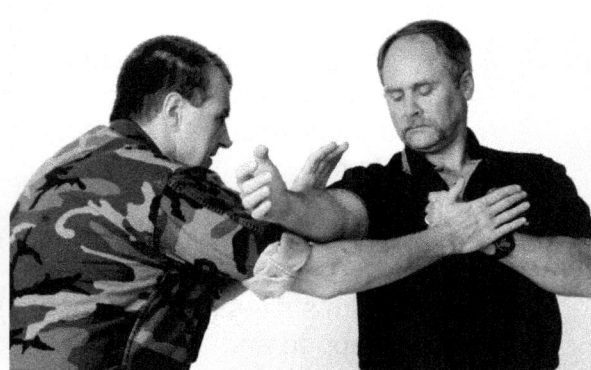

Single and double hand, palm strike blocking are vital defenses.

Partner Drills

As established in *Training Mission One*, we have Solo Command and Mastery exercises and partner drills. The trainer with mitts may stay still, then move, then also add flashing the mitt, or a kicking shield. The mitt should be held by the trainer at the prescribed target height. The instructor chooses how many reps per set to execute. Partners are essential for skill development exercises and combat scenarios.

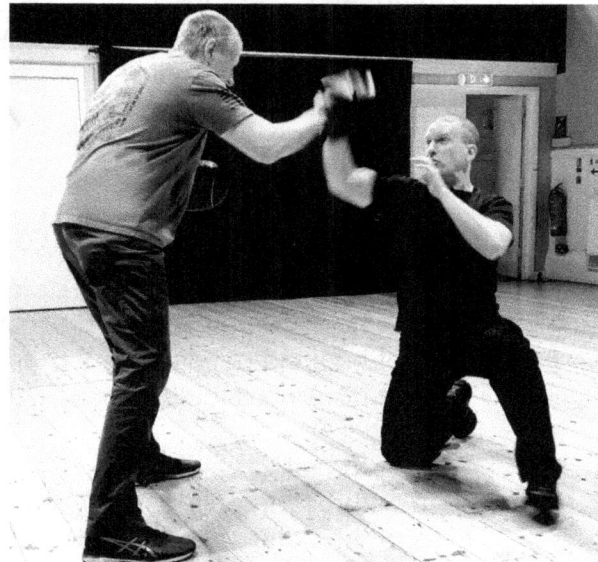

Jethro Randolph, our lead agent in the United Kingdom, gets his knee-high palm strikes in.

The Partner Drill Workout List
The mitt should be held by the trainer at the prescribed target height. The instructor chooses how many reps per set to execute.

Standing workout
- Sets of hooking palms from 12 o'clock.
- Sets of hooking palms from 3 o'clock.
- Sets of hooking palms from 6 o' clock.
- Sets of hooking palms from 9 o'clock.
- Sets of hooking double hand, ear claps.

- Sets of thrusting palms from 12 o'clock.
- Sets of thrusting palms from 3 o'clock.
- Sets of thrusting palms from 6 o' clock.
- Sets of thrusting palms from 9 o'clock.
- Sets of thrusting double hand, strikes/pushes.

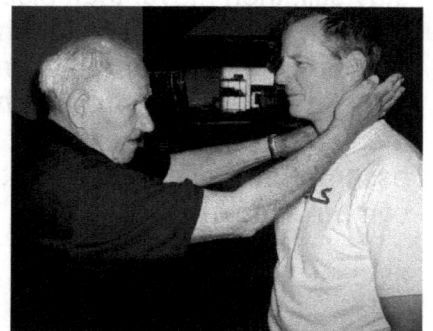

- Sets of thrusting right web hands to throat height.
- Sets of thrusting left web hands to throat height.
  Note: Carefully and wisely select a pad and position to hit.

- Sets of palm strikes (thrust or hooks) while your arm is wrapped and "while held."
- Sets of palm strikes (thrust or hooks) while his arm is wrapped and "while holding."

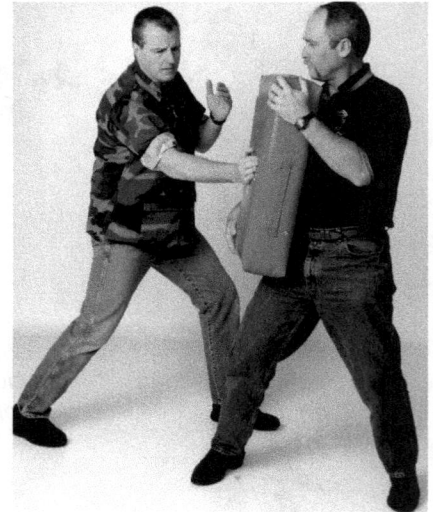

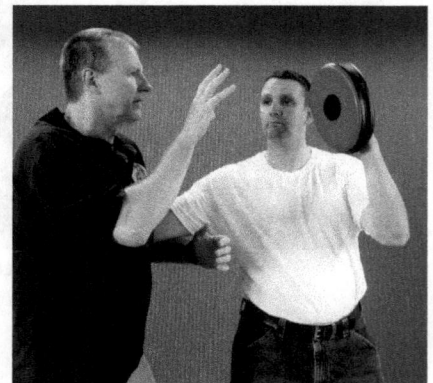

Kneeling workout
Kneelers fight people in 3 directions, above them, equal height to them, and below them, which is the topside of a ground fight. Targets therefore may be anything, like:
- blocking/passing leg kicks.
- knee shots.
- groin shots.
- takedown push pulls.

- Sets of hooking palms from 12 o'clock.
- Sets of hooking palms from 3 o'clock.
- Sets of hooking palms from 6 o' clock.
- Sets of hooking palms from 9 o'clock.
- Sets of hooking double hands.

- Sets of thrusting palms from 12 o'clock.
- Sets of thrusting palms from 3 o'clock.
- Sets of thrusting palms from 6 o' clock.
- Sets of thrusting palms from 9 o'clock.
- Sets of thrusting double hand, strikes/pushes.

Palm strikes while holding the arm of the trainer.

One of my earliest instructors, retired South African Commando Ben Mangles demos double palms to the arteries.

Bottom side ground
Your opponent/trainer may be three different vertical heights over you:

    1: Sitting atop you, torso up, head high. (See right.)
    2: Torso half-way up/half-way down.
    3: Down, chest to chest, or almost chest to chest.

He may also be 3 "heights" horizontally.

    1: High on your chest.
    2: Down around your belt line/belly. (See right.)
    3: Between your legs. (Or one leg in, one out.)

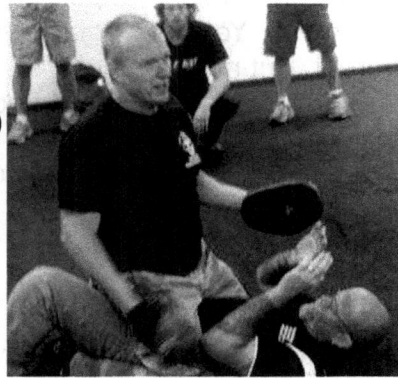

Big Dawg Kerwood gets ready to palm strike some mitts.

He could be kneeling.

    1: Just off to your left or to your right.
    2: Near your head, near your feet.

He could be standing over the downed, grounded on your back.

    1: Over you, leg split, like the classic mugger. (Or one leg in, one leg out.)
    2: Standing to your left or right, near head or feet.

Given the options and the targets, instructors should pick a position and remember that we are trying to develop generic power strikes for all these situations, that may well cover the options.

    - Sets of hooking palms from 12 o'clock.
    - Sets of hooking palms from 3 o'clock.
    - Sets of hooking palms from 6 o' clock.
    - Sets of hooking palms from 9 o'clock.
    - Sets of hooking double hand, ear claps.
    - Sets of double hooking palms from 12 o'clock.
    - Sets of double hooking palms from 3 o'clock.
    - Sets of double hooking palms from 6 o' clock.   >< | These may be useful in ground escape motions. |
    - Sets of double hooking palms from 9 o'clock.

    - Sets of thrusting palms from 12 o'clock.
    - Sets of thrusting palms from 3 o'clock.
    - Sets of thrusting palms from 6 o' clock.
    - Sets of thrusting palms from 9 o'clock.
    - Sets of thrusting double hand, strikes/pushes.
    - Sets of double thrusting palms from 12 o'clock.   >< | These may be useful in ground escape motions. |
    - Sets of double thrusting palms from 3 o'clock.
    - Sets of double thrusting palms from 6 o' clock.
    - Sets of double thrusting palms from 9 o'clock.
    - Sets of thrusting right web hands to throat height.
    - Sets of thrusting left web hands to throat height.
    Note: Carefully and wisely select a pad and position to hit.

Bottom side, on your right side
Be wise and take care on how you position your shield, mitt. One might even use a heavy bag laid on the floor. Experience this non-sport reality. You are down on your right side. Left side up. You may or may not like the results in terms of power. Everyone will be different. But now you know.

Sets of high (or head) hooking palms, left hand.
Sets of medium (or arms or torso) hooking palms, left hand.
Sets of high (or head) thrusting palms, left hand.
Sets of medium (arms or torso) thrusting palms, left hand.
Sets of web hand strikes to throat, left hand.

Bottom side, on your left side
Be wise and take care on how you position your shield, mitt. One might even use a heavy bag laid on the floor. Experience this non-sport reality. You are down on your left side. Right side up. You may or may not like the results in terms of power.

Sets of high (or head) hooking palms, right hand.
Sets of medium (arms or torso) hooking palms, right hand.
Sets of high (head) thrusting palms, right hand.
Sets of medium (arms or torso) thrusting palms, right hand.
Sets of web hand strikes to throat, right hand.

Palm strike - The 3 Elevation, Focus Mitt Drill
This drill produces a workout for standing, kneeling, bottom ground, bottom right side, bottom left side, and ground top. *The 3 Elevation Drill* is a "commandment" drill.

Step 1: Trainer holds mitts as trainee palms strikes. Trainer simulates a knee kick.
Step 2: Trainee drops to his knees (one or both) Trainee hits some standing mitts, held low or high. Trainer simulates another knee kick.
Step 3: Trainee drops on his back, trainer steps over trainee for a series of hits, then sits on trainee for a series of hits. Trainer then rolls to the right.
Step 4: Trainee rolls to the left side for a series of hits. Trainer rolls on back.
Step 5: Trainee gets atop trainer for a series of hits. Trainer pushes and rolls left.
Step 6: Trainee rolls to the right side for a series of hits. That set is done.
Step 7: Trainee safely escapes, gets up. Series starts over.

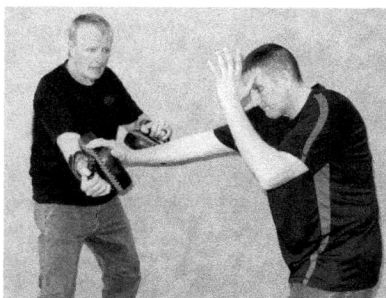

Standard "kick-boxing" format, for starters.

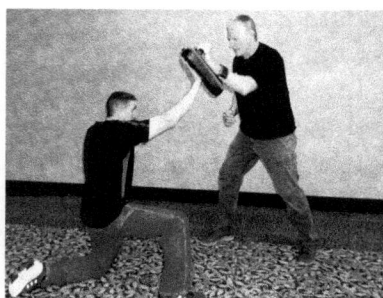

Trainee's anticipate kick to leg causes drop to knees.

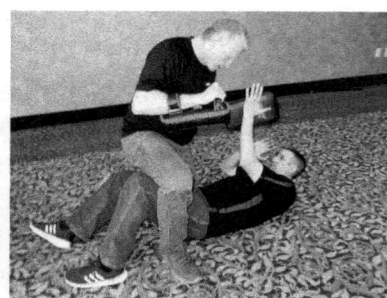

Trainer's anticipated kick to knee causes drop to back.

Stop Six Module Palm Strike Applications in Scenarios.
Smart ways to emphasize the palm strike within the *Stop 6* collisions. Expressed through the stalking/mad rush format or the bully format. In the Stalker/Mad Rush, the trainer charges in expects a trainee response on the forearm contact.

Stop 1: Since there is no official physical contact in Stop 1, let's review the interview and other related stance positions from which to deliver palm strikes.

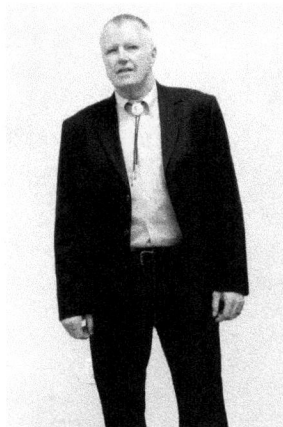

Hands down stance. Spring up for attack or hit low. This is also the "bus stop stance."

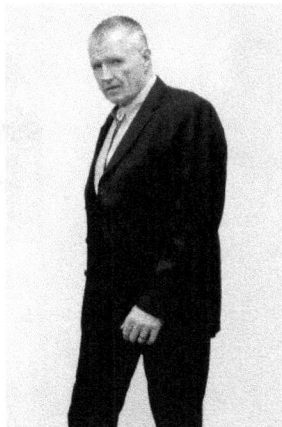

Hands down stance. Generate power from a casual body twist.

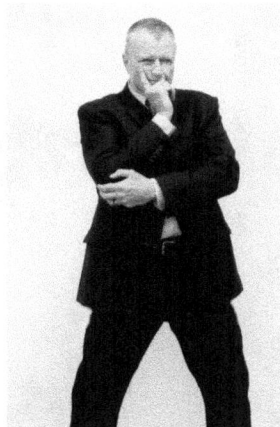

Inquisitive thinker. Hands held high naturally.

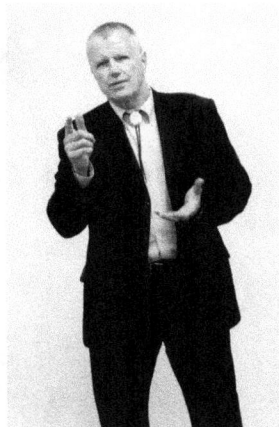

The conversationist. Hands held high naturally.

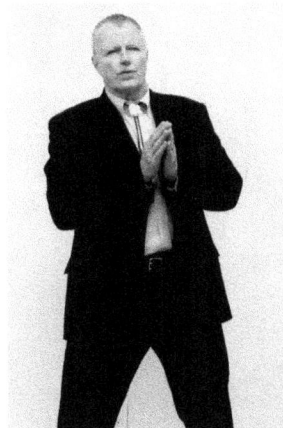

The prayer hands. Gets the hands naturally up.

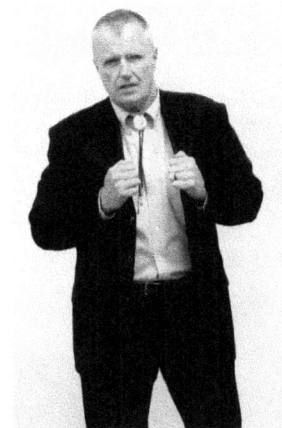

The lapel grabber. Casual looking and hands up.

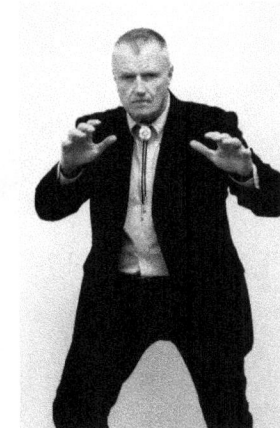

Any ready position.

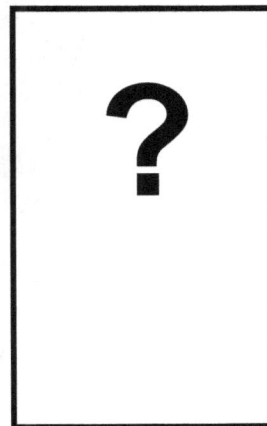

Your own developed, tested favorite.

Stop 2: The Stalker and Mad Rush Attack Drill

The trainer stalks, then charges in and grabs. As this is *Stop 2* training, the trainer stops there and the trainee immediately responds. Gets a release and hits, or hits and gets a release. Since this is a palm strike study, at least one strike must be a palm strike. Kicks too? Trainee takes stunned attacker to the ground in a *Level 2* basic takedown.

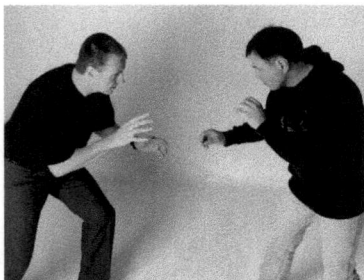

The trainer stalks...

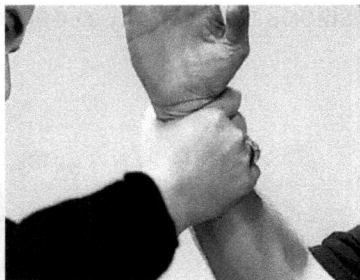

...and stops at a Stop 2 grab.

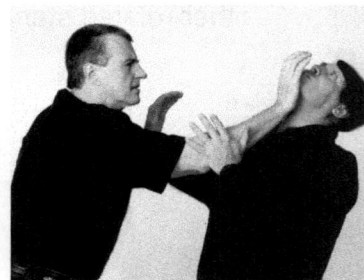

Trainee gets a release and palm strikes, as many times, and where, as needed.

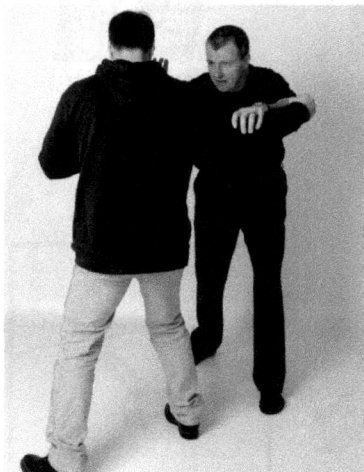

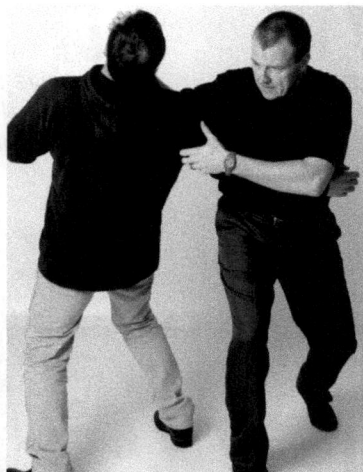

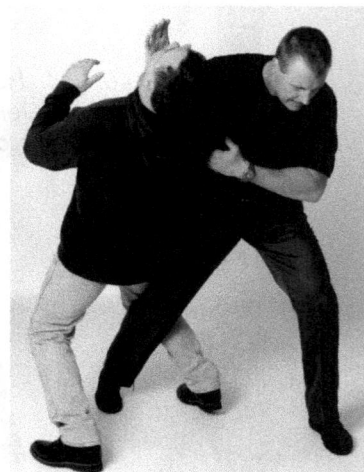

Trainee stuns, then begins any takedown. Here, a leg sweep.

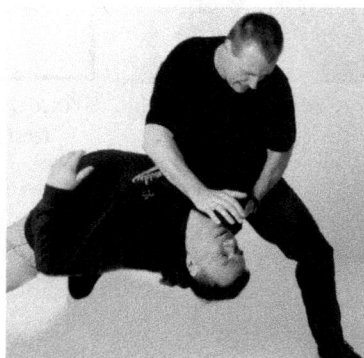

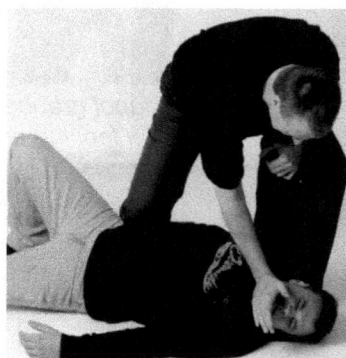

Trainee finishes, as appropriate for the situation.

Stop 3: Stalk, Mad Rush and the Forearm Collisions

The trainer stalks, then charges in forearm deep with forearm contact. As this is a *Stop 3* problem the trainer stops at a forearm collision and once there the trainee immediately responds. Since this is a palm strike study, at least one strike must be a palm strike. Kicks too? Trainee takes stunned attacker to the ground in a Level 2 basic takedown.

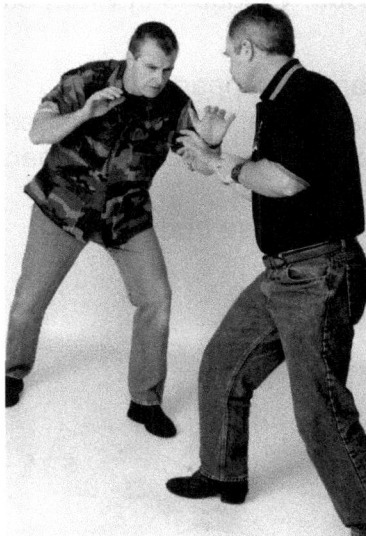

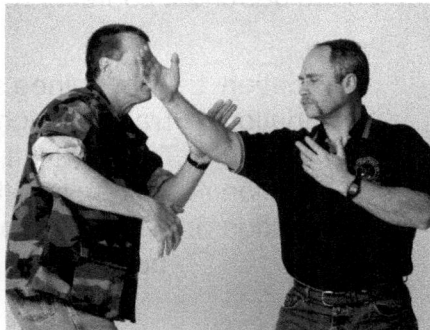

Forearms collide (or are forearm deep. The scenario must include at least one palm strike to exercise the option.

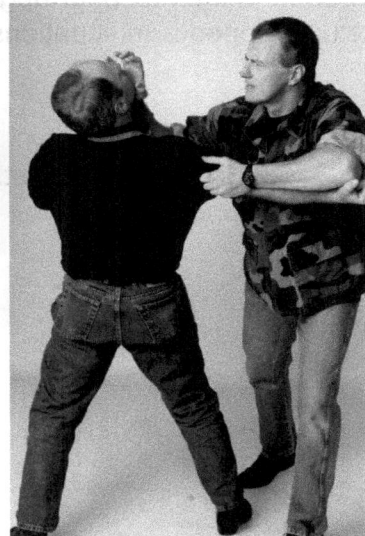

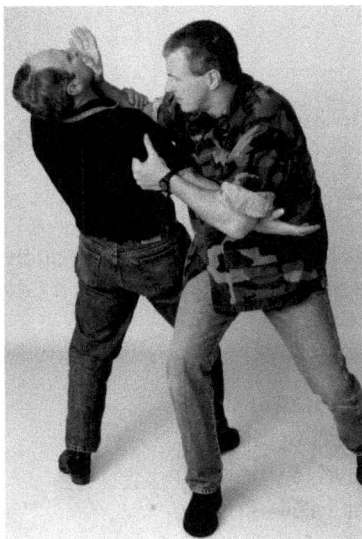

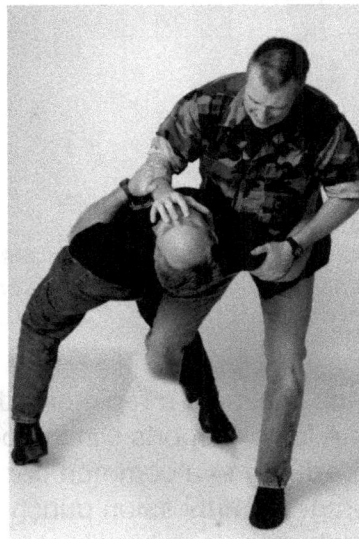

Stop 4: Stalk, Mad Rush and the biceps, shoulder, line/neck collisions

The trainer stalks, then charges in forearm deep with forearm contact. As this is a *Stop 4* problem the trainer stops at this collision and once there the trainee immediately responds. Since this is a palm strike study, at least one strike must be a palm strike. Kicks too? Trainee takes stunned attacker to the ground with any Level 2 basic takedown.

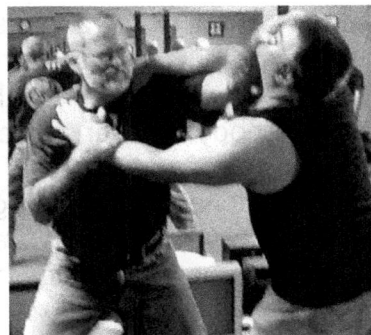

Stop 5: The Stalker, Mad Rush Attack and bear hugs and shoulder/chest collisions
The trainer stalks, then suddenly charges in, purposely causing a very close, torso collision. The trainee disconnects and strikes back, using palm strikes and other strikes, and takes down the attacker. The trainee may use the leg sweep or rear pull presented in *Training Mission One,* or any takedown from their experience, to finish a scenario. There's three fundamental bear hugs and shoulder/chest contacts with four variations of wrapped or unwrapped arm situations:

1: Chest-to-chest.
2: Shoulder-to-chest. ><
3: Chest-to-back.

Variation 1: Both trainee's arms wrapped.
Variation 2: Trainee's right arm free, left arm wrapped.
Variation 3: Trainee's left arm free, right arm wrapped.
Variation 4: Trainee's both arms free.
Variation 5: "Chest Bump!" This close body contact but no arms wrapped.

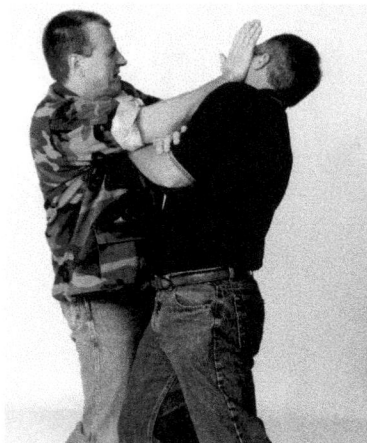

Close, chest-to-chest contact example. No arms wrapped.

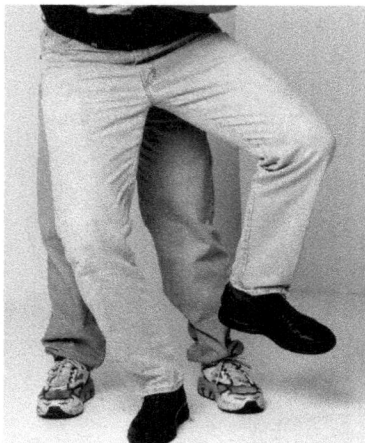

The classic (and Level 2) foot stomps are a suggested back to chest solution.

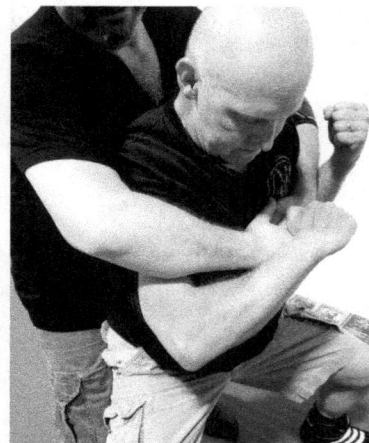

One such escape might include a Level 2 finger break.

A sports clinch is almost a regimented, very close, chest-to-chest situation. A formal, sports clinch does not often appear sporty-picture-perfectly in a common bar room brawl, supermarket-rage, road-rage, beauty salon punch-up, poker table scuffle, domestic violence, arrests, "street" fights, unless one, or certainly two of the fighters have sports related boxing, Thai boxing or MMA training, which about 99 percent people don't.

In sport boxing, the act of clinching in boxing, it's an act or instance of when one or both boxers hold the other about the arms or body in order to prevent or hinder the opponent's punches. It often happened when boxers tire, too.

All clinches are bear hugs but not all bear hugs are clinches. (This will be dissected in *Training Mission Five,* our core mission now concerns using palm strikes in all the *Stop 6* problems.)

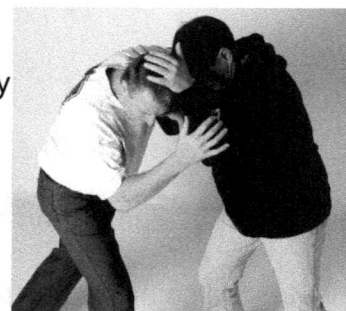

Stop 6: Stalk, Rush to Ground/Floor/Cement/Carpet/Cobblestone/Mud/Tile etc.
Trainer and trainee crash to the floor, be it from a trip or a takedown. The trainee may be on the side, on the back or topside?

   a: Palm Strikes: The trainee gets disconnected enough to do palm strikes and other strikes, and takes out the trainer, or gets up and stomps the trainer? Or escapes? Anything to finish a scenario.

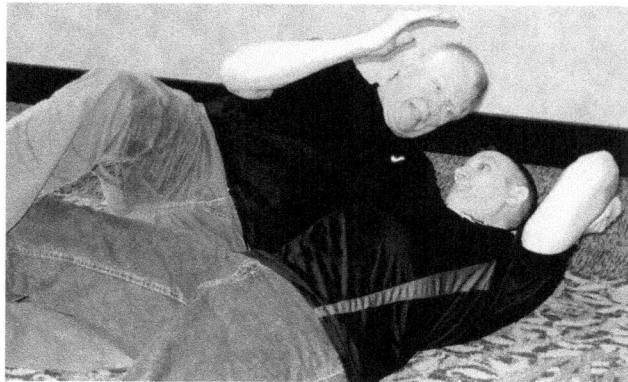

   b: Face Maul: The trainee gets disconnected enough and palm strikes the face, attaching to it for a ripping, face mauling. This usually really distracts the attacker and they try to stop the face maul. Grabbing your forearm is a common result. Meanwhile try to inch out of his attempted trap with other strikes, and take out the trainer, or get up and stomp the trainer? Or escape? Anything to finish a scenario appropriate for the situation.

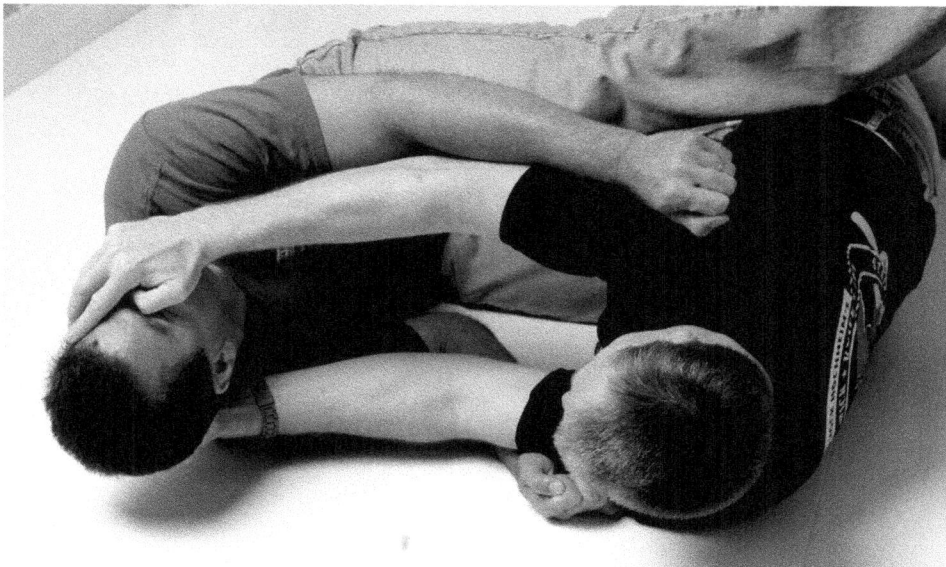

Level 2 Kick Module: The Stomp Kick

Standing targets, the instep and shin. A suggested target for a standing foot stomp is the "shoe lace" area of the foot. Many fragile bones. While all foot stomps are stomp kicks, not all targets are the foot. A target could be any body part with enemy bent, kneeling or grounded. Two standing "stances," "bus stop" and "fighting-ready." Your toes will point off to 2 or 10 o'clock-ish. List a number of reps per sets.

Solo Command and Mastery and Partner Drills and Exercises
Place a mitt or a shield on the floor.

1: Bus stop/neutral stance.
- sets to 12 o'clock right foot.
- sets to 3 o'clock right foot.
- sets to 6 o'clock right foot.
- sets to 9 o'clock right foot.

- sets to 12 o'clock left foot.
- sets to 3 o'clock left foot.
- sets to 6 o'clock left foot.
- sets to 9 o'clock left foot.

2: Fighting ready stance (right forward, then left forward).
- sets to 12 o'clock right foot.
- sets to 3 o'clock right foot.
- sets to 6 o'clock right foot.
- sets to 9 o'clock right foot.
- sets to 12 o'clock left foot.
- sets to 3 o'clock left foot.
- sets to 9 o'clock left foot.

3: The stomp kick statue drill
- Facing in.
   left stomps left foot, ankle.
   right stomps left foot, ankle.
   left stomps right foot, ankle.
   right stomps right foot, ankle.

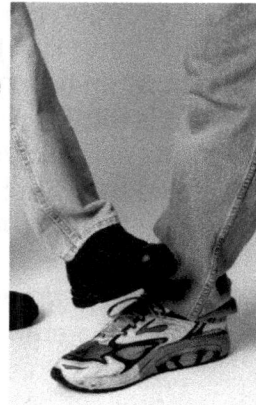

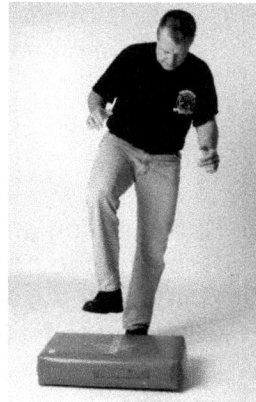

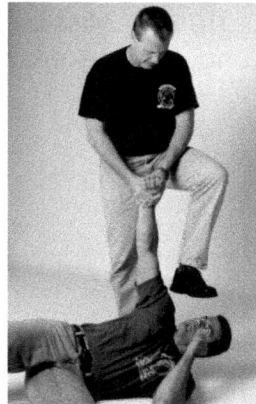

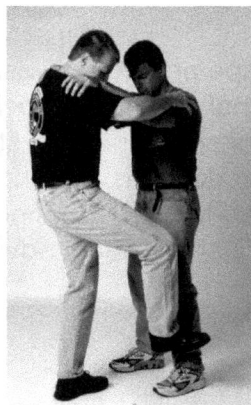

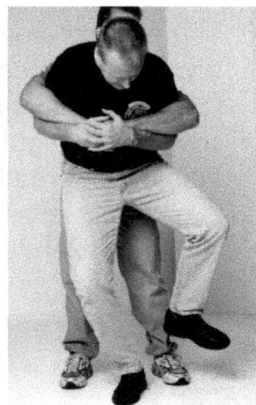

- Facing out.
   left stomps left foot, ankle.
   right stomps left foot, ankle.
   left stomps right foot, ankle.
   right stomps right foot, ankle.

4: While grounded

The stomp kick looks like a common thrust kick when grounded. If possible rise up on your hands into a crab walk position. This generates thrust and allows for a little target acquisition, or chase movement.

- sets of grounded right leg, thrust kicks from a crab walk.
- sets of grounded left leg, thrust kicks from a crab walk.
- sets of grounded left leg, thrust kicks from on your right side.
- sets of grounded right leg, thrust kicks from on your left side.

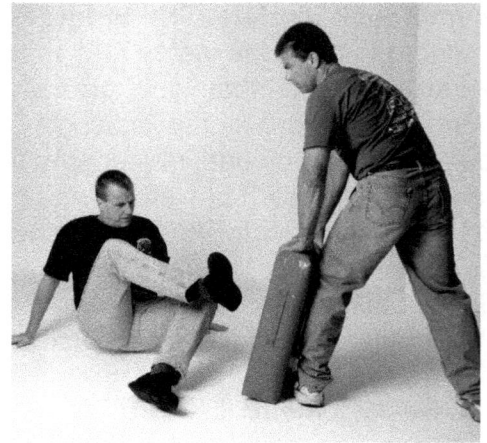

5: Kick sparring (kicking in motion)

Combine the prior, front snapping kick with a stomp kick. As we advance, each introduced kick will be added. I found some kick boxing sparring invaluable. I also found value in isolated kick sparring. It will be officially introduced in later *Training Mission* books. This is valuable for footwork exercising too.

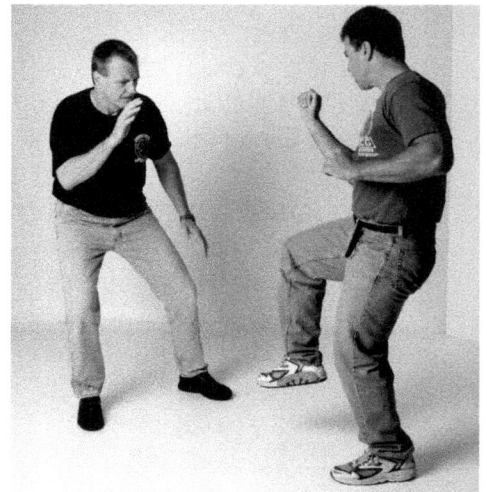

6: The escape stomp

If you need to escape and do not wish to be followed by a criminal you have knocked down, you might consider an ankle stomp. This might greatly reduce his chasing speed and is certainly less-than-lethal. This is not a repetition work out exercise, just important advice.

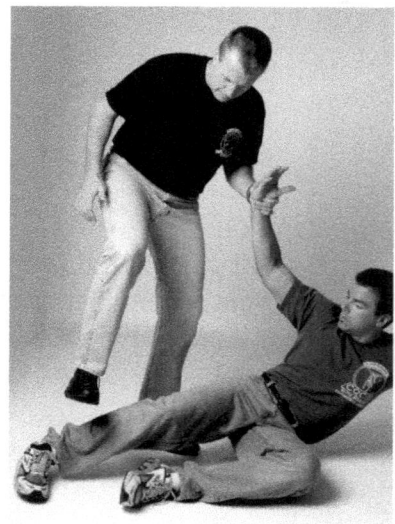

Stomp Kick Summary

The stomp kick can manifest itself in many situations. It is certainly not always a vertical application when standing or kneeling. It can slant out as needed, until it be comes a full-on standing thrust kick, which will be covered later in the *Training* Mission series.

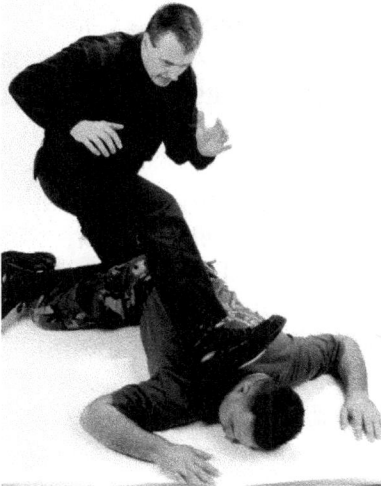

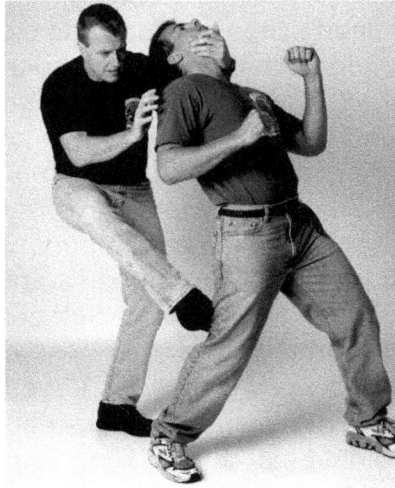

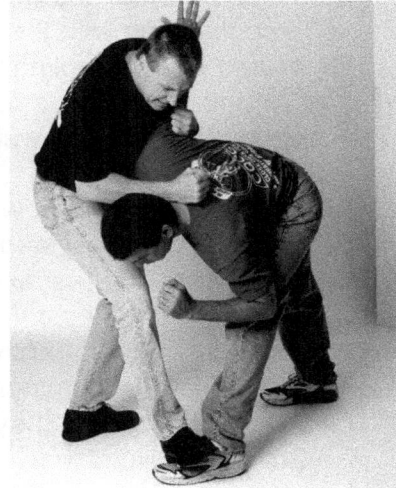

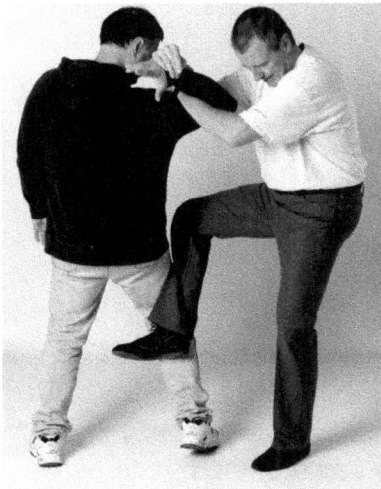

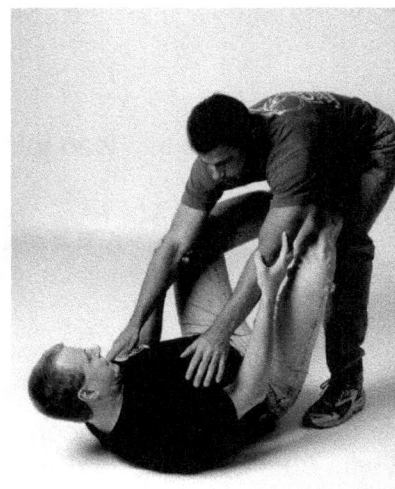

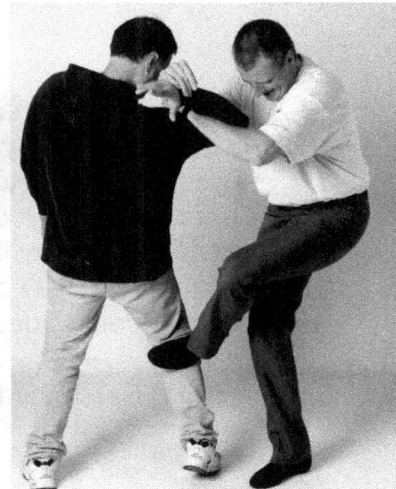

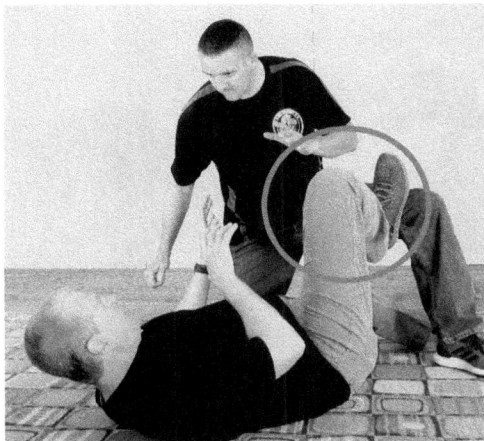

A stomping, thrusting kick motion is used in groundfighting too, such as to shove a leg away.

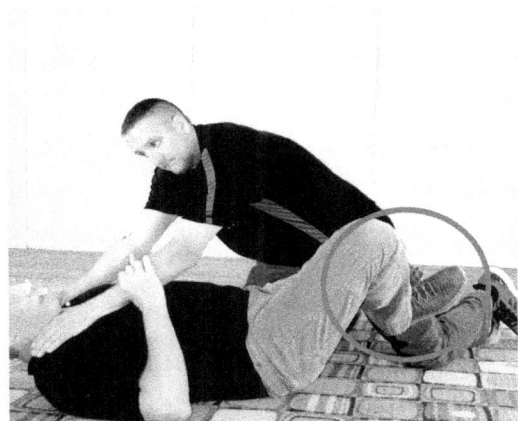

Unarmed Level 2, Stop 2 Grappling: Finger and Wrist Grappling

It is the duty of every martial person to learn each joint and the directions they go in and the directions they don't go in, standing through on the ground, whether they think they are studying "survival fighting" or "arts/sports." This joint, directional knowledge comes from many martial sources.

In conjunction with the defined scope of *Stop 2*, its orderly progression, we will study finger and wrist grappling as it fits with the topic. In order for an opponent to grapple, he has to grab you with his hands (and fingers). These finger catches, twists and rips are educational, handy, as well as sometimes, even fight stoppers, whether afoot or down on the ground.

What we cover here, what I have found to be important is often from the Wally Jay *Small Circle Jujitsu* system, early Remy Presas *Modern Arnis* and *Aiki-Jitsu* as three main sources. The rest are from various experiments and collections. The following "Big Ten," finger examples could almost be a book of their own. Lots of explanation. Lots of photographs. Experiment with these, but they are best learned in a hands-on, (no pun intended) class or seminar. Simply put? Rip, twist, kneed and/or break a finger (or two?). Like all martial things, they may or may not work like you expect.

Ground applications. Take note that any of these finger "rips/twists" can be used in ground fighting, to damage or temporarily control a person. (there are no submission, win, tap-outs in the so-called "street-fight." It's just break, damage or wait.

Finger Cranks and Breaks

The fingers twist 5 ways. Every direction can lead to a crank or a break.
   - twist all the way to the right.
   - twist all the way to the left.
   - bend all the way in.
   - bend all the way out.
   - bend side-to-side.

Example 1: Catch the Bully Pointer
> We'll start here with the Simple concept of catching the "pointy finger."
> It might start with bully or might be from any catch of the one finger.
> Catch it. Bend it back over the knuckle.

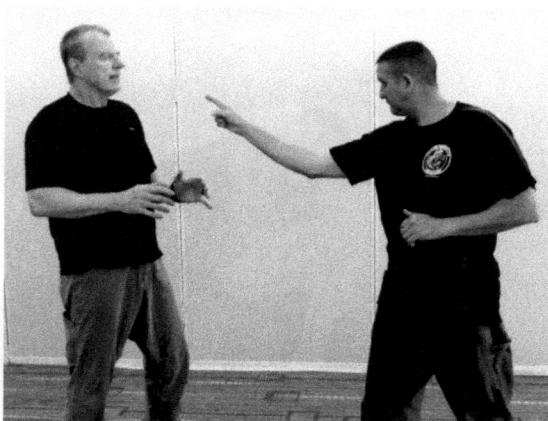

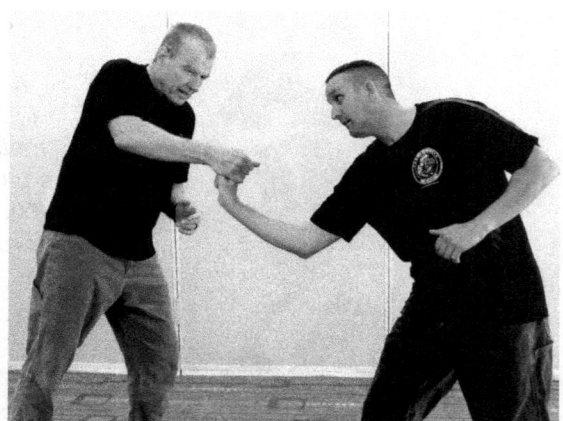

Example 2: The military finger twist-break strategy.
        If you get that pointy finger, or any finger, you can twist the finger till it
        breaks at the palm knuckle. Old military methods suggest breaking
        the trigger fingers.

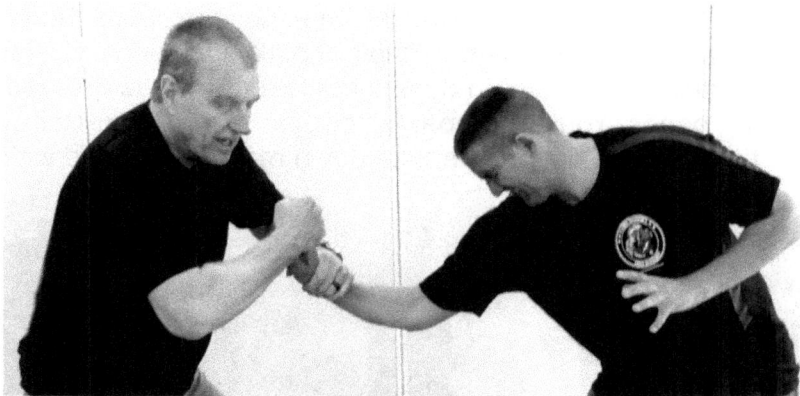

Military finger, twist break. (On the trigger finger?)

The so-called "pointing" finger is also the trigger finger. It is not uncommon,
standing or on the ground, when grappling to countering pistol pulls, that you grab
at the gun pull from the holster and catch the trigger finger outside the holster,
waiting for the trigger to enter into the trigger guard of the pistol. If possible, some
suggest this enables the catcher to control the gun draw to some extent. Exercise
this situation in training.

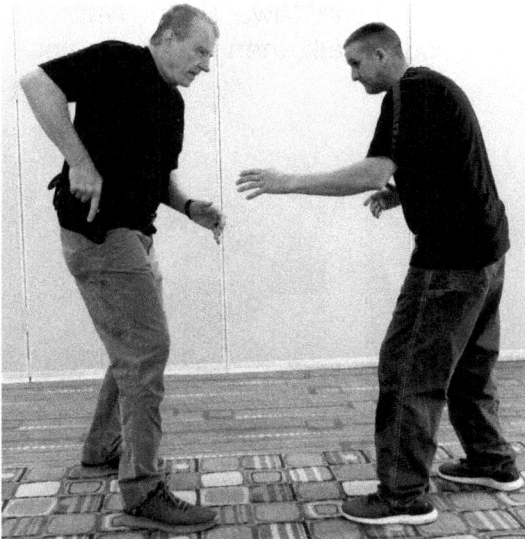

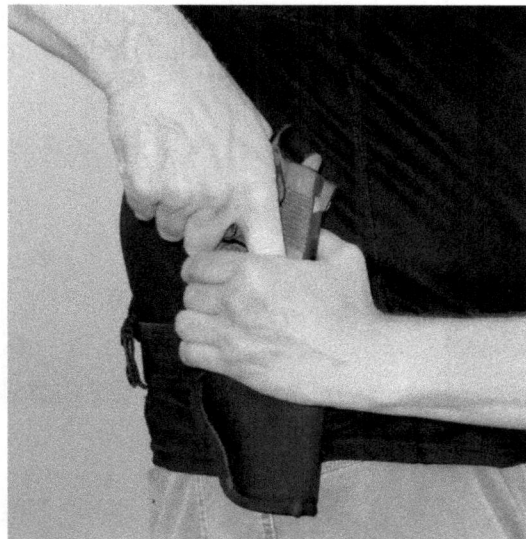

Example 3: Pinky lock versus his "handshake-style" grab on your forearm.
From what many call, "same-side" grab. As with all such grab events, do you hit him first? Dodge his punch? Yank out? What? That is all situational and a legal issue. But in this section, we are exploring finger locks and breaks right now, for concept only.

The trainee does a curl which usually exposes the trainer's pinky to a grab. Slip the thumb in and get pinky lock and/or break the pinky or control his hand to an outer wrist take down, as detailed in the upcoming pages. You will probably need on-scene instructor guidance in getting the take down. The take down may be assisted with kicks to the knee area.

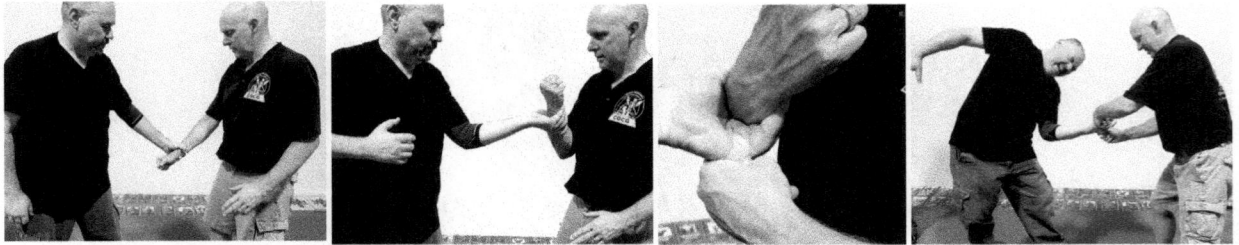

The common grab. The "curling" up of the grabbed hand. Grabbing pinky exposed. Thumb insert on the pinky. Outer wrist throw principle, guided/helped by the pinky.

Example 4: Pointy finger lock versus his guard arm grab, to the infamous "duck walk.

His palm down grab of your guard arm. As with all such grab events, do you hit him? Dodge his punch? Yank out? What? That is all situational and a legal issue. But we are exploring finger locks and breaks right now.

The trainee makes a full, hand grab of the trainer's pointy finger. Crank it back, but pull the knuckle area inward toward you. While cranking this, pull him down to the classic duck walk, then flat on the floor.

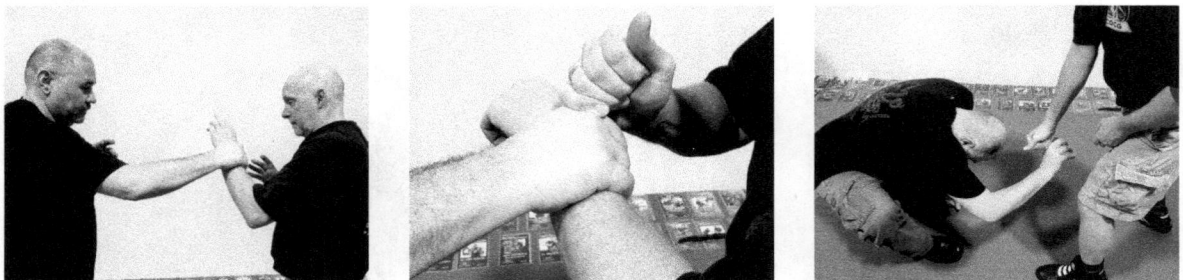

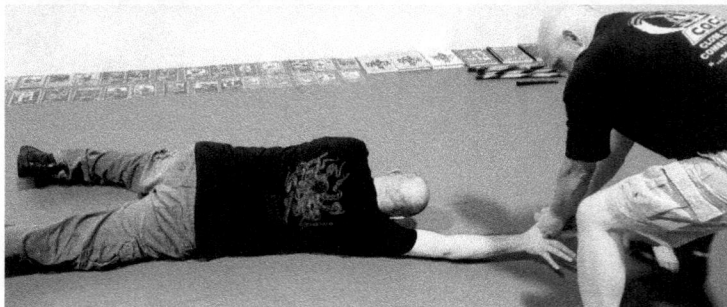

Example 5: The Underhand Wristlock, catching the ball of the thumb catch.
He grabs both your wrists. As with all such grab events, do you hit him? Dodge his punch? Yank out? What? That is all situational and a legal issue. But we are exploring finger locks and breaks right now.
Sweep one hand under the other grab. The sweeping hand clutches the ball of the thumb of his hand, (or vice versa). Twist to outer wrist throws, as detailed in the upcoming pages.

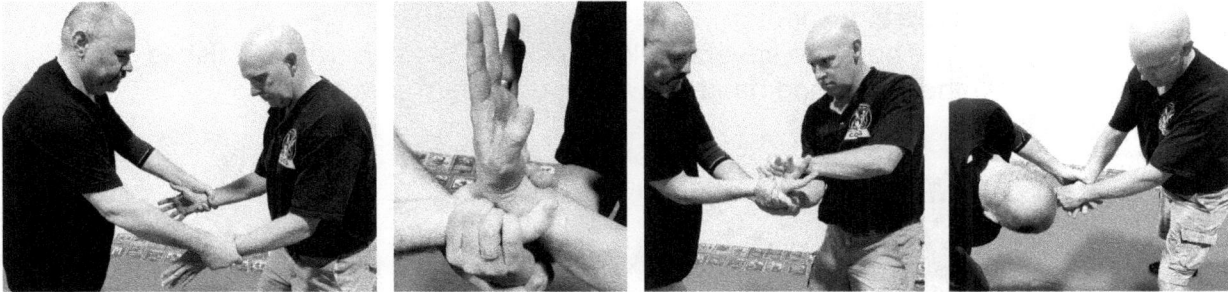

Example 6: Catching the foolish, yet common, thumb's up grip
The thumb's-up, threatening, stick holder! Solve this problem with a "thumb-catch" and "golf club grip" sweeping pulldown. Many stick bearers and threateners think nothing of holding a stick with a thumb up on the shaft. During the threat, snatch his thumb, and thank the thumb inward with a mopping motion.
If you get two hands involved, with a mopping motion, it's a powerful takedown as you "mop" inward and down.

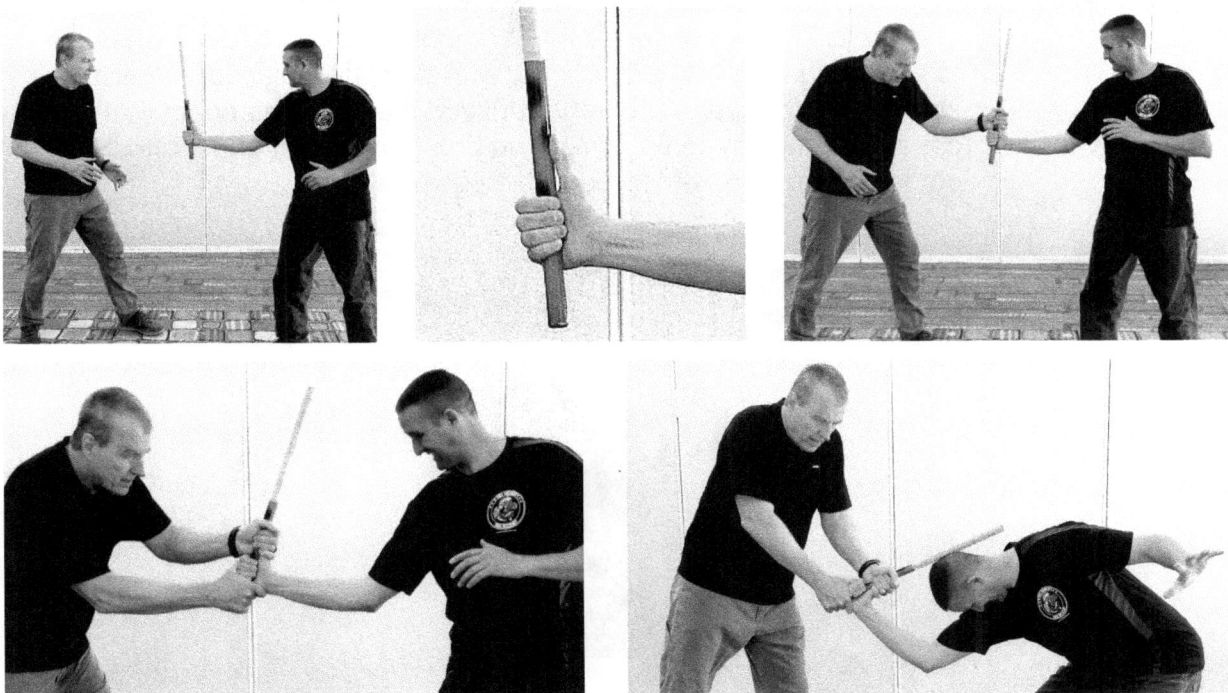

Example 7: Finger torture the choker
As with all such grab events, do you hit him? Dodge his punch? Yank out? What? That is all situational and a legal issue. But we are exploring finger locks and breaks right now.

Part 1: He grabs you in the common, two hand, front choke. You cross-grab the point finger and yank it back from your neck-shoulder area across your torso and down to the opposite side hip. This should be very painful and either break the finger, or cause the attacker to drop to a knee!
There are several follow-ups here but one simple finish is to twist the finger and hand outward, pulling him away.

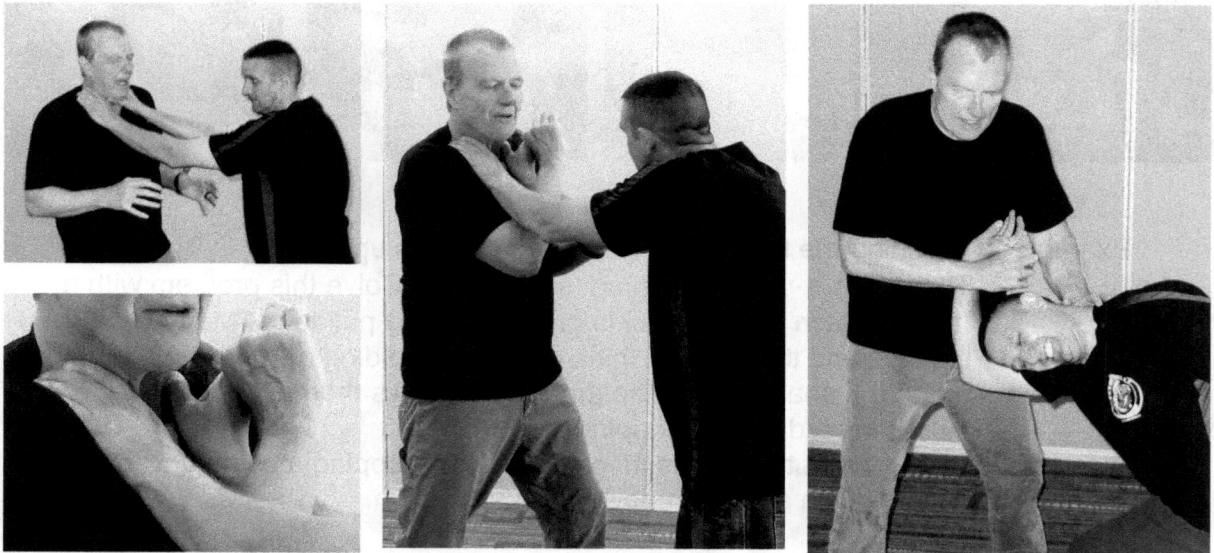

Part 2: This happened to me. Without the long details, I was able to access the pinky of an attacker with his poorly placed, forearm choke from the rear. I broke his pinky at the knuckle and, in that case, he let go immediately, got up and freaked out about his dislocated finger.

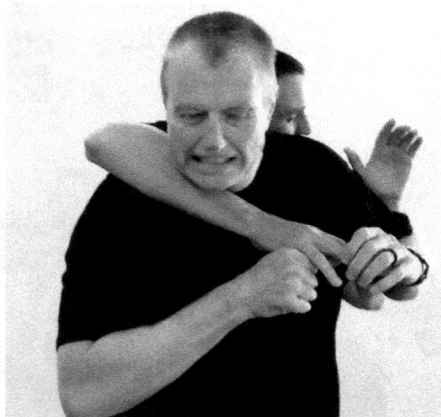

Example 8: Escape a bear hug

As with all such grab events, do you hit him? What? That is all situational and a legal issue. But we are exploring finger locks and breaks right now. From the classic your-back-to-his-front position. Try to get a finger or two and bend it back. If fingers are tight? King Kong hammer fist the back bones on his hand. This should loosen his fingers. Get one and bend it back. Try this standing and on the ground.

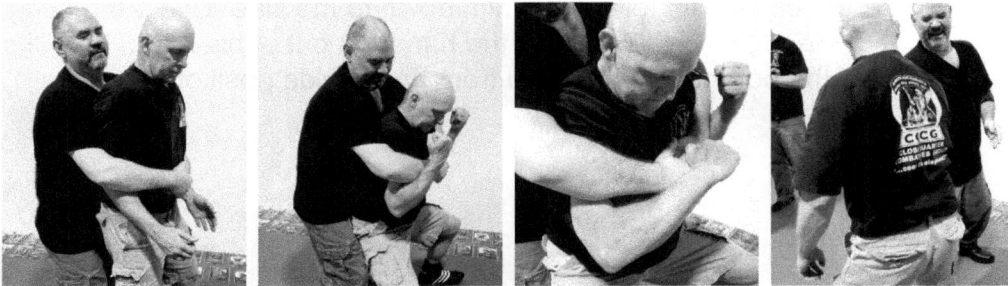

Example 9: Standing versus pistol mugger

This is meant to spread the concept of a pistol trigger guard, finger catch. The attacker has a one hand grip, extended within your reach. Your hands are up in submission, surrender. When the time is ripe, you double hand snatch the gun while avoiding the barrel, and bend the pistol back over his trigger finger. Turn the pistol in such a way as to "mop" him down to the floor. If you just pull the handgun out of his hand, he may still have the potential, where-with-all to charge you. If you yank/mop him to his knees, you have more time to get the pistol into useable position.

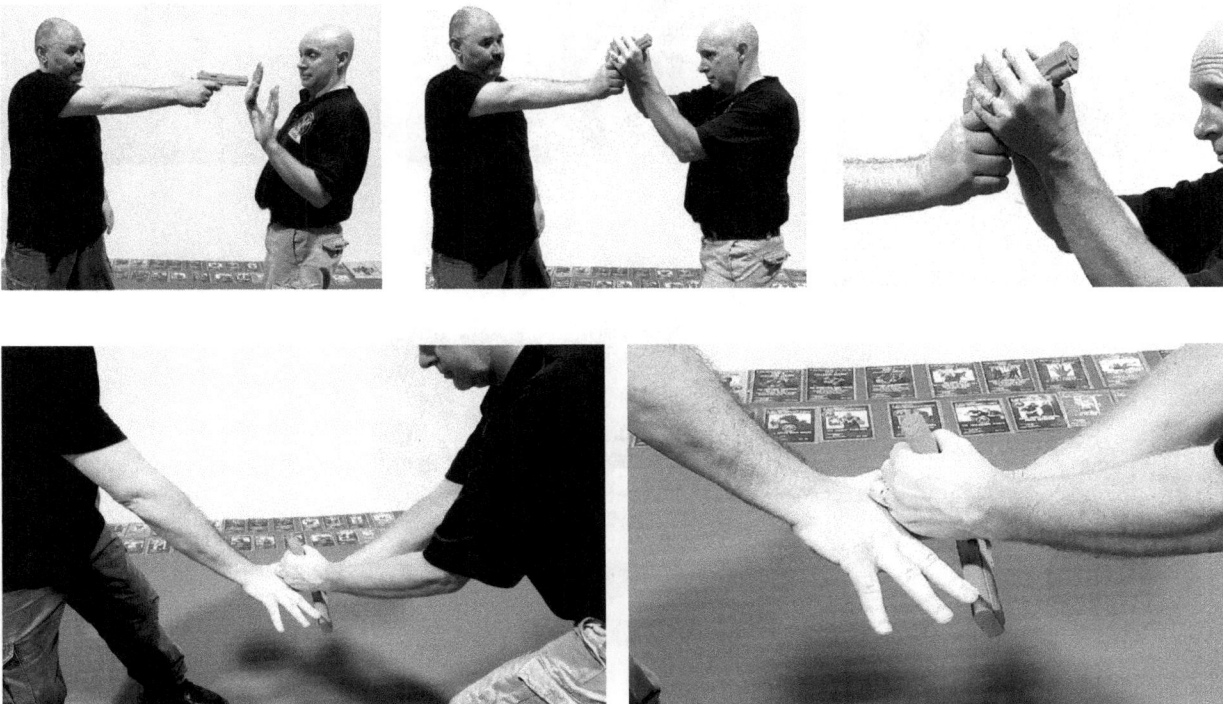

Example 10: Grounded versus pistol mugger

This is meant to spread the concept of a pistol trigger guard, finger catch, but many times in the history of crime, a domineering mugger has stood over a quaking victim, however stupid this position is. The attacker has a one hand grip, extended within your reach.

Your hands are up in submission, surrender. When the time is ripe, you double hand snatch the gun while avoiding the barrel, and bend the pistol back over his trigger finger. Crank him to the side so as to either break his finger or take him down to the side. Use a thrusting kick if need be. If you just pull the handgun out of his hand, he will still have the potential to fight you from his topside position.

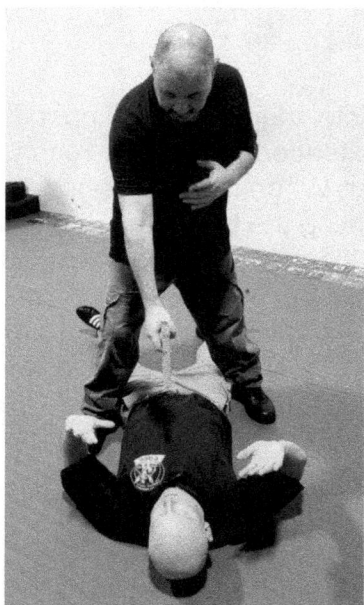

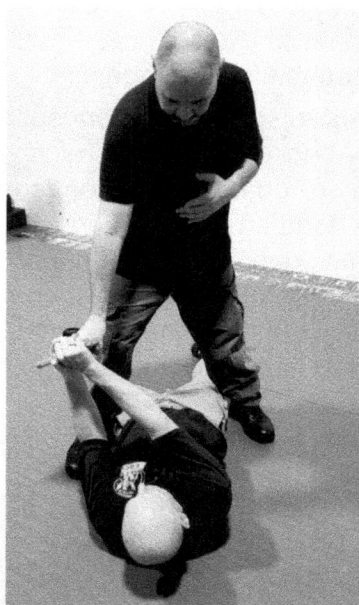

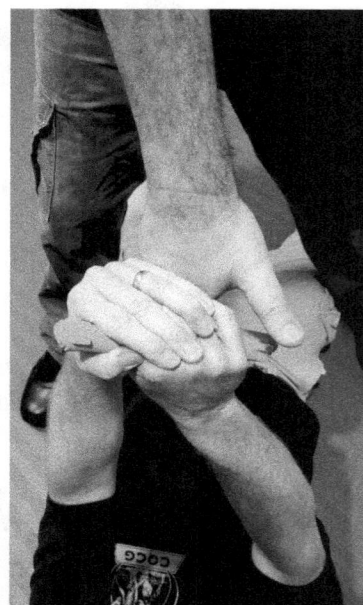

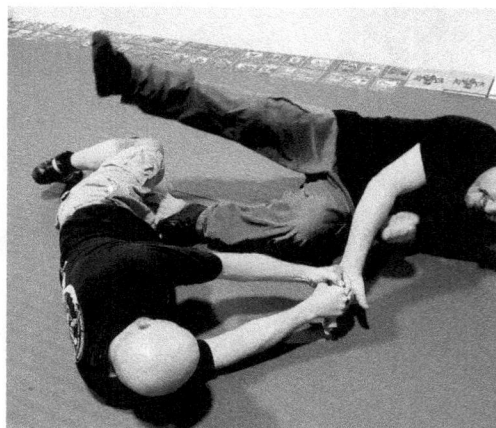

Example 11: Rattlesnake Drill, Finger Cracker

In order to grab you, to wrestle with you, they have to put their hands on you. And you may have the opportunity to get to their fingers and apply all the bends and twists shown here. As with all such grab events, do you hit him? Dodge his punch? Yank out? What? That is all situational and a legal issue. But we are exploring finger locks and breaks right now.

In the drill, a trainee is down on his or her back. The trainer is atop, and they begin to wrestle, to get a flow of activity. The trainee perceives a grab and reaches for a finger or two and attacks it at about 20 percent of the move. The trainer then stops.

The trainer then gets into another topside position and repeats. The trainer stops with each capture.

This teaches the trainee that finger attacks are viable and possible. Breaking an attackers finger in a ground fight may or may not cause the reaction you expect.

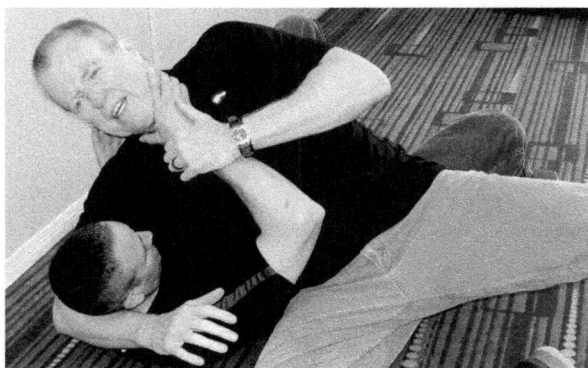

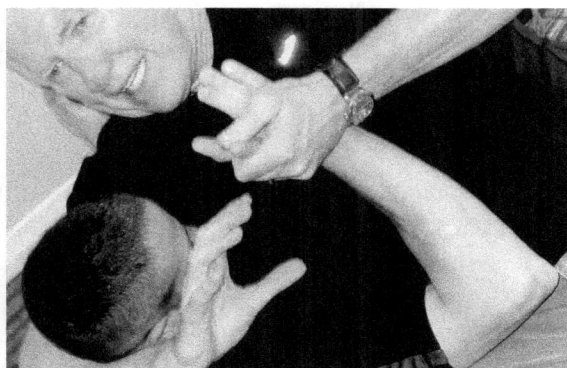

One of the most important "roll" drills you can do for survival ground fighting, along with the eye attack and face maul, is the finger break exercise. Let the roll get started, then the trainee seeks out the fingers. More on these methods in Stop 6 ground fighting of the Stop 6.

Counters to finger locks

      1: Early phase counters

          - yanks outs.

          - hit the locker with the free hand.

          - push, pull out.

      2: Mid phase counters

          - hit the locker with the free hand.

          - push, pull out

      3: Late phase counters

          - leap ahead of the direction he is taking you.

          - roll ahead of the direction he is taking you.

Wrist Grappling
Cranking and Ripping the wrist is a *Stop 2* topic and is here for this course continuity. It should not be prioritized over your other selected, favorite grappling or takedowns. I think every martialist should know about "wristlocks", because they indeed have been used successfully. As a police officer I know that many times when you get a "wrist throw" attempt, you often just rip something in the suspect's wrist (and arm) because they do not know to fall in the safest direction, as trained people do.

Wrist Cranks and Breaks
Like the fingers, the wrist twists 5 ways. Every direction can lead to a crank or a break.
- 1: twisted all the way to the right.
- 2: twisted all the way to the left.
- 3: bend all the way in.
- 4: bend all the way out.
- 5: bend side to side.
- these directions equate to:
   * all the way out? The outer wrist throw (horizontal or vertical).
   * all the way in? The inner wrist throws horizontal or vertical).
   * all the way in or out? The 2 goosenecks (horizontal or vertical).
   * side-to-side? The S, V, Z or center locks.

Lecture Point 1: Big hand clap-grab versus fine motor-skilled detailed grabs. Several martial arts want ridiculously detailed, pinpoint grabs on the hand to twist the wrist, that just can be done in real time fights.

Lecture Point 2: The "upside-down, "handshake" demo. In order to explain to new people the best crank of the outer wrist crank, I will let them see and do the upside-down hand grab. The wrist is at the "breaking point."

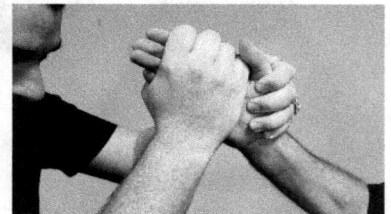
A solid and catch.

Lecture Point 3: Chop the wrist area to get a bend. If you are trying to get a bent wrist and the wrist won't, you might have a chance to hammer fist or edge-hand strike the wrist and/or lower forearm area to get a bend.

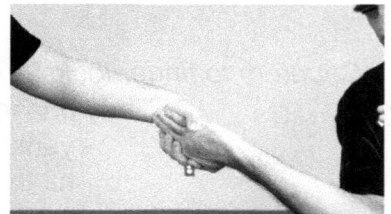
The upside-down handshake.

Lecture Point 4: Vertical and/or horizontal forearm. The captured forearm may be vertical or horizontal.

Lecture Point 5: Ground applications
Take note that any of these hand or wrist "rips/twists" can be used in ground fighting, to damage or temporarily control a person.

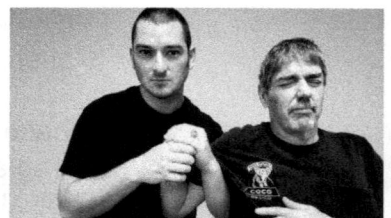
All the goosenecks.

Wrist crank scenario samples to learn from:

Example 1: 3rd party rescue, outer wrist crank/throw
> I like to start the study of wrist cranks with the 3rd Party rescue, because it offers the best version of cranks for an out wrist crank/throw/attack. Once practitioners get this down, they understand the mechanics. The more they are out of this scenario side position, the less effective and tricky the wrist cranks are.
>
> A third party witnesses a suspect pulling a weapon while suspect is facing a third party. The trainee charges in grabbing with two hands, the hand holding the weapon. Or, the case of a pistol, one hand on the gun, one on the hand. Or, both hands on the gun. The trainee violently pulls the weapon hand up and out to the suspect's rear. The weapon often flies out of the suspect's hand, but if not, it must be disarmed.
>
> I learned this in military protection classes and training from the US Secret Service. Nine out of 10 people are right handed and because of this, many suspects are "observed" from their right side.
>
> Option 1: Do this versus a knife-draw-attack.
> Option 2: Do this versus a single hand pistol draw.
> Option 3: Do this versus one limb of a choke.

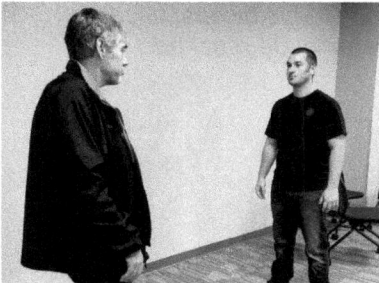

An assassin stalks a VIP.

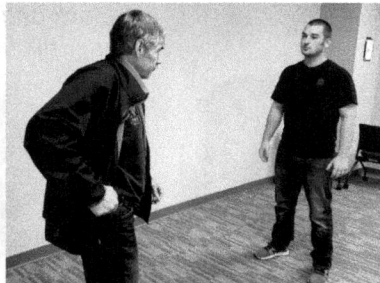

A 3rd party protector sees...

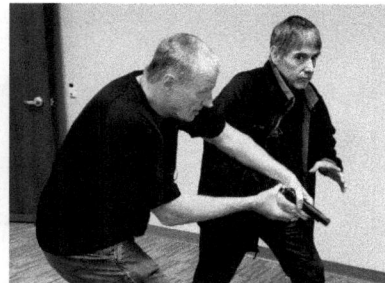

...a weapon draw and moves in.

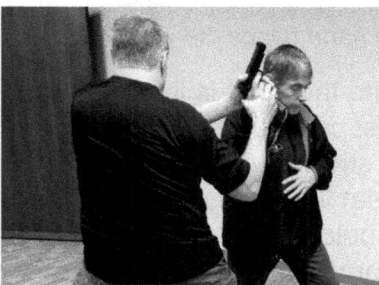

Pulls gun up and off target.

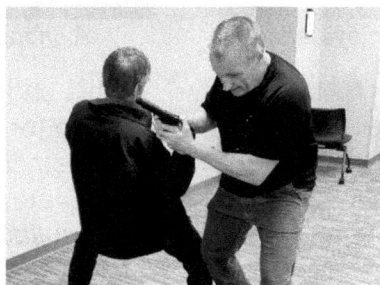

Vertical outer wrist throw.

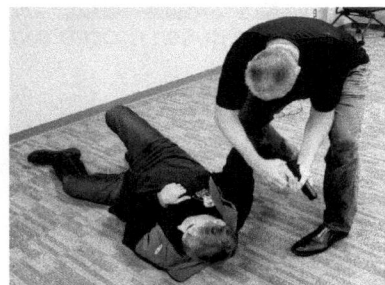

"Rides the gun down." Disarm.

Example 2: Outer Wrist/Twist Throw #1

There are vertical forearm versions and horizontal forearm versions. In terms of a horizontal forearm, this is not very high at all on my personal, to-do list, but people have successfully done this. I have only once, opting for other moves. But, as a martialist you must be able to explain it's pros and cons. It really requires elbow control too.

This is one of the wrist throw scenarios I had to learn for a Filipino black belt test. It involves several factors that are interesting. The opponent punches. You dodge the punch, split-armed, he can't reach your head and you can't reach his head, so, you punch the biceps. then bounce off the biceps with an eye attack. Your attacking hand comes in to strike the lower forearm and/or wrist, getting a bend at the wrist. You get the outer wrist takedown, assisted by kicks to the knee area. This is a Filipino Martial Arts scenario I had to learn for testing.

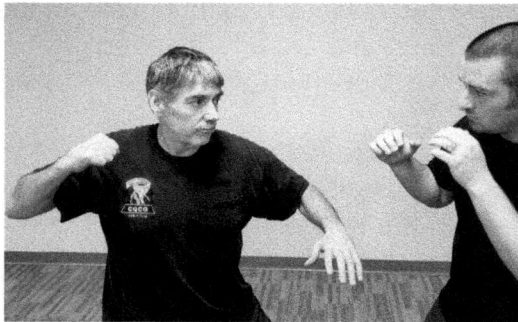
He's punching!

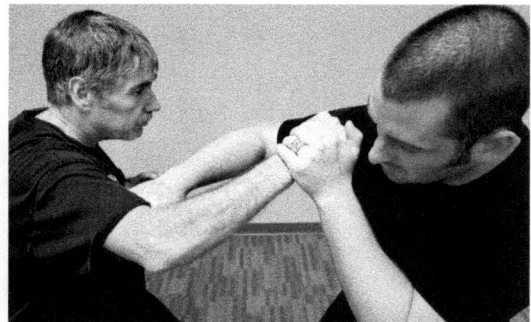
A block and punch to his biceps, because his face cannot be reached.

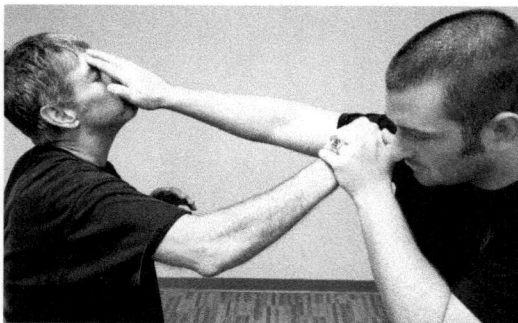
The punch ricochets into an eye attack.

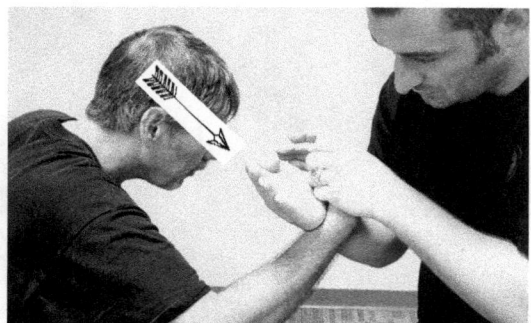
A chopping hand bends the wrist.

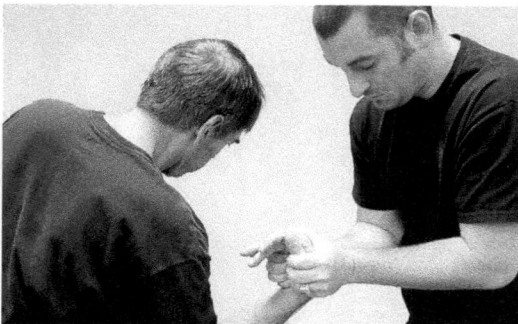
Stunning set-up for a outer wrist throw.

This chop into the wrist is important and a set-up for wrist cranks when the suspect is isometrically strong.

The late, great Wally Jay of *Small Circle Jujitsu* would push down on the outside, top segment of the back of the hand, in a very small circle of the wrist, in comparison to the bigger circles used in traditional martial arts.

Example 3: Outer Wrist/Twist Throw #1 Versus a knife attack

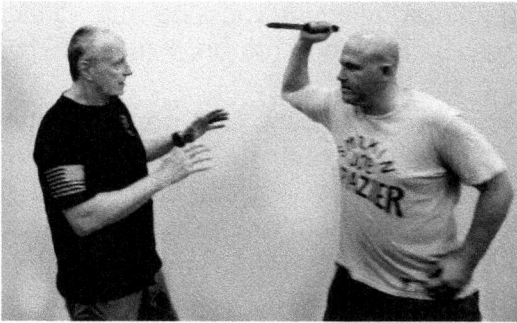
The classic overhead, reverse grip attack.

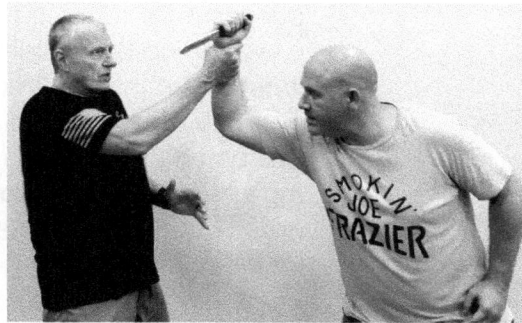
The "cross grab".

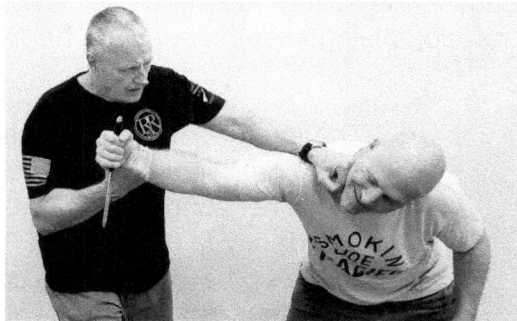
Hit him if you can as soon as possible.

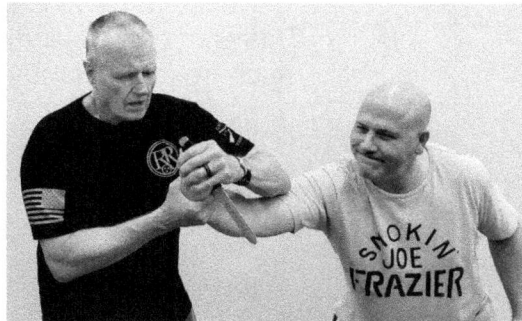
The other hand "caps" off the top of the grip.

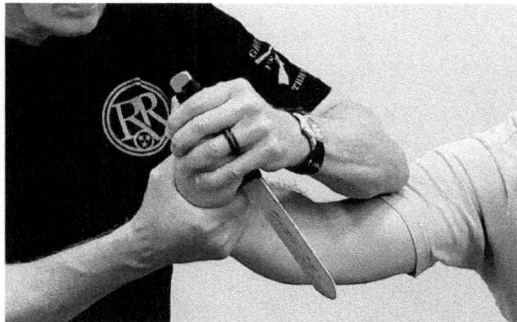
Have a closer look.

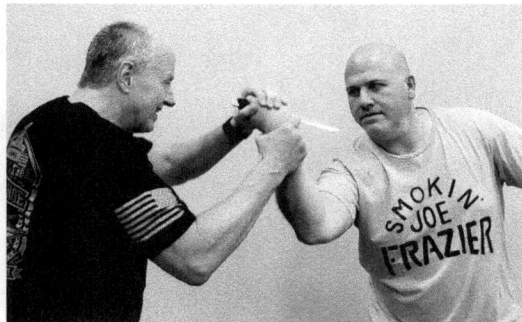
Violently twist out the wrist, across then...

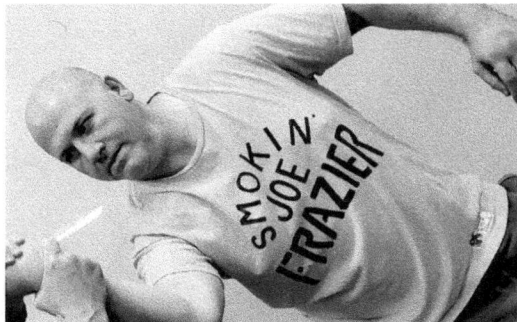
...over and down.

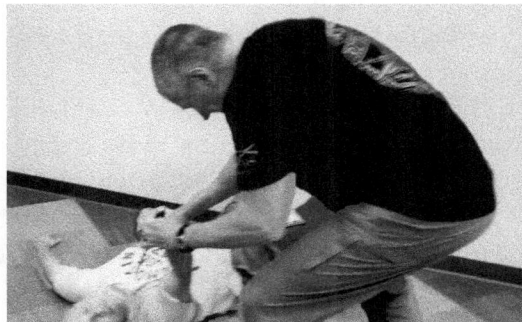
Finish as legally as possible.

Example 4: Inner Wrist Crank (with elbow positioning)

This is not very high at all on my personal to-do list, but people have successfully done it. But, as a martialist you must be able to explain it's pros and cons. It really requires elbow control too. You are twisting the wrist to the inside direction of his body.

I have used several practical applications. One application is picking this catch up inside some *Stop 4* arm wrestling. The other is in interrupting same-side, pistol or knife quick draws. For the purposes of this progression, for the concept, I shall document the "arm wraslin" version. In later *Training Mission* books when we cover unarmed versus pistol and knife threats we'll use this concept against half-drawn quick draws, an bent arm, hand down position, in great detail.

A circular twisting that causes the suspect to bend over forward. This is not easy versus a non-complying suspect because he has so much freedom of movement.

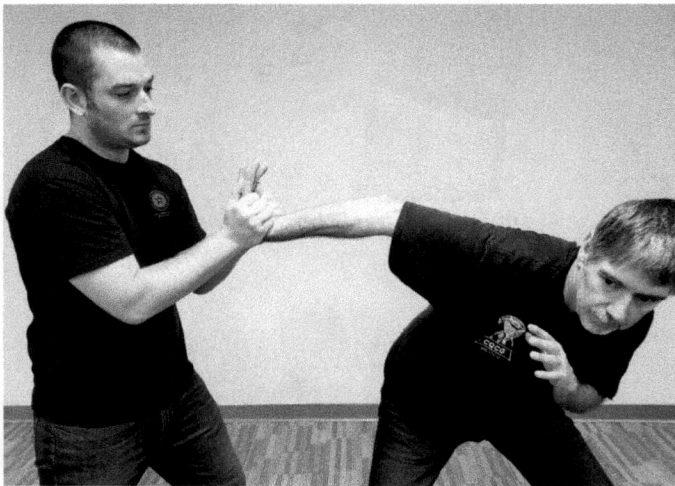

The straight arm, inner wrist, circular crank requires...a straight arm, and resisting people have a natural tendency to quickly bend at the elbow and other joints as to prevent hyper-extensions. This elbow bend screws your wrist-screwing potential up!

In various FMA systems I studied, if one got the inner wrist twist, they quickly snap-kicked the face for the next attack.

If you continue to twist and he continues to bend forward, controlling the elbow is once again a big deal. It is vital to control the elbow as quickly as possible, by your hand, by your forearm or by your torso.

The inner wristlock takedown must lead to many accompanying steps to be successful. Just twisting the wrist inward is very incomplete.

This wristlock is not one of my favorites, but still one that a martialist must know about and be able to discuss its pros and cons.

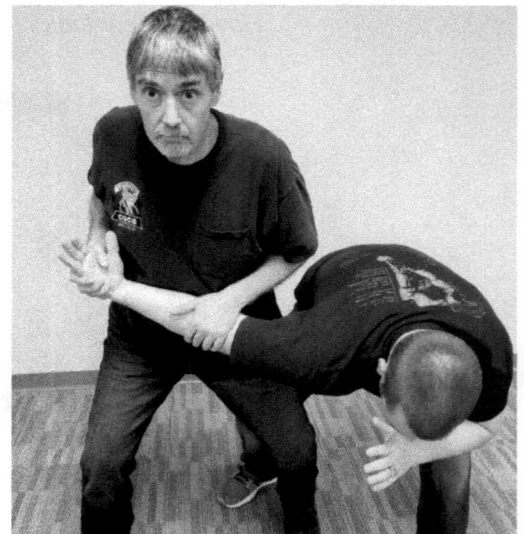

Example 5: The center wrist lock

This is called many things. The "center lock," the "extended wrist lock," the "Z wristlock", or "S wristlock," or "V wristlock lock," because of the arm position.

It is as though the trainer will be making an imaginary car turn. His left hand makes a right turn with the steering wheel. His right hand makes a left turn with the steering wheel. That is his eventual position for this lock-crank. There is a bend at the elbow and a bend at the wrist. It is the most painful wristlock to most people. If you don't control the elbow, and the elbow raises high, you must change locks.

Your palm is on the back of his hand. Your other hand should hold the elbow at his palm level or a bit lower. You twist his palm forward, tightly, like taking a lid off a jar, toward his nose.

This can be done standing and on the ground, for the releases we emphasize in the book, and weapon retention.

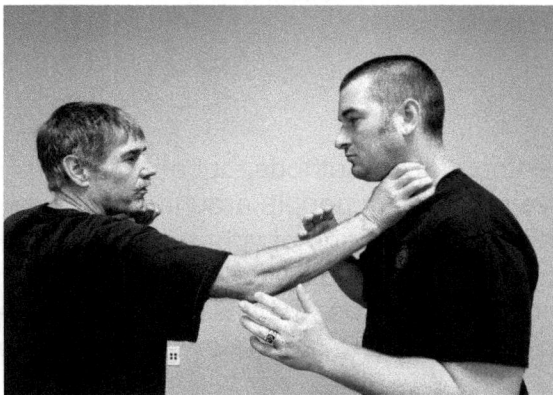

A throat grab, for example.

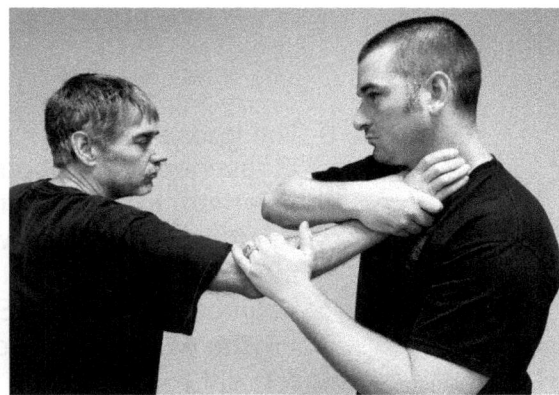

The center lock acquisition.

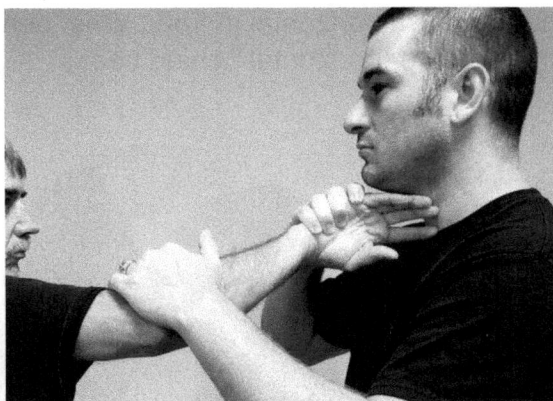

His right hand is made into the left steering wheel turn, so to speak.

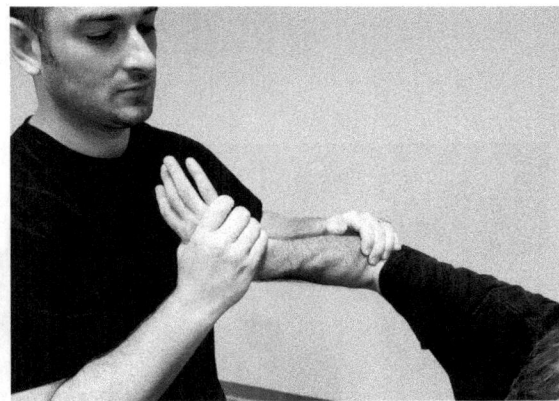

The slighty bent hand is twisted toward his nose. The elbow is kept just below the trainer's wrist level.

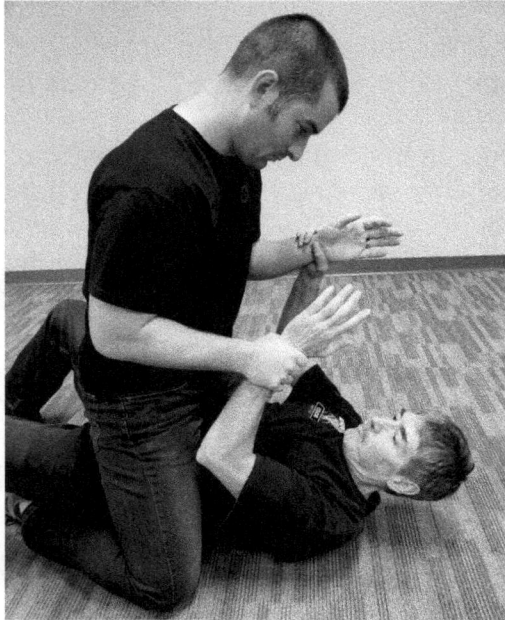
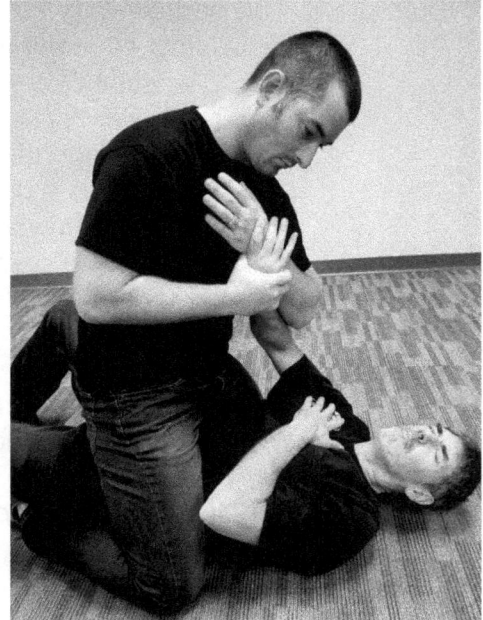

This is particularly painful when the suspect is captured on the bottom-side ground.
He has no mobility or freedom to escape.

Example 6: The goosenecks
    Goosenecks are popular law enforcement methods, but anyone can use them to shut down or move recalcitrant people around. It involves the freezing the elbow by cradling it in the bend of your arm, and cranking down on the knuckle area of the hand, usually palm down but could at times be palm up. Sometimes the elbow bend, by way of compressing the wrist, can force someone onto the ground. (I have seen it done for real.)

    There are three main ones:
        1: Elbow in crook of arm. Forearm vertical. Wrist bent.
        2: Elbow in crook of arm. Forearm horizontal in front. Wrist bent.
        3: Elbow in crook of arm. Forearm horizontal behind back.
          Wrist bent.

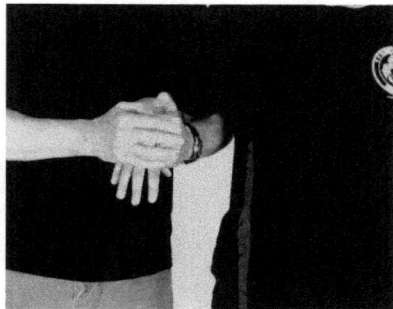
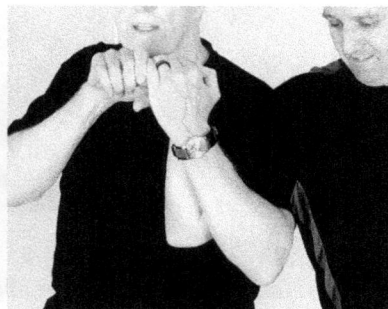
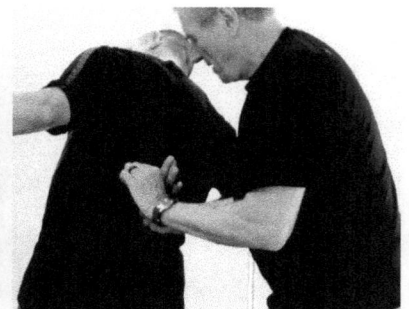

Horizontal goose.

Vertical goose. Hand twisted to the side to enhance capture.

"Cup and saucer" goose. With added finger lock.

Wrist Lock/Crank Flows

There are two kinds of locks in the world. One lock that must lead to another lock because the first one is not a "finisher" and one cannot hold a person frozen in a lock crank forever. And a second kind, a lock crank that leads to a takedown. There are more frozen locks than takedown locks. That is one reason why martialist must learn how to flow from one to another. A lock flow is a series of locks that make sense in movement. One way the chain makes sense is that the next move covers the most probable counter/escape the lock would make to escape the pain of the first lock. (It might be hard for a locker to predict what any person would do, especially an untrained person. You can guess, but it's hard.) The equation reads:

> Event 1: Locker locks.
> Event 2: Lockee tries to escape (what's his most common move? His most
>   common directional way out?)
> Event 3: Locker tries to thwart this escape with another lock.

A lock flow is also useful in showing/teaching a person the ins and outs of a particular joint crank. An experiment. A comprehensive study. These are the reasons why I suggest every practitioner work on lock flows standing and on the ground. Not to a tap-out submission, as they are fairly useless in real fights, but to build knowledge and experience in grappling.

This is a wrist lock, flow that I learned from JKD legend Larry Hartsell in a seminar ages ago. It's 1-2-3 simple and people have a better understanding of the Center, V, S or Z lock, whatever you wish to call it.

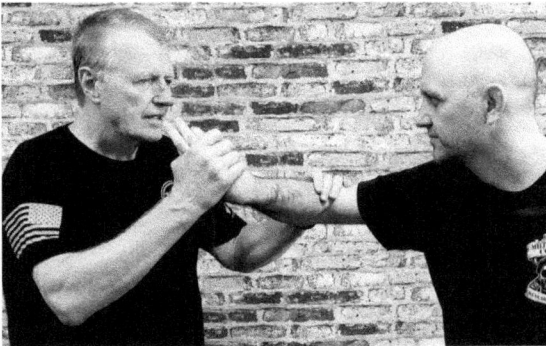
The classic center, V, S or Z lock.

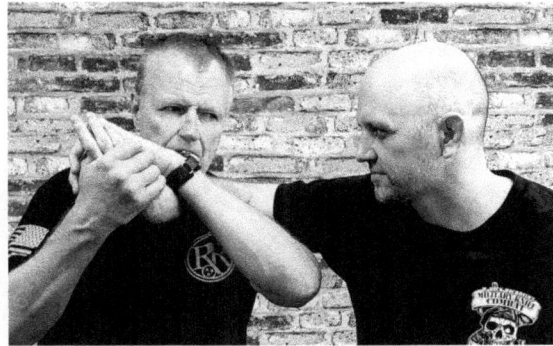
Inner arm sweeps in and up and helps the crank toward. This is a very painful catch.

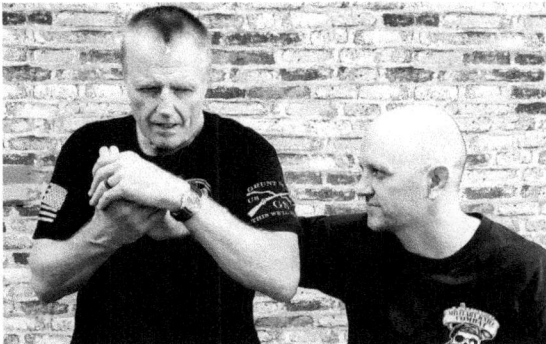
Then, the elbow is captured.

You can use this lock flow, as I must present something here for you, but the martial world is full of standing and ground lock flows concerning wrists, and many of them are acceptable studies.

Counters to these wristlock problems.

I could write a medium sized book on the these counters and escapes and the topic would be overwhelming to the mission of the book. Come see us in seminars or watch my joint crank video listed on the next page.

General counters to wrist cranks
>1: Early phase counters.
>>- yanks outs.
>>- hit the locker with the other hand.
>>>* hit main, locking limb.
>>>* hit both locking limbs.
>>>* head or body of locker.

>>- push, pull out.
>>- early escapes unique to the capture.

>2: Mid phase counters
>>- hit the locker with the free hand.
>>- push, pull out.
>>- slap releases to capturing limbs.
>>- mid escapes unique to the capture.

>3: Late phase counters
>>- leap ahead of the direction he is taking you.
>>- roll ahead of the direction he is taking.
>>- late escapes unique to the capture.

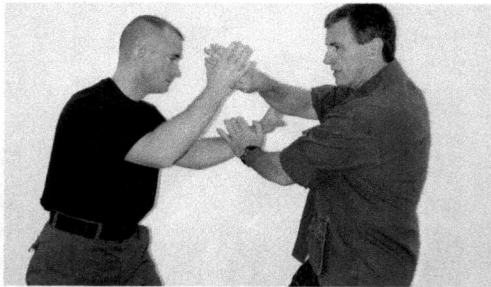

Mike Gillette rushes in and we get a chaotic Stop 3 collision.

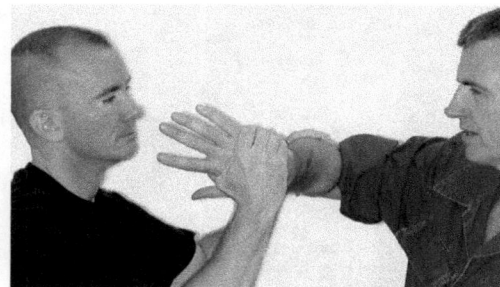

He happens to see a center lock brewing.

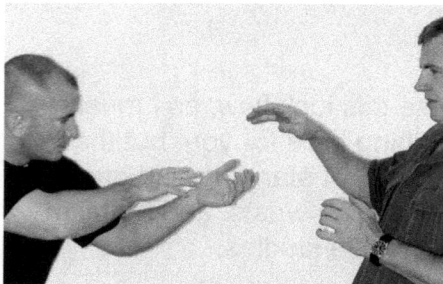

Early phase: I yank out. Get back.

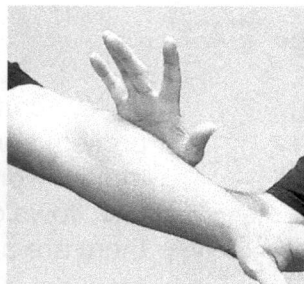

Mid-phase: I slap release

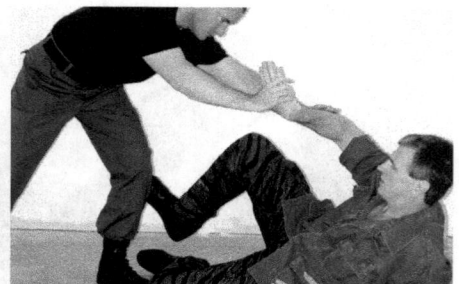

Late phase: I drop ahead of the takedown, going to where I want.

A late phase escape example is, I know I am locked in and I am going down. Down right where he wants me. So I move fast and ahead of the capture where I can do some damage. *NOT* where he wants or expects me to go. With this center-lock crank I drop down and inward to his center, to attack his legs and groin with kicks. Look over the various wrist locks and there end destinations and see where you are forced to go, and where you can actually go before the inevitable and what return damage you can deliver in a smarter ending spot.

Suggested reading and viewing for Force Necessary Hand! Level 2...

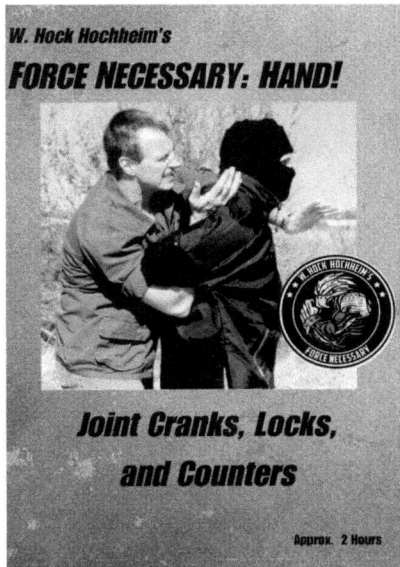

Joint Cranks, Locks
and Counters video.

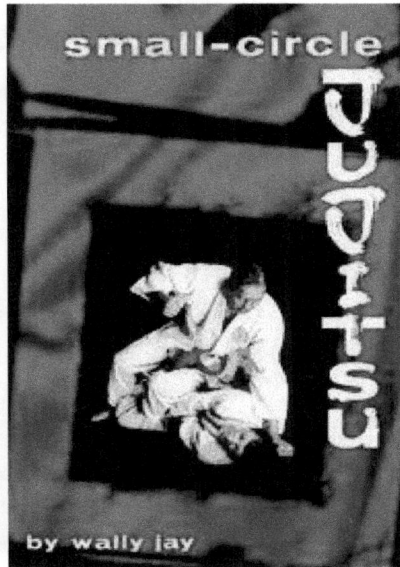

The great Jay book, as
organized by Mike Belzer.

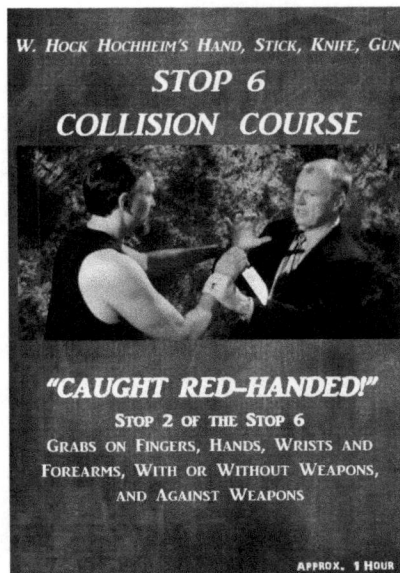

Stop 2 video.

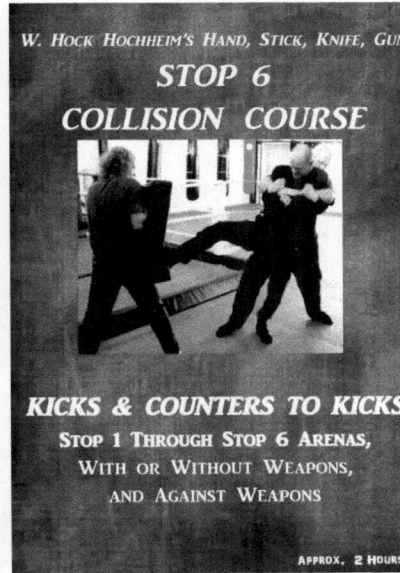

Kicks and Counters video.

FN: Hand Addendum 1: The B.P.P Grab Drill

This is just a support drill to build grabbing skills. We use the Block, Pass and Pin Drill for a variety of skill developments, and in the Stop 2 study this is great developer. One might have to learn this in person with a trainer. (It is not a requirement, but you'll be glad to master it.)

Series "0" The Introduction: The review of the 6 "block, pass, pin" events.

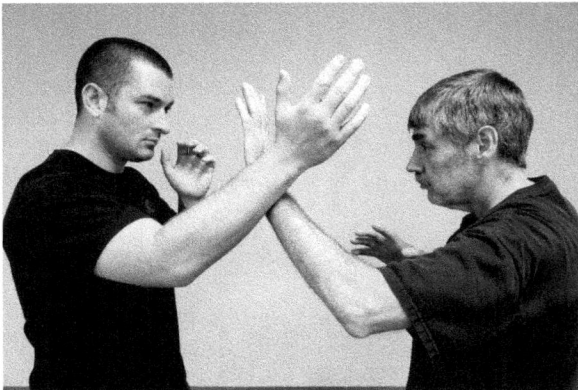
Event 1: He strikes. You block.

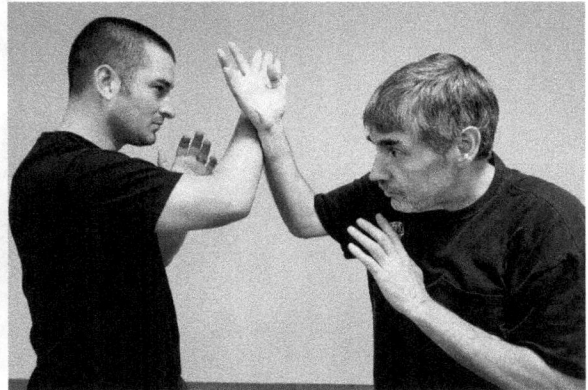
Event 2: Your right limb scoops under his strike. Your right passes him over.

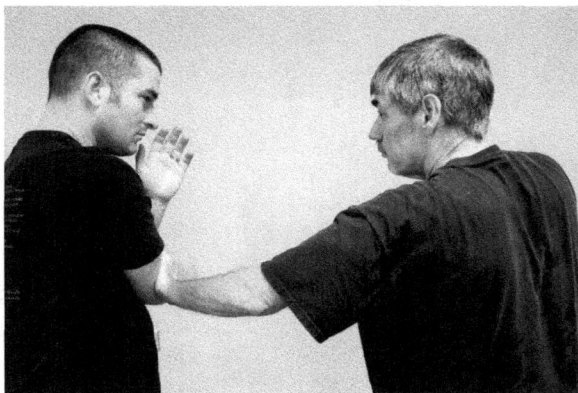
Event 3: You pin on the elbow.

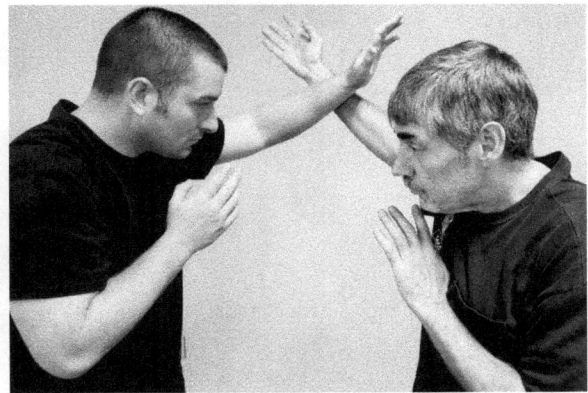
Event 4: You strike. He blocks.

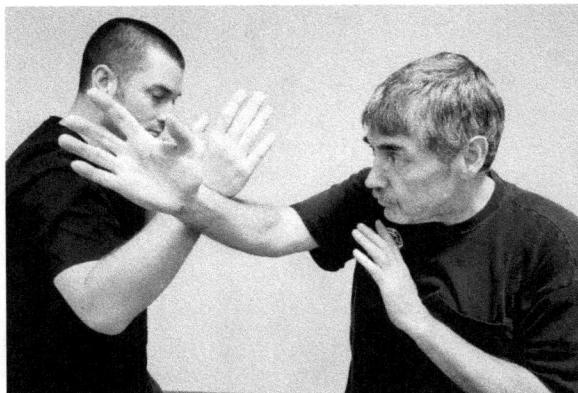
Event 5: He passes your strike over.

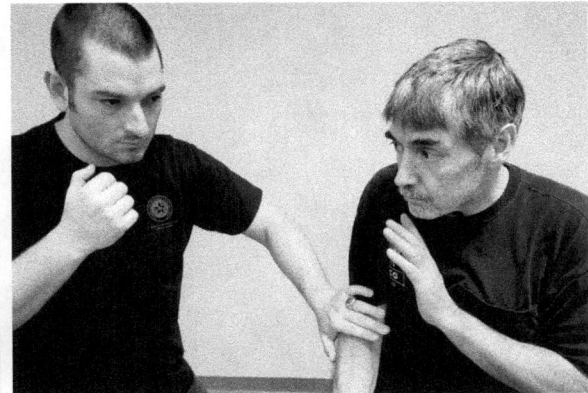
Event 6: He pins on your elbow.

Series 1: The same side that blocks, then grabs.

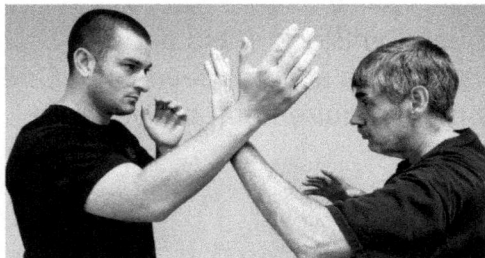

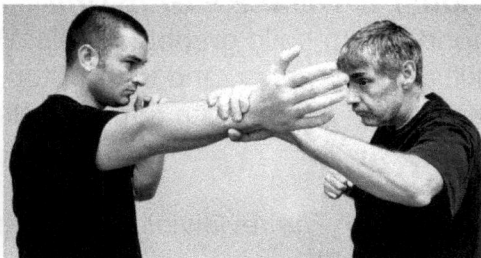

Event 1:
He strikes. You block with your left limb. This block turns into a grab.

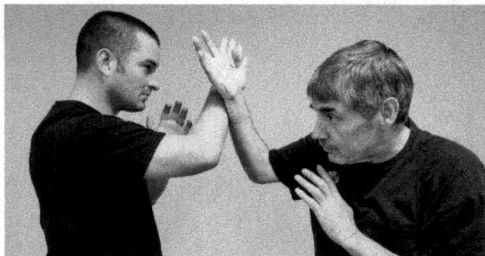

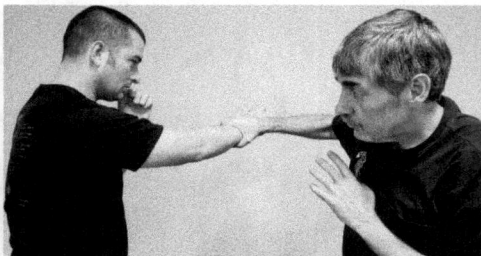

Event 2:
He strikes and you pass. You pass with your right limb. This pass turns into a grab.

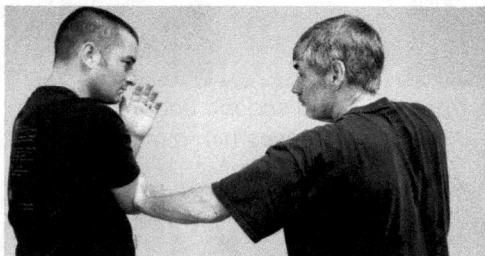

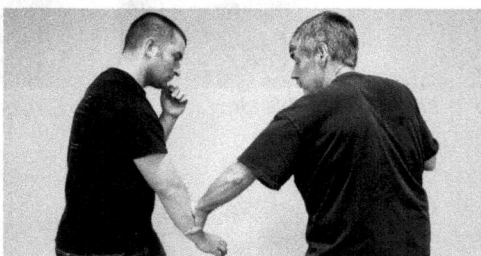

Event 3:
He strikes. You block. You pass with your right limb. Then you pin the elbow with your left. Your left hand slips down the forearm and grab.

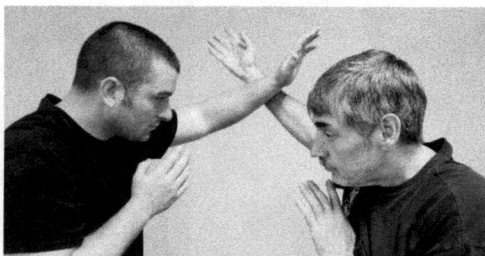

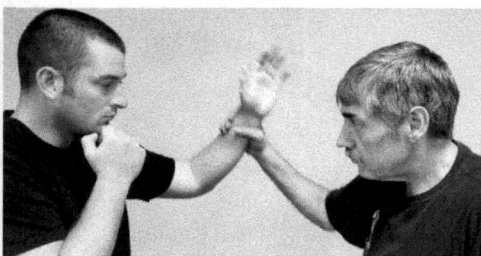

Event 4:
Block, pass, pin. You strike. He blocks. Your blocked hand shifts down, thumb comes out, hand goes back up for a grab.

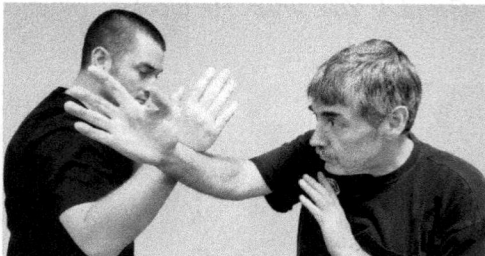

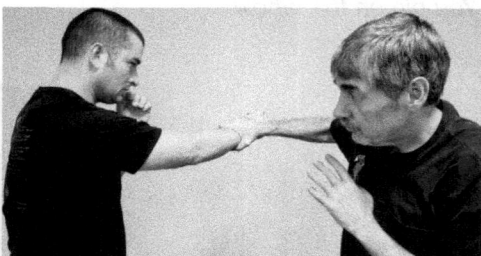

Event 5:
Block, pass, pin. Block, pass. You strike. He blocks. He passes. You grab his pass. Looks like event 2.

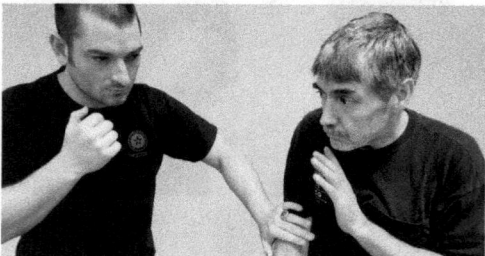

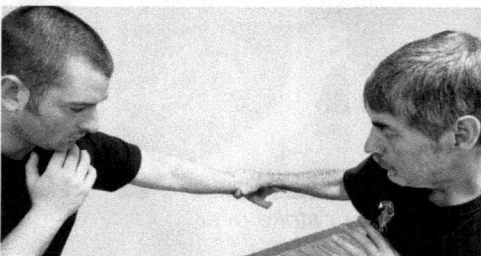

Event 6:
Block, pass, pin. He blocks, pass and he pins you elbow. You turn your hand palm down. Slide it horizontally until you grab his former pin.

Series 2: The same side that blocks, then grabs. The other hand hits.
Work through the 6 events, this time, when the blocking hand grabs, as simultaneously as possible, strike the face, throat, whatever, with whatever strike you chose.

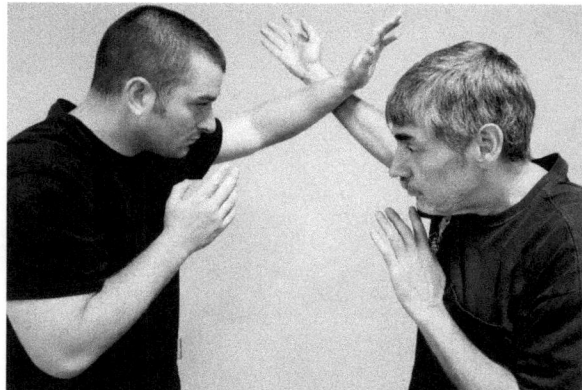

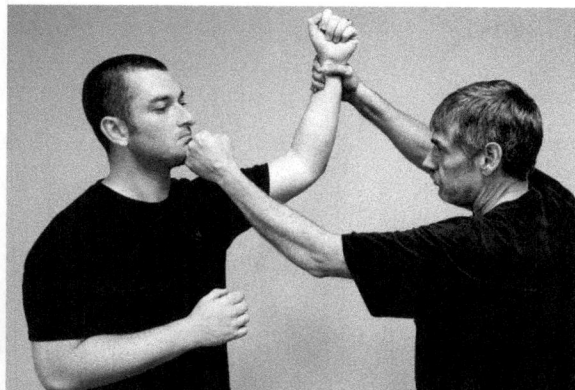

Event 4 sample - contact, same side contact. Contact turns into grab and punch.

Series 3: The other hand reaches over and grabs.
Work through the 6 events, this time, the same side blocks but the other hand reaches over and grabs.

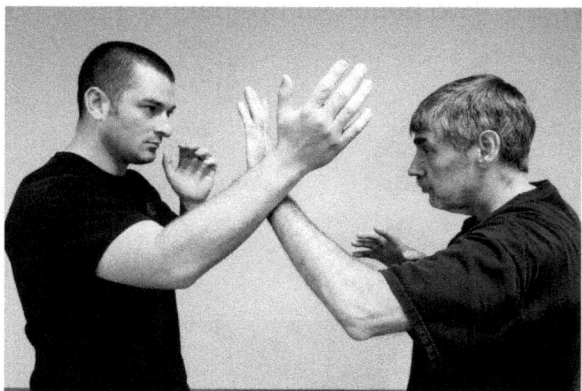

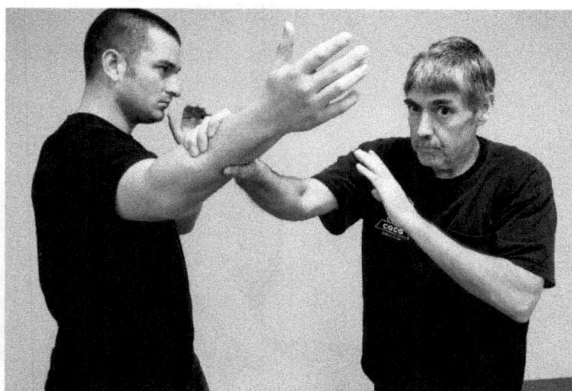

Event 1 sample - same side contact, and other hand reaches across and grabs.

Series 4: Both hands grab the strike.
In this series, there is contact and both hand grab.

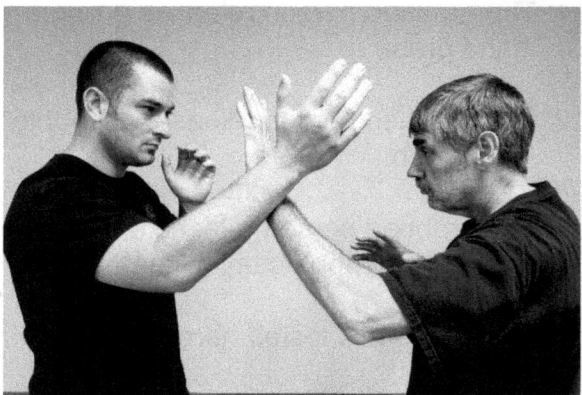

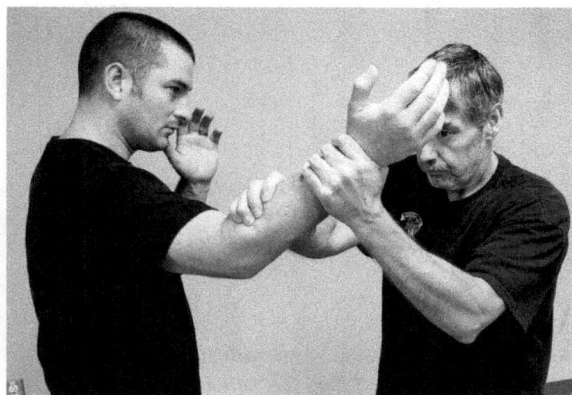

Event 1 sample - same side contact, and both hands grab.

Series 5: The Split Grab. This is challenging for some. The same side contact produces the above grabs, but in this series, the other hand seeks out his "other hand" and grabs that other hand! Then splits on all 6.

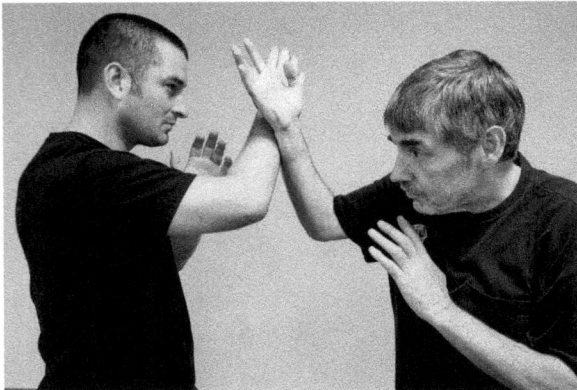
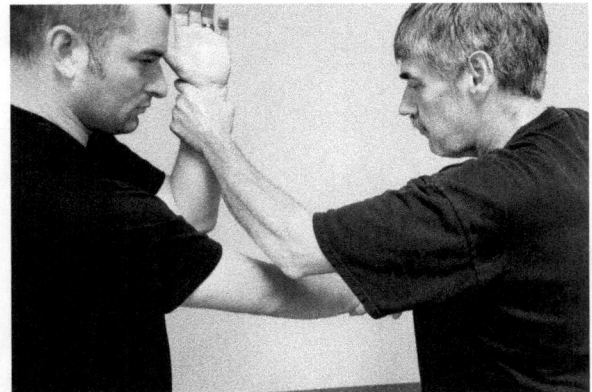

Event 2 sample - contact, the left hand scoops under and passes. The left hand now grabs the passed right and the free right hand seeks out his left wrist for a capture.

Series 6: The Release! The grabbed person releases a single hand grab, and double hand grabs. Using whatever release we covered in prior pages, get the release. This is also the time that grab strength gets tested. Two hands on one. Two hands on two hands.

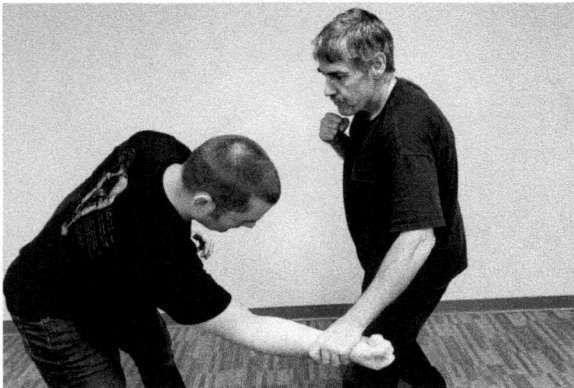

Achieved grip strength is tested here.

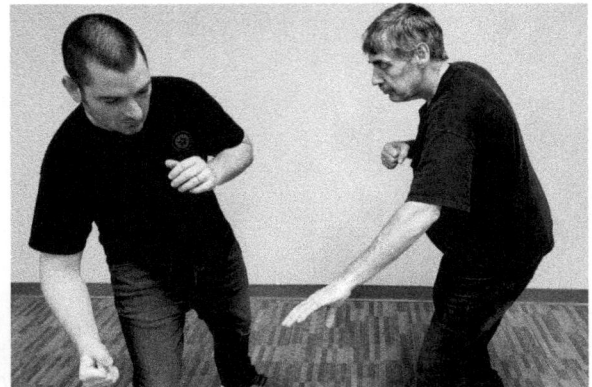

Work the releases previously listed releases on the 6.

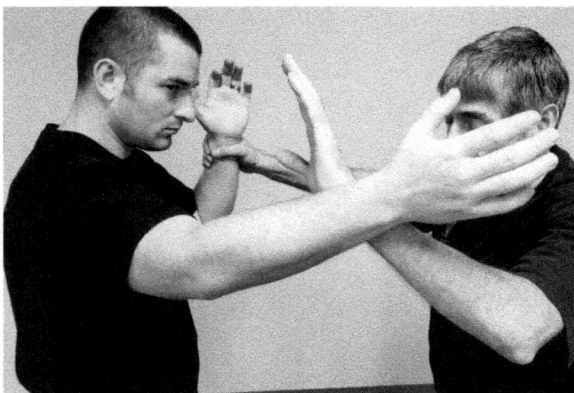

Ernesto Presas called this 'Double Unlockings," practice, getting free of two grips.

On all 6 events-
1: The grabbed person releases a single hand grab.

2: The grabbed person releases a double hand grab.

3: The grabbed person release a split grab with a "double unlocking."

4: Grip strength is tested here.

Series 7: Grabs versus a stick.

The stick attack is stopped, grabbed and disarmed on events 1, 2, 3, and split grabs 1-6. Action is taken on "his" events 1, 2, 3 as there is no sense grabbing his empty hand on events 4, 5, 6 when and while he has a free, loose stick to hit you with. However with the split grab series, you are grabbing the free hand *AND* the stick hand. The disarms? Remember we will cover all the how-to disarm topics in later *Training Mission* books. This book and *Stop 2* is just about the grab developments. Of course in classes and seminars, experiment with everything you see fit.

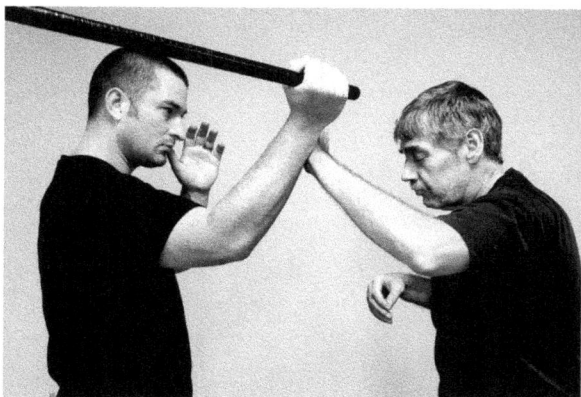

Run the 6 events. Blocks turn to grabs on events 1, 2 and 3. (Why grab the empty hand on 4, 5 and 6! The stick hand is free!

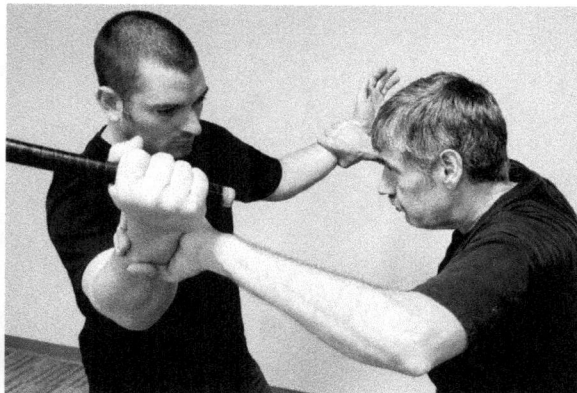

Split grabs 1-6. Run the 6 events. Blocks turn to grabs on all 6 events, as the weapon hand is also caught. Experiment with follow-ups.

Series 10: Verus a knife.

The knife attack is stopped, grabbed and disarmed on events 1, 2, 3, and split grabs 1-6. Action is taken on "his" events 1, 2, 3 as there is no sense grabbing his empty hand on events 4, 5, 6 when and while he has a free, loose knife to hit you with. However with the split grab series, you are grabbing the free hand *AND* the knife hand. The disarms? Remember we will cover all the how-to disarm topics in later *Training Mission* books. This book and *Stop 2* is just about the grab developments. Of course experiment with everything you see fit in workouts, classes and seminars.

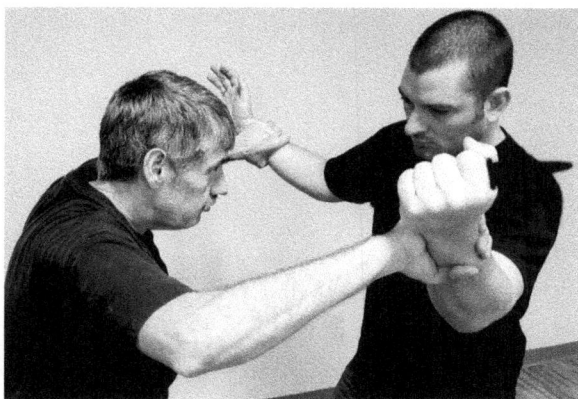

Series 11 and On: Invent, experiment with variations.

   Note: This Grab exercise will best be passed onto you with personal hands-on, instruction, as true step-by step analysis, might take hundreds and hundreds of photos and a thousand words and a long training film. I hope what is presented here will inspire you to try it. This is a fantastic support, skill developing drill, once you "grasp" it.

FN Hand Addendum 2 - The Handshake "Trick"

In the olden days, old school Japanese Jujitsu called techniques, once loosely translated into English, as "tricks." And the handshake trick involves the deceptive move of going for the handshake and turning it into a wrist or forearm grab, from which many grappling follow-ups occur.

The handshaking hands interlock by way of the thumbs being up. If you move into the handshake with your thumbs up and then at the last few seconds, drop your thumb, your hand will pass his hand deeper, setting up the potential for the wrist or forearm grab. Once acquired, other related arm captures may begin.

In the old, US Army military police academy a handshake was taught as a trick to tie up a right-handed suspect's weapon-side hand, preventing him from a quick draw and in some cases, allowing an officer to disarm a handy knife or pistol from a body carry site.

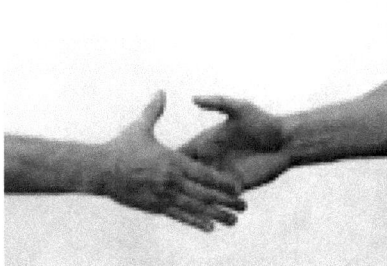

Coming in for the shake.	*Thumbs up ends the movement.*	*A thumb down passes through.*

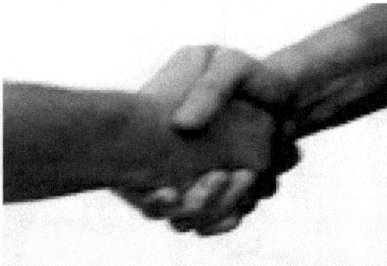

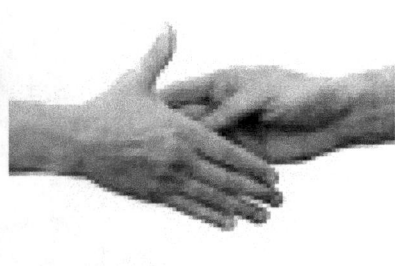

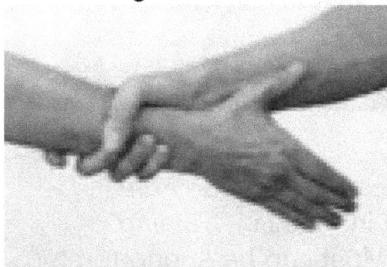

And the wrist/forearm is grabbed.	*This grab sets up whatever the following moves are.*

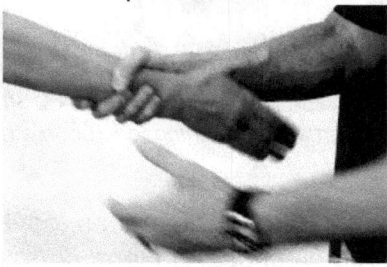

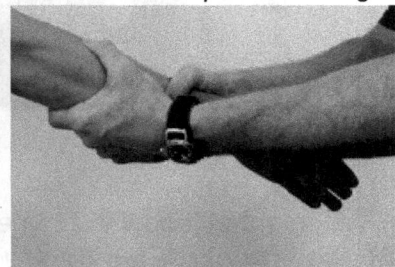

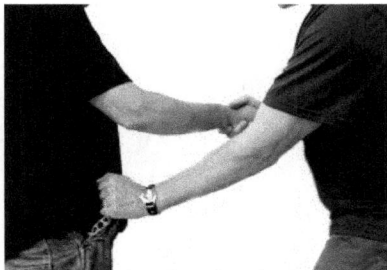

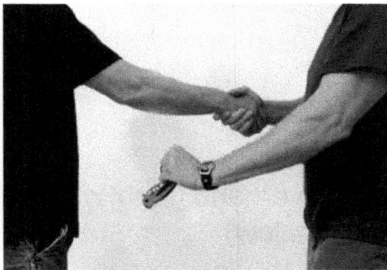

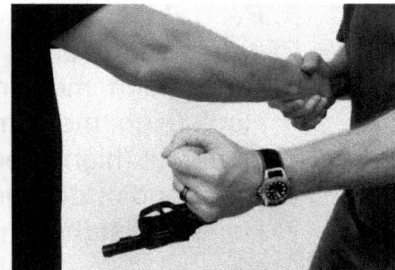

Old school police training used the handshake to prevent quick draws and for weapon disarming. Remember, some of these the pistol will pull out from him (or you), upside down.

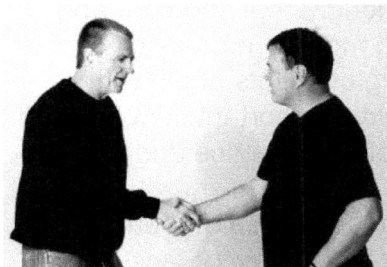

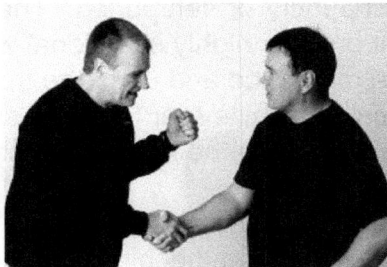

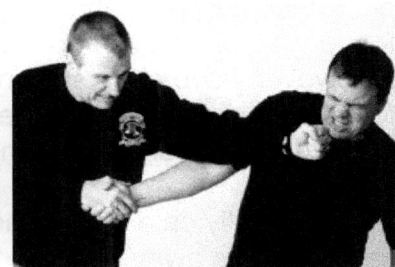

And needless to add, this can set up a strike.

FN Hand Addendum 3: Cable Machine Workout

The need to strike with force. You can hit heavy bags and pads held by training partners, but you can build strong power other ways, especially when you train alone.

A while back I taught a seminar at *Doc Sheldon's Private Training Center* in the Cincinnati, Ohio area. The place is loaded with equipment, and I saw a cable machine in one corner of the gym. As an aside to the seminar, I showed some folks the workout I've never stopped doing with cable machines since the 80s, that I thought was fairly common knowledge. But no one there had seen it before. They found it inspiring. Since, others around the world said the same thing. So for the record, here it is. This book is a good place to introduce the cable machine concept since all strikes we will study now and henceforth require power and force support exercises.

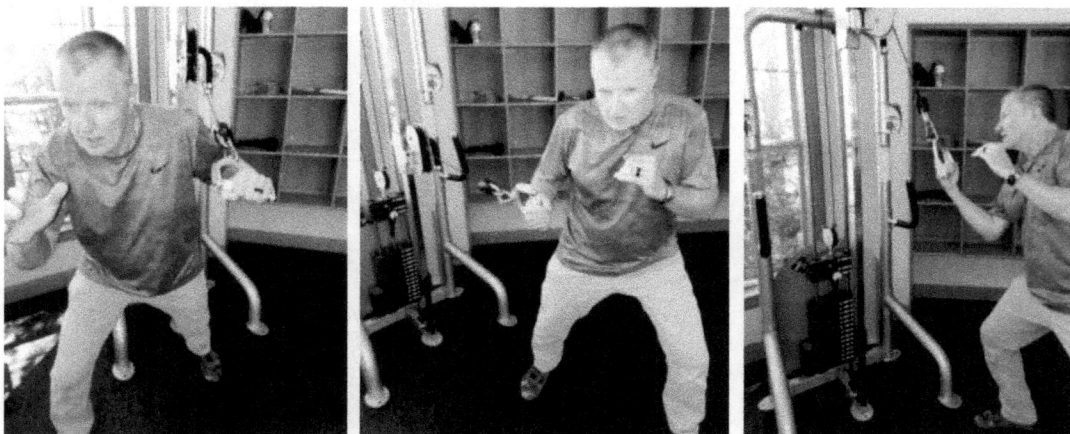

Cable machine training to support striking.

We might all know the big essential, generic strikes, covered in detail in *Training Missions books, Stop 6* and *Force Necessary: Hand courses.* Most can be supported by cable machines.

    1: Palm strike.
    2: Jab (high, medium, low).
    3: Cross (high, medium, low).
    4: Hook (high, medium, low).
    5: Uppercut (high, medium, low).
    6: Overhand or descending overhand (high, medium, low).
    7: Hammer fist (high, medium, low).

There were eras in the US military that never taught an official jab or official cross, but rather just called them "right punch" or "left punch." They thought that shoulder and foot positions weren't important or were highly situational when moving in chaotic, combat. I, however, have always seen a difference and used the training concepts of jab with its foot/shoulder forward and the cross with its rear foot/rear shoulder important, if at least not for training purposes alone. And I see the need for such isolated practice and development.

Technically on a cable machine, you are always "pulling" on the handle and pulling cable weights away from the "tower" of the machine. But if you face away, or face toward the tower, it creates differing exercises. To define this particular exercise process I explain that when you stand facing the machine, the cable is pulling you into it, pulling your hand into the machine. When you are facing away from the machine, you are pushing the handle away from the machine. No matter, you always are pulling the weight rack up.

This is how I like to define the exercises for clarity. Push-Pull. Face-away, push. Face in, pull. I would like to add that you can use these same cable machine methods with palm strikes for all you anti-punchers out there. But only in the "pushing outward" method.

You have to close your hand to grip the handle when facing toward the machine. Don't hyper extend your wrist! Use reasonable weights. Emphasize the palm heel as much as possible when doing the palm strikes and the knuckles as much as possible when
punching.

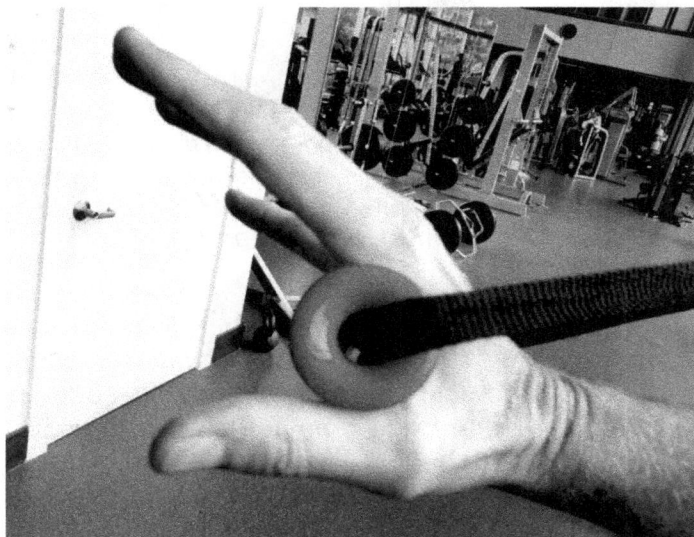

Take care not to hyper-extend your wrist. Take care to emphasize your punch or hammer fist.

If you shadow box with hand weights, you are abstractly building the path for punching. Abstract because you have to remember that your hand, arm and shoulder are battling up and down gravity with that hand weight. The more the weight and the more the hand extends, the more you are building/fighting vertical gravity and building those related up-down muscles. With a cable machine there is no up/down gravity, just the machine pivot point behind or before you at the prescribed height. Some people shadow box with mere 1 or 2 pound weights, and this is so light there is not much "gravity" fighting at all. But more hand weight? You are losing goal effectiveness. Vertical muscle building? Or, horizontal muscle building?

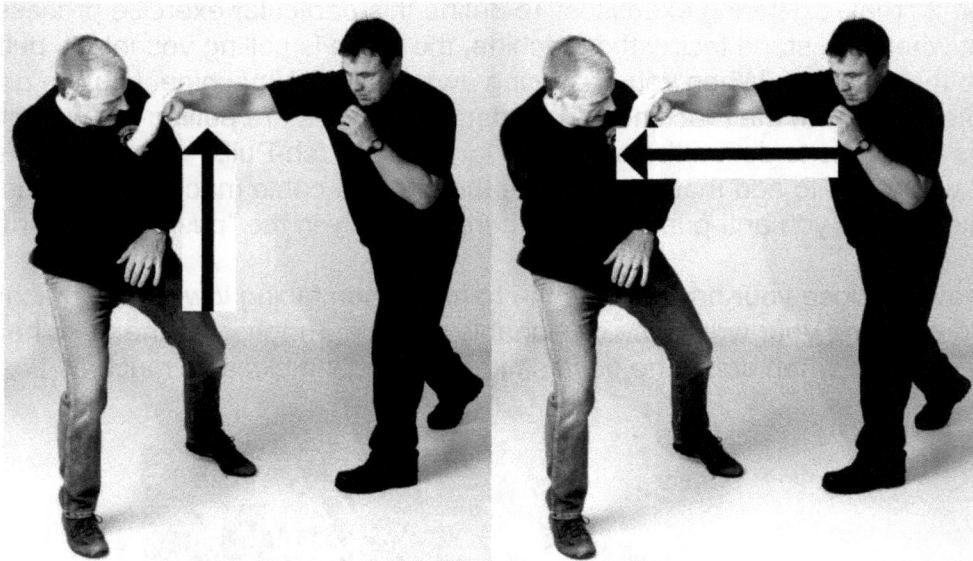

Randy Roberson (my first private student from the late 80s) throws a training punch. If he had a weight in his hand, he would be countering vertical gravity and getting some abstract development. To really maximize the horizontal development, he needs a cable machine.

I think this cable machine method develops striking power and speed. I do a set of 25 reps with each strike, in the pull and push directions, when this segment comes up in my workout rotation, which can be once or twice a week (for 40 years now, give or take sickness, medical operations, and travel). It takes about 20 minutes of non-stop motion. The next day my arms are somewhat sore as well as my back muscles, what with all the torso twisting. It can be aerobic, but if you switch your feet a lot with the uppercuts and hooks, it adds to the workout.

People like to do various exercises with those big rubber bands, but they can be limiting in range when attempting all the below listed strikes, and you have to hook those bands onto something! Will the hook be the right height? How will you hook it? Meanwhile, the ubiquitous cable machine will offer the range and the heights, and quick-change resistance. It's all about the push-pull.

Long ago, fitness and sport experts suggested that you must develop the pushing and pulling aspects of functional movement. One way is breaking movements down in isolated exercises. For example, in football practice years ago, they made us run up and down hills. Running down the hill as fast as you can, made you run faster than you ordinarily would. You can feel the extra speed as you struggle to keep up with yourself flying down hill. You also experience what it feels like to be faster than you normally are. Remember that feeling. Emulate it.

The same is true when you work strikes with a cable machine. When you face the machine and punch, the cable weight pulls and should make you move faster. Just a little! Like running down the hill and falling, don't overdo this and yank yourself into an injury. Strike and let the cable weights make you a bit faster. And, when you retract, you also get that benefit. With this advice, I stand facing the machine and facing away, back to the machine.

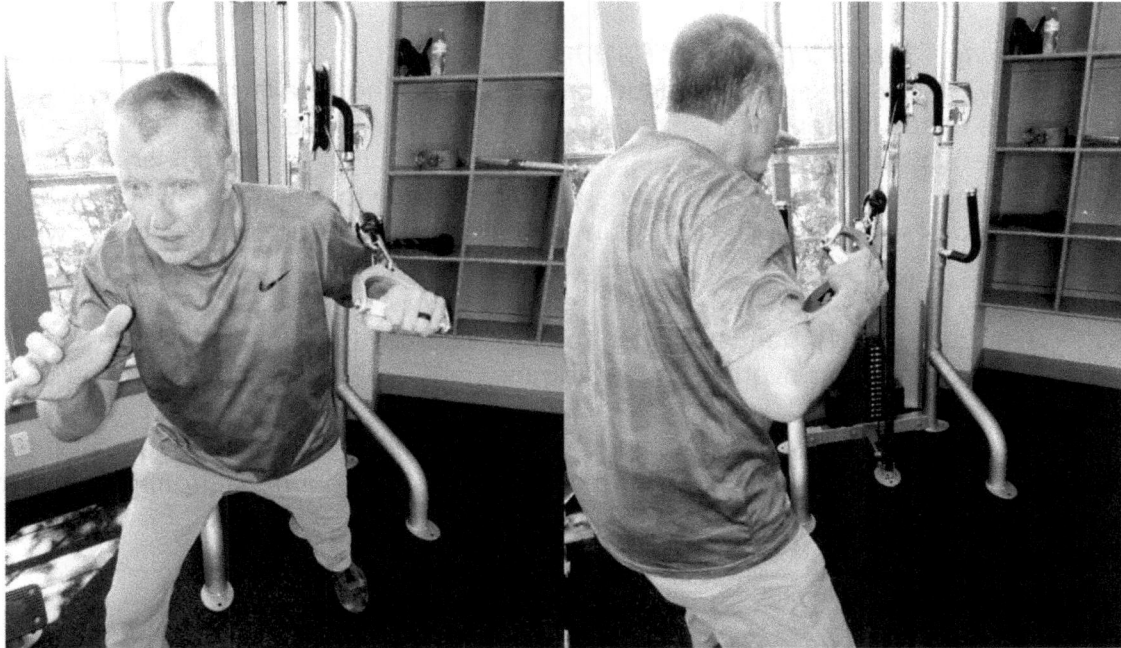

*The cross punch. Do 25 facing out. You are always "pulling" the weight rack up,
but pulling or pushing the cable. Don't forget the lower, straight, stomach punch.
Set the height adjustment low.*

I don't do these with heavy plates, but you can build up to anything you want, I guess. Just try to remember:

1: Don't hurt your wrists!

2: Whether punches or palm strikes get the right positioning for your hand, the best hand-to-handle position. When punching, try to get your knuckles involved in the pulling and pushing. When palm striking, try to get your palm heel involved in the pushing. (You can't face the machine and "pull" the palm strike because your hand is open.

3. Always try to keep your free hand up and open. Don't get sloppy and let that other hand drop.

4. Keep your mouth closed, teeth together as a matter of routine. You can still expel "martial" air. Reread the breathing chapters in the first half of the book.

5: For up and downs strikes like uppercuts, you face the machine. For other exercises, face both toward and away from the machine for sets.

6: Set the best height adjustment on the machine to maximize your goal.

Descending Overhand (Punch or Palm) strikes.
You know the descending overhands, or you will see the details in *Training Mission Five.* This essay is a primer inspiration for training. The strike can be very successful and is used in MMA and UFC fights. If you want to get that slight hooking motion at the end (one used to hit behind the ear) You may have to reduce the weight a bit as the wrist goes a little funky with the turn and slight hook. Experiment with the weight.

   * A set of right overhands pushing the handle away from machine.
   * A set of left hand overhands pushing the handle away from the machine.

   * A set of right overhands pushing the handle with a slight hook, again face away.
   * A set of left overhands pushing the handle with a slight hook, again face away.

   * A set of right overhands pulling the handle facing the machine.
   * A set of left overhands pulling the handle facing the machine.

   * A set of right overhands pulling handle with a slight hook, again facing in.
   * A set of left overhands pulling the handle with a slight hook, again facing in.

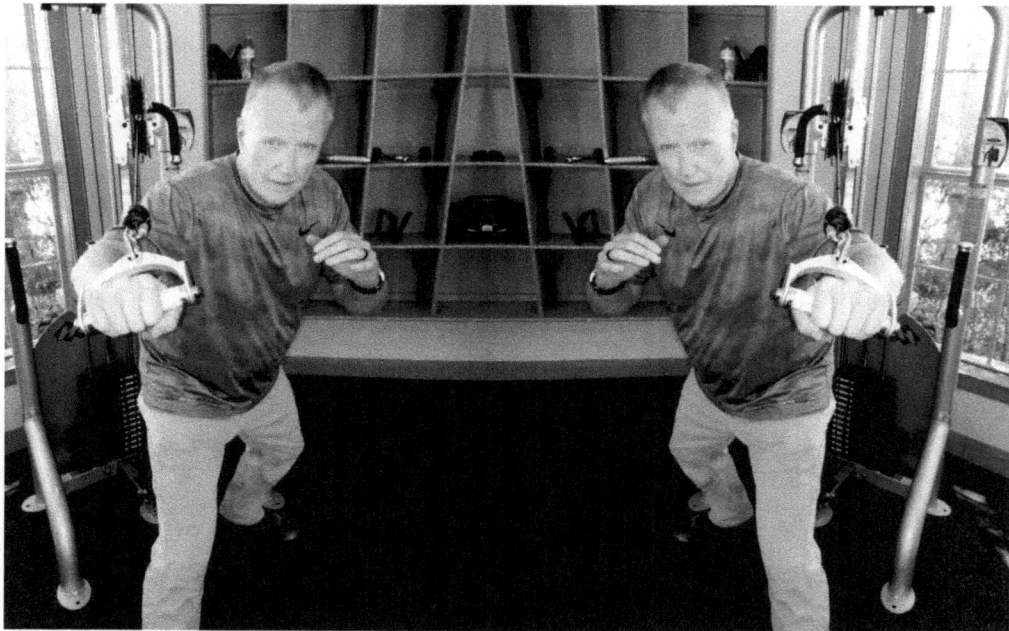

Descending overhands. Right and left hand. Right and left leads.
Pushing away from the machine. Then turn around, face the machine and pull.

Hooks (punch or palm strikes) (High hooks, medium hooks or low hooks)
For punching, you obviously close your fists tightly. For palm strikes, the hand is open and you hit with the parts of your hand, appropriate for the target. Ear claps? Flat palm of the hand. Behind the ear shots or lower? The heel of the hand.

* A set of right hooks pushing away from the machine.
  - high setting.
  - medium setting.
  - low setting.

* A set of left hooks pushing away from the machine.
  - high setting.
  - medium setting.
  - low setting.

* A set of right hooks pulling away from the machine.
  - high setting.
  - medium setting.
  - low setting.

* A set of left hooks pulling away from the machine.
  - high setting.
  - medium setting.
  - low setting.

(You can use a lot of footwork doing these.)

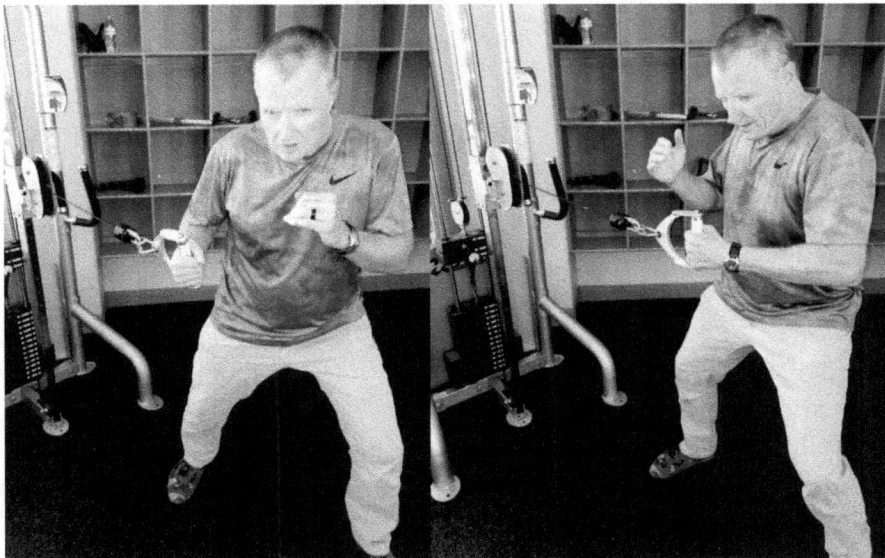

The hooks. Right and left hand. Right and left leads. Pushing and pulling. High hooks. Medium high hooks. Low hooks. Both directions.

Uppercuts (Punch or Palm)
You will face the machine, setting the height adjustments. Also think about the height of your target. Torso shovel hooks? Chin? Open hand palm strikes to the groin?

  * A set of right uppercuts pushing the handle up.
  * A set of left uppercuts pushing the handle up.

  * A set of right uppercuts pulling the handle down.
  * A set of left uppercuts pulling the handle down.
   (You can use a lot of footwork doing these.)

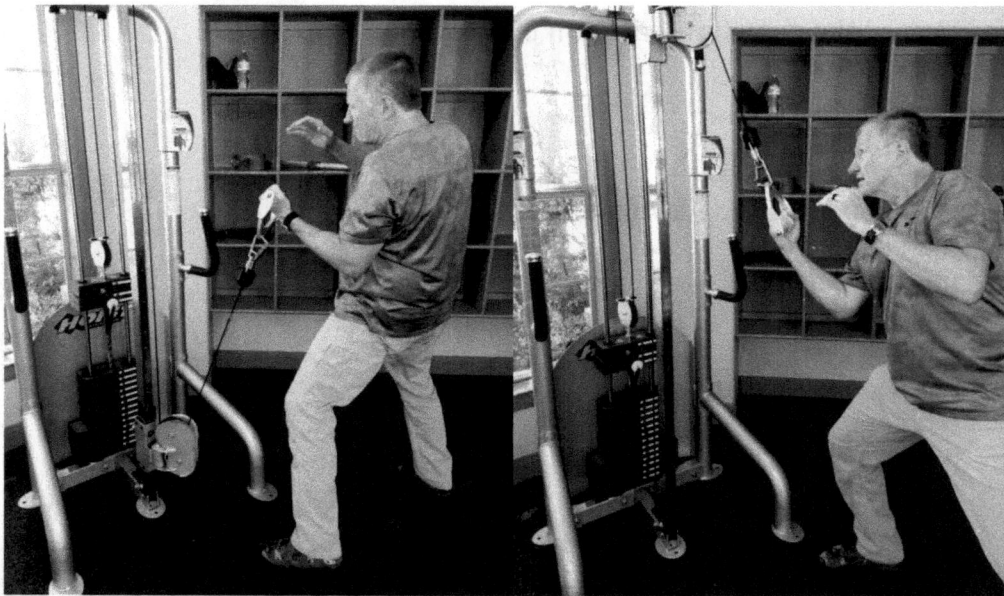

Uppercuts. Right and left. Pull the handle up. Pull the handle down. Think of various target heights.

Hammer fists (top of the hand and bottom of the hand).
Hammer fists are great and natural strikes. You have to find the best handle or rope at the gym to use. A good gym has this variety usually laying on the floor, waiting to be used.

  * a set pulling down diagonally.
  * a set pulling up diagonally.
   (You can use a lot of footwork doing these.)
   (Vary the angles. You know from common sense now
    what to do.)

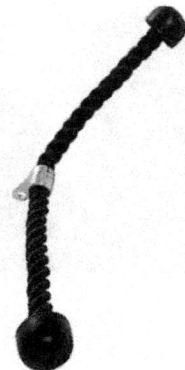

Combinations (Palm, hammer fist and punch)
Set the gear-pulley-pivot points at various north-south heights and the "arms" at various distances apart. Invent combinations of the above, in both push/pull directions!

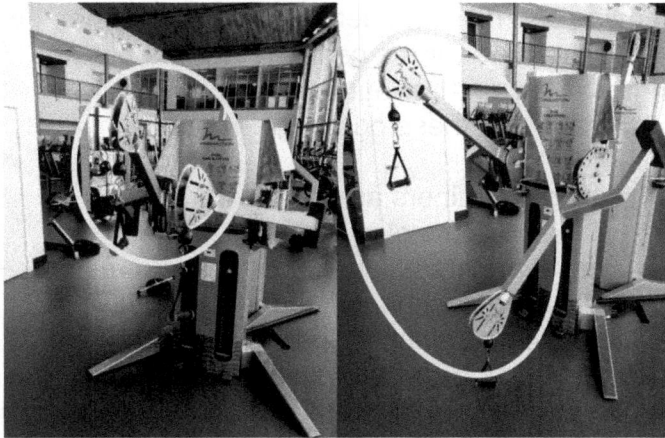

Some other points.
Of course you should still hit the bags if you can. But, as I have aged, hitting things that don't give-way much is a problem. And I don't wear big boxing gloves, nor wrap my wrists, as I don't want to become dependent upon them. I do not want to become a boxer. I do not train boxers. I train non-sport survivors. Your next criminal encounter will be a bare-knuckle event. Heavy bag impacts cause me and many other older vets follow-up wrist, shoulder or back pain. That impact goes somewhere back up into you. There are various pieces of equipment that "give" sufficiently. Traditional makiwara pads hardly give if hung on a wall.

I have old martial arts friends who can't hold a cup of coffee from arthritis today from unforgiving impact training. Think of modern, safer ways to toughen your hands and fists. (You'll find more about this in the *Training Mission Five* material.)

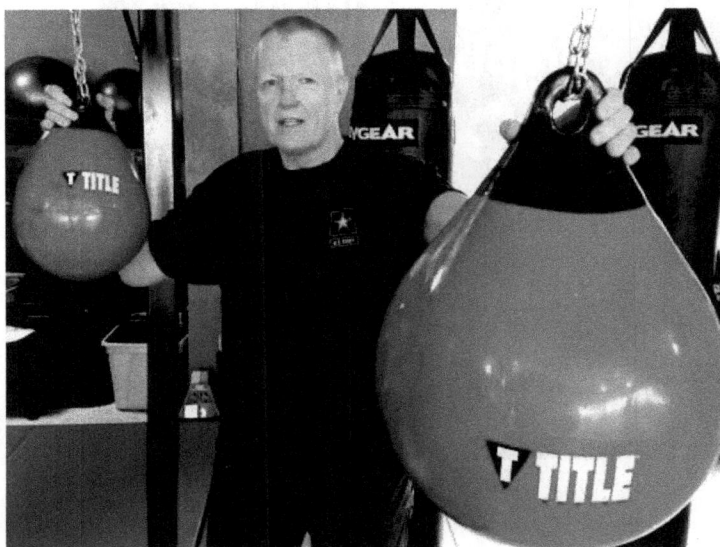

These bags are filled with water. They give-way and at times even feel like real body impacts.

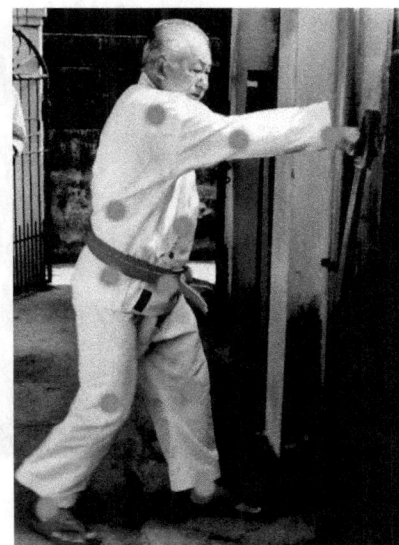

These impacts go back into you somewhere.

Cable machines also have straps for your ankles and the rest of your legs. You can also rig yourself up for cable, kick (and knee) work. Through the years I have done snapping, hooking kicks/knees with cable machines. Back and forth. But, as I have gotten older with bad hips and deteriorating backbone discs, I can no longer do these under the cable weight without follow-up pain. I want to warn you that your regular muscles are not accustomed to working at these odd angles so take it easy at first.

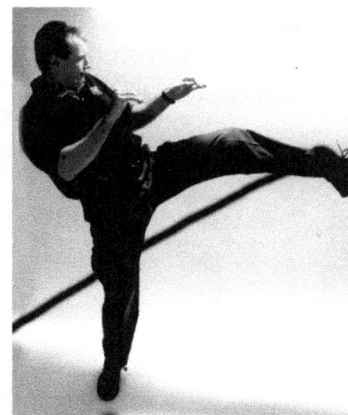

Kicking with cable resistance.

You will be looked at by gym trainers as unsafe, uncool and crazy. I am sure there will be a fitness gym guru that will tell people I am killing you with these ideas. I just don't think I am. But, after you start blowin' and goin,' changing footwork with each strike, they tend to leave you alone.

In this exercise vein, as usual, as natural, you will do this and get over-confident and keep adding the weight plates. More, more, then more. Then you will hurt yourself. Then you will heal, recoup, rebuild, add, add again, get over confident, hurt yourself again, heal again, recoup again...you get the picture. This is the life we have chosen. This is the lifetime routine. Get used to it or die uncoordinated, fat and out of shape.

These cable exercises have been very beneficial to me. It's one more thing I can do in a typical, solo gym workout that leans toward functionality.

Note: By the way, I also do the normal cable machine exercises too!

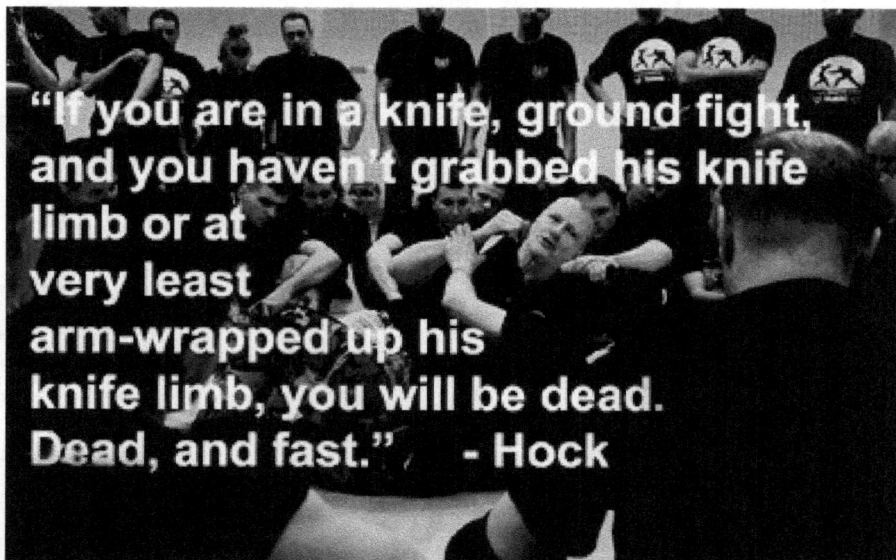

"If you are in a knife, ground fight, and you haven't grabbed his knife limb or at very least arm-wrapped up his knife limb, you will be dead. Dead, and fast."   - Hock

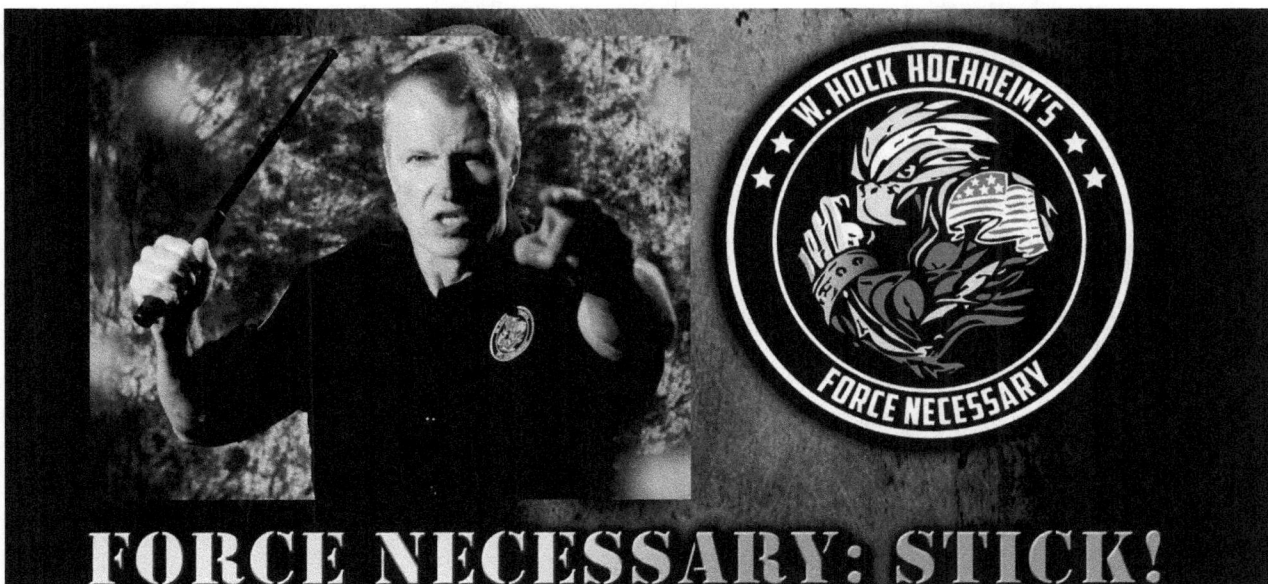

CHAPTER 20: FORCE NECESSARY: STICK – LEVEL 2

Review Training Mission One, Stick Level 1

Commonalities of Hand, Stick, Knife, Gun
Examine Stop 2 as explored within the Level 2 stick context.
Examine the "What" question as explored within the Level 2 stick context.
Examine the Footwork Drill #2: The In and Out Drill, as detailed in Part 1.
Examine the grip releases from Part 1.
Continue studying your local self defense laws.

Physical Performance Requirements

Problem-solving impact weapon retention.
- protecting the belt and holster/sheath.
- protecting the drawn stick when being presented and while being used.

Problem-solving the Stop 2 version of the Ambush, Dodge, Evasion, Counter Exercise.

Problem-solving the Tangler Exercise.

Two of the Stop 6: Grabs on Fingers, Hands, Wrist and Impact Weapons

In Stick Level 1 we drew the stick under various stressors, under the Stop 1 parameters of a hands-off, somewhat distant showdown. However, to introduce some training stressors we had some contact. The main thrust here in Stick Level 2 is solving the *Stop 2* problems with a stick, but we will leave *Stop 2* confines a time or two to be topically comprehensive when the subject matter calls for it. The overall essence of the Level 2 study is about retention and the "In the Clutches Of" drills. Familiarization of that topic covers a lot of important, problem-solving.

You are about to draw your stick, or have drawn the stick and the enemy grabs your weapon-side limb or the weapon itself. You may grab his weapon-bearing limb too, or not. Remember, when you are holding a stick, the enemy might be:

- empty-handed.
- holding a stick, or sheathed stick.
- holding a knife or a pocketed or sheathed knife.
- holding a pistol or one holstered or tucked.
- holding a long gun, or has a long gun slung/attached to his body.

What - Stick of the Ws and H Questions?

Look at the beginning of this book to study the overall "what" questions. Specific to the stick, here are some "what-stick" things to consider:

"What stick will you buy and/or carry?" Expandable? Fixed? Small? Big?

"What stick training course will you take?

"What is your mission?" What, if any, mission do you have?

"What will you be wearing that either covers or conceals your stick?"

"What are your the local laws about impact weapons? Carrying? Brandishing? Using?

"What do you expect to accomplish with your stick?

"What is your "weapons continuum" Are you also carrying other weapons too?

"What is the weapons disparity?" Disparity is defined as, lack of similarity or equality; inequality; difference: a disparity in age; disparity in rank. And a disparity of weapons, such as stick versus knife or versus a pistol.

"What happens next? After you used that stick, what happens next? Redemption? Jail? Law suit?

Continue to try and collect, and answer the "what-stick" questions.

Footwork #2: The In and Out , "While Holding Stick" Footwork
As previously covered in the first part of this book, practice the in and out footwork pattern while holding an impact weapon, one hand, two-hands, saber grip and reverse grip. You do not have to strike only on the forward step. Also strike on the back step.

Series 1: Left foot is anchored in the axis. Right foot works in and out at about 2 and 4 or 5 o'clock. All while holding a stick in one hand or two-handed grips.

Series 2: Right foot is anchored in the axis. Left foot works in and out at about 10 and 7 or 8 o'clock. All while holding a stick in one hand or two-handed grips.

Note: Do the following exercises solo in the air, on a heavy bag or war post.

Series 3: Solo quick review of *Stop 1*: Step in and out and draw the stick.

Series 4: Solo one-hand grip:
- step in and out with single-hand slash with a saber grip.
- step in and out with single-hand tip stab with a saber grip.
- step in and out with single-hand pommel stab with a saber grip. >< * right-hand. * left-hand.
- step in and out with single-hand slash with a reverse grip.
- step in and out with single-hand tip stab with a reverse grip.
- step in and out with single-hand pommel stab with a reverse grip.
- step in and out with single-hand, reverse grip, pommel stab.
- step in and out and block.
- step in and out and block, and any strike combination.

Series 5: Solo two-hand grip:
- step in and out with two-hand grip shaft thrust/shove.
- step in and out with two-hand grip and any shaft hook.
- step in and out with two-hand grip, and any right tip hook strike.
- step in and out with two-hand grip and any left tip hook strike.
- step in and out with two-hand grip block.
- step in and out with two-hand grip block and any strike.

Series 6: Combinations:
- step in and out with any single-hand strike and two-hand strike combination.

Series 7: Freestyle:
- freestyle blocks and strikes while moving in and out.

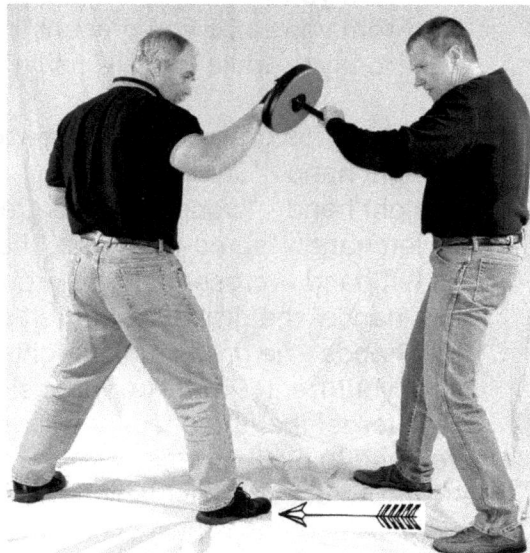

Impact Weapon Retention

Retention begins at the carry site. You can purchase a carrier that will limit the removal of your baton/stick, but it will never fully ensure that an opponent won't strip a stick from your belt line or pockets or carry site. Tactics become the last, best option.

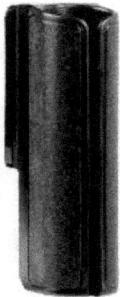

A breakaway sheath sample. The closed baton breaks out the opening, either by your hands, or your enemy's hands.

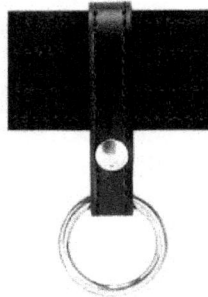

A very common baton, carrier loop. The baton has a rubber grommet and slips down into the ring, stopping at the grommet. Any opponent can also pull this stick out.

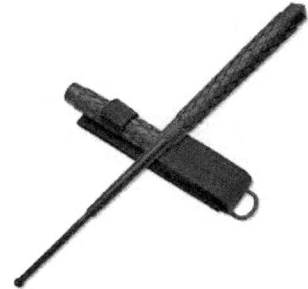

There are many versions of sheath carries. None really offer any significant retention capabilities.

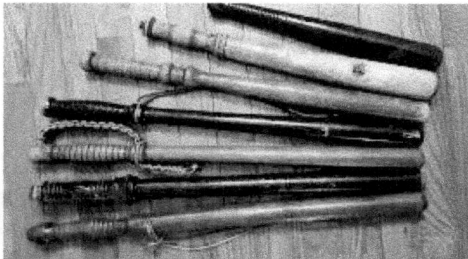

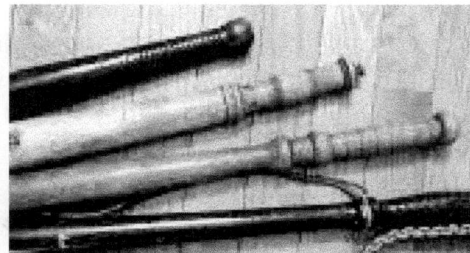

Many new and old batons have retention straps that a person can wrap around their hand or wrist. Note the pommel caps that help against the stick being pulled straight out of the hand.

* Your impact weapon may be removed:
- 1: From its carry site (where is that on you?)
- 2: From you while attempting to touch and draw your weapon.
- 3: From you while you are drawing the weapon.
- 4: From you while you present the weapon.
- 5: From you while you are using the weapon in strikes and blocks.

* Understand his grabs for your weapon. and weapon-bearing limb.
His right hand - "same-side grab," he grabs at your left side weapon with his right hand.
His right hand - "cross-grab" he grabs at your right side with his right hand.
His left hand - "same-side grab," he grabs at your right side weapon with his left hand.
His left hand - "cross-grab" he grabs at your left side with his left hand.
Both hands - he grabs at your left side weapon with both hands.
Both hands - he grabs at you right side weapon with both hands.
From your front. From your right side. From your left side. From your back.
Don't forget that the attacker will usually try to strike you or grab you too. Deal with that.
We need to place priorities to:
- "protect the belt." which could be any carry site, but with a stick, usually the belt.
- "protect the drawn stick" when its removed from the belt.

Retention challenges

And attacker can come at you, trying to take your impact weapon from your front, back, right, left, from above and from below. They will go for your belt carry or your pulled, produced, weapon. Full ambush or full frontal assault.

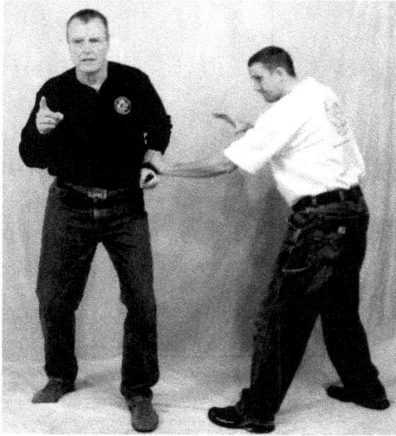

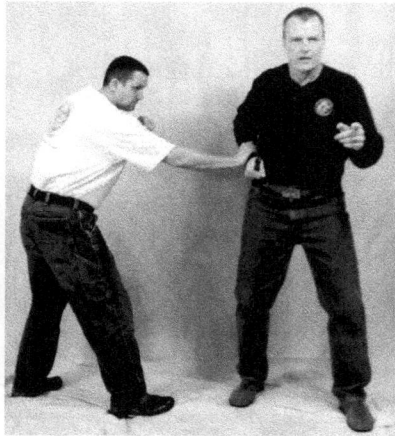

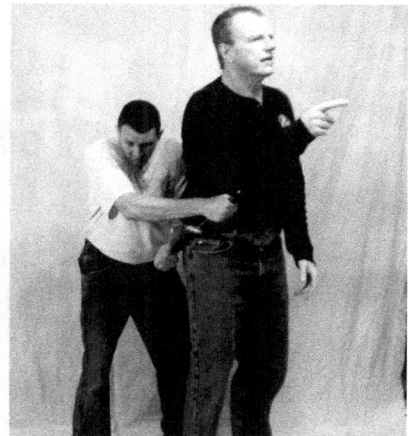

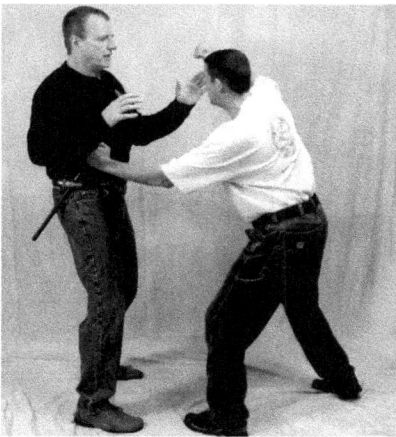

So, we hope you have a safe and retainable holstering system for your impact weapon. The most common counter to a belt-line attack, take-away is to get at least one hand on your stick in a "death-grip," keeping it in place, on your belt line. Using two hands on your stick opens you up to his fisticuffs, forearm strikes and elbows. You need to strike him with yours, so you need not grab your stick with two hands. Keep one free to fight.

Also it is advisable to use your body (and footwork) to dynamically move in the best direction to get a release while you are striking him in the face and neck. More on this later.

Getting your stick grabbed when it is out, has another set of options we'll explore that includes the "In the Clutches Of" drill series. Don't forget the strike the attacker as a priority solution. Strikes and kicks are defined in the *Force Necessary: Hand* progression.

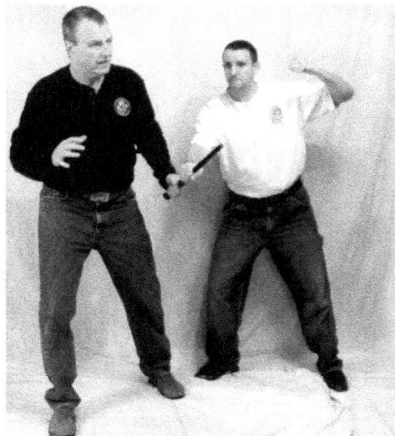

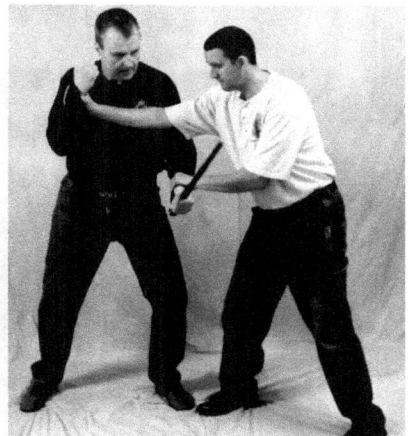

Stop 2 Basic Retention Problem Solutions, "Protecting the Belt."
Various police and military agencies around the world do not carry handguns and have expandable batons on their "stong side" instead. Here is a "protecting the belt" collapsed baton movement. Switch sides.Our first level of protection is keeping the impact weapon in its common carry site. The belt. And then keeping the stick safe in the first stages of common belt draws.

* The opponent grabs at your impact weapon while it is on your carry site:

       Sample Solution 1: Grab his grab to secure your weapon and strike his face and throat repeatedly until he desists.

       Sample Solution 2: Grab his grab and stomp and kick his feet and legs. Execute a powerful body twist in the best direction to free him from your weapon.

       Sample Solution 3a: Protecting the closed or "collapsed' expandable baton.The opponent sees your hand drop to another very common carry site on your body for a stick. Your hand grips your unexpanded baton. His hand lands atop your hand.

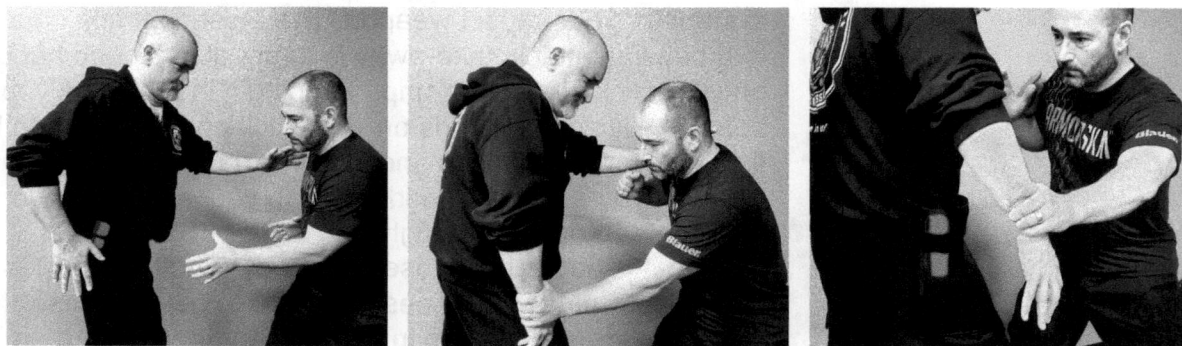

He sees you are dropping your hand to the closed baton on your belt. He grabs only your hand. You remove your hand from your weapon. The weapon is no longer involved! You must step back and away from the grip with the in-and-out footwork pattern of this level.

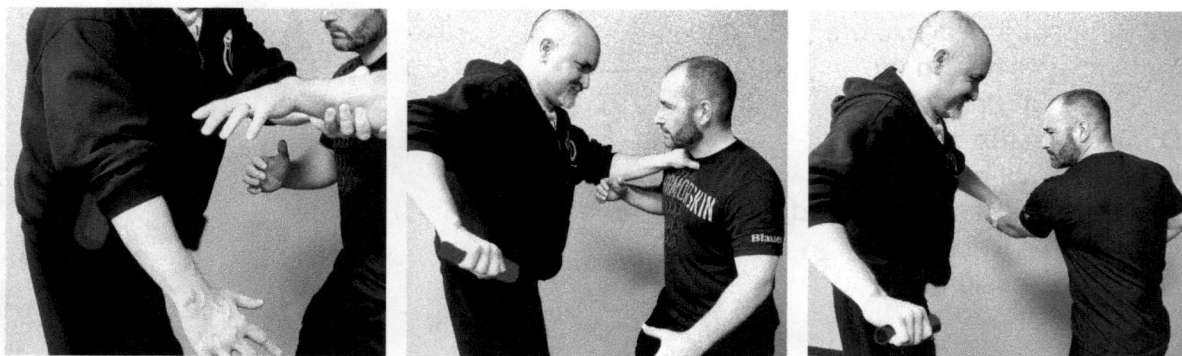

You push-pull, slap-release his grip on your hand, as you pull the baton. Draw if still needed. Or release his grip, but hang on as an option and arm drag to the side for a clearer path to draw.

Sample Solution 3b: Protecting the fixed baton/stick. This follows the same steps as with the previous, collapsed, closed expandable baton.

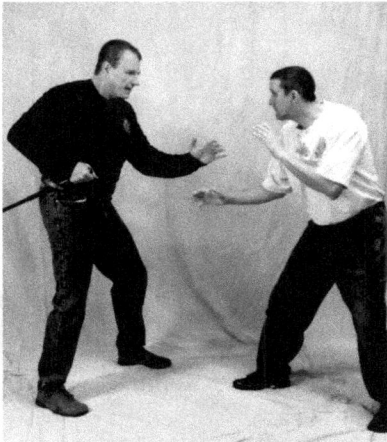

He sees the movement to a stick draw.

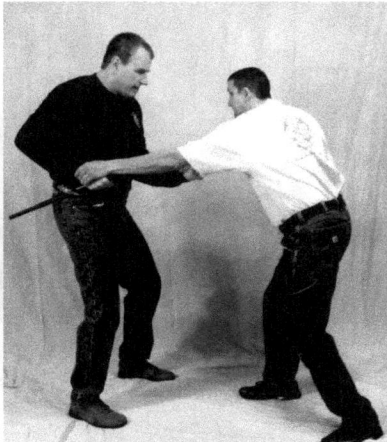

He tries to stop it. But only gets his hand on your hand.

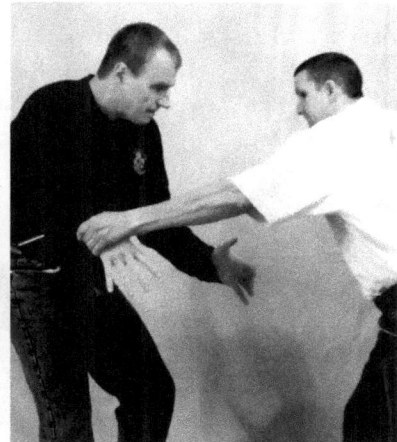

You let go of the stick, move your hand away and step back.

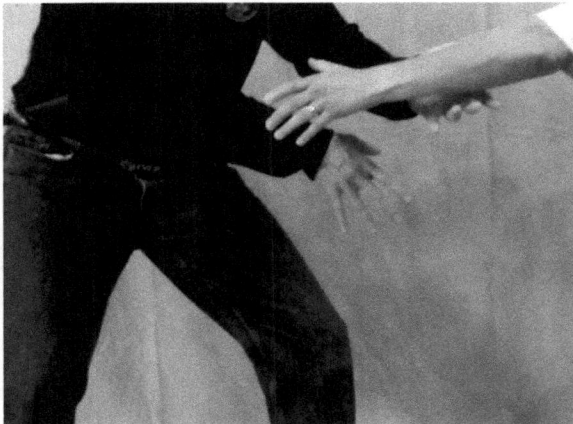

You slap release.

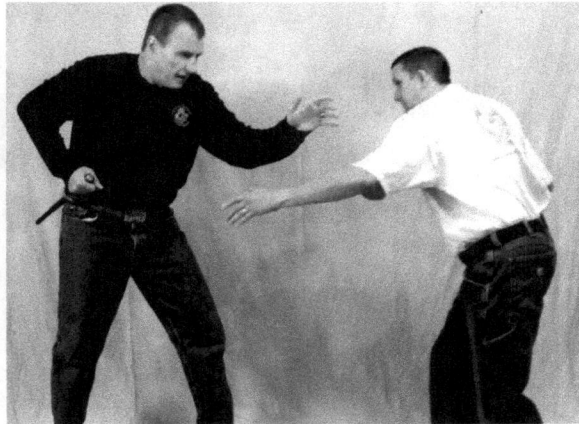

You regroup and decide to draw or not.

Sample Solution 4: The opponent grabs your arm as you begin to pull your weapon. Slap-push the grab off of you.

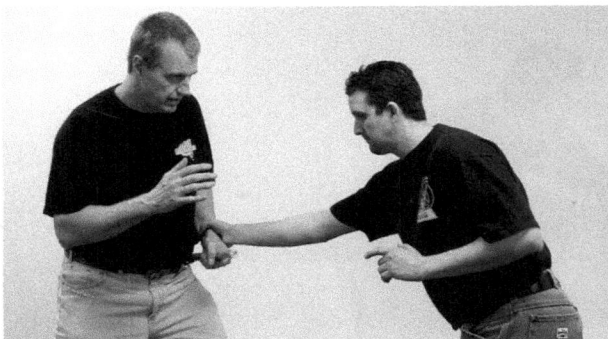

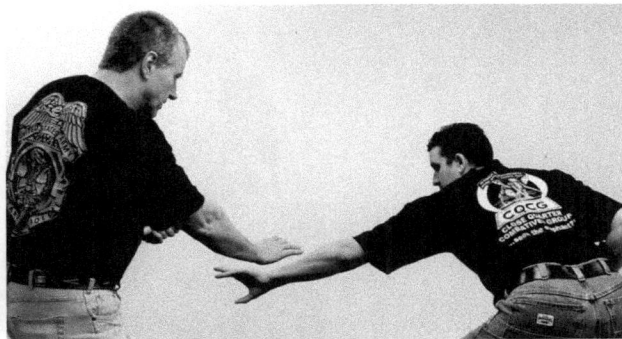

Discover the best direction for a release and slap-push release.

Sample Solution 5: If a sufficient amount of the handle is exposed, circular releases using the handle. Draw stick.

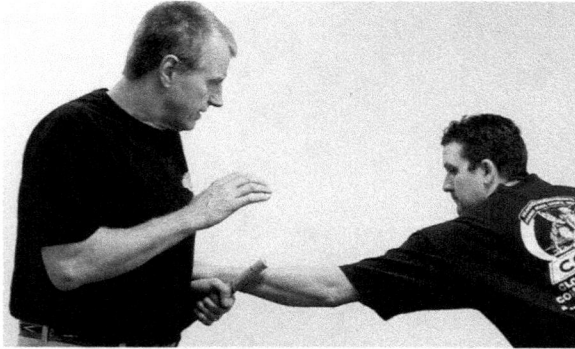

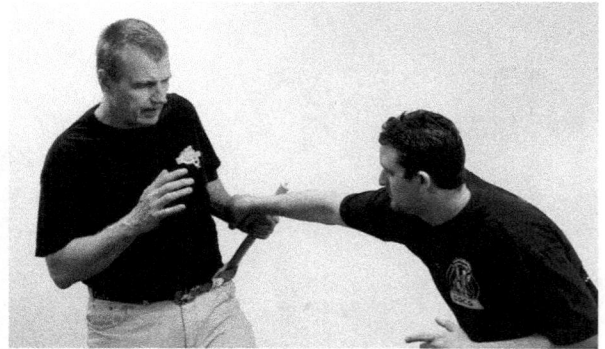

Use the exposed end of the stick to circle his wrist and push. Assist with a slap hand.

Sample Solution 6: A cross-over grab. Elbow roll over the hand grab. Draw stick.

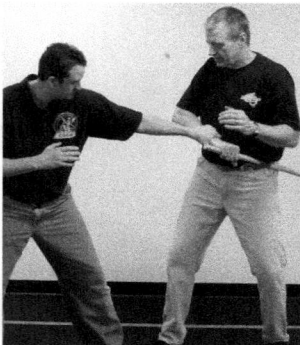

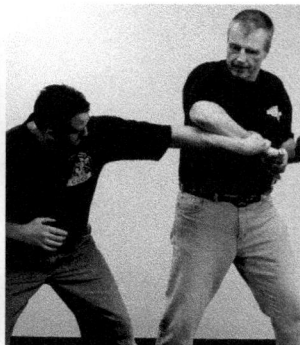

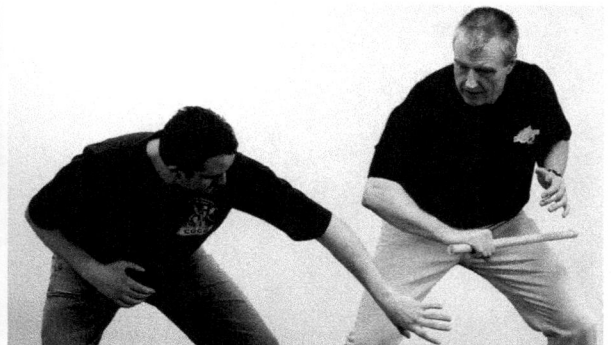

Elbow up. Elbow over his forearm, in as close to a center lock as possible. Elbow down.

Sample Solution 7: Powerful arm movements, torso twists combined with more slap-outs. These motions can also include the complete draw of the weapon.

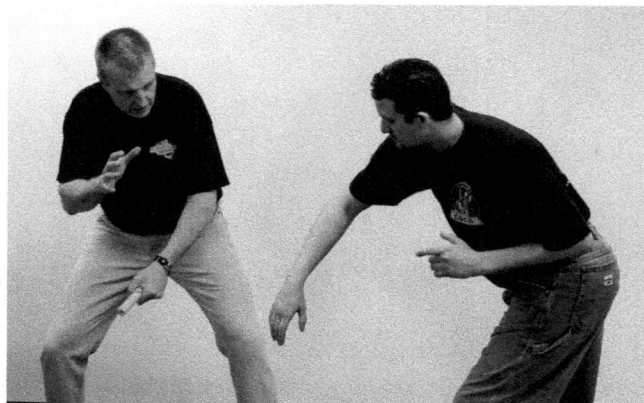

Basic retention problem solutions, "Protecting the drawn stick."
The stick is now fully out and subject to one-hand and two-hand grabs of the *Stop 2* realm. Arm-wraps on your stick and so forth are closer in and officially *Stop 4* problems, but in the interest of being topically comprehensive, we will cover them here in Level 2.

The opponent now grabs your produced stick:
- when it is drawn and presented.
- before or after you hit him?
- with one hand, right or left, or with two hands, in various configurations on the combat clock. Your stick may be horizontal or vertical or in between.
- your stick may be out and up, as in a classic police pose, or pointed down.
- your stick and arm may be in an inward-slash, ready position or a backhand ready position, or up and down positions.
- your weapon and weapon limb may also be grabbed during and after the stick attack.

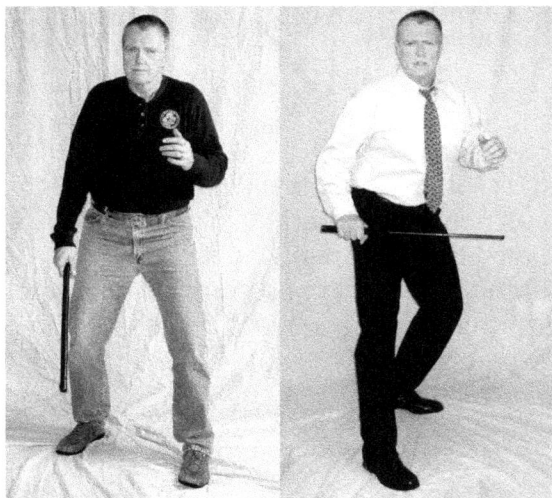

Stick out now, you will be attacked as you are in various ready positions.

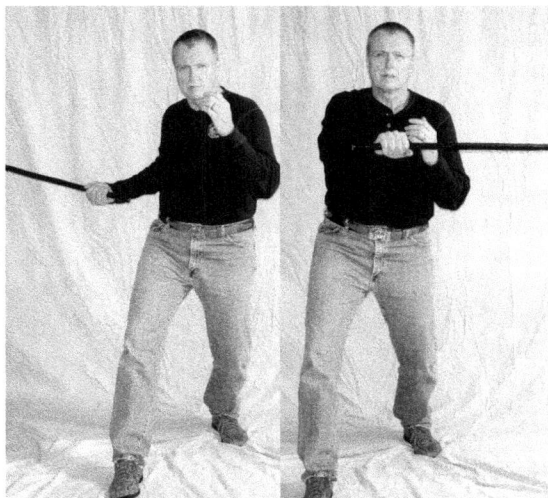

You will be attacked before, during and after your various weapon hooks and thrusts.

Sample Solution 1: The hand switch vs. a limb grab. Pass the baton with the same focus and intensity as if in an Olympic relay race.

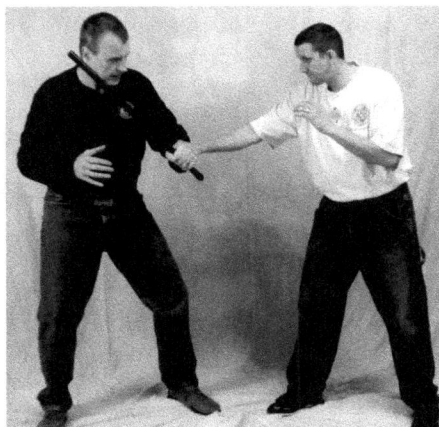

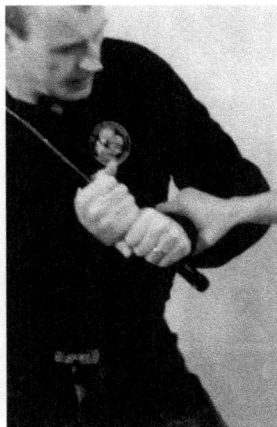

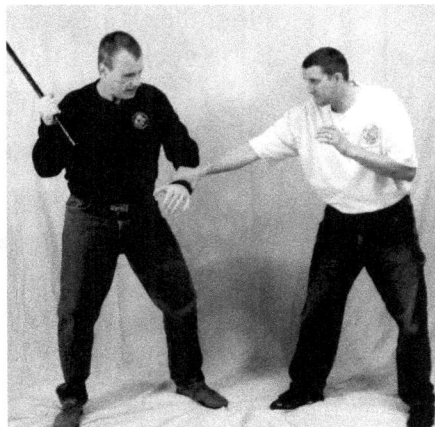

Sample Solution 2: A good grip

One mistake is to not hold your weapon properly. Solidly. This seems to be obvious, but there are some training systems that fail to emphasize this, or they do mention proper grips, yet slip into bad grips.

We dissected the various one and two hand grips for holding sticks in *Training Mission One*. Grip strength on the stick is important, especially when hitting. There is a naive, ignorant negligence when someone hits twice, real fast, with a small, wrist-based motion. The tendency is to open fingers, cheerleader, baton twirl the stick for the second shot. This will be powerless and probably one will lose their stick on the second impact.

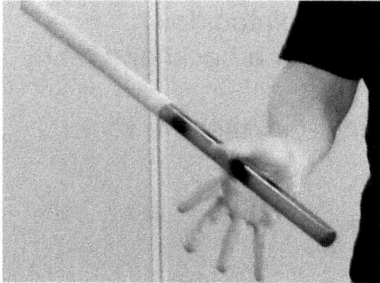

Do not "high school" cheerleader your baton for the second fast hit.

Can you imagine this lame, fingertip grip block actually stopping any attack?

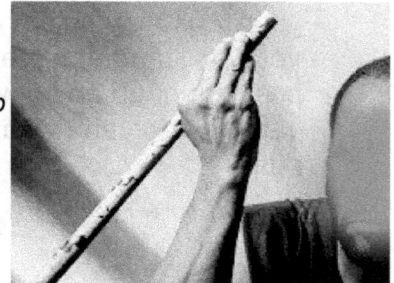

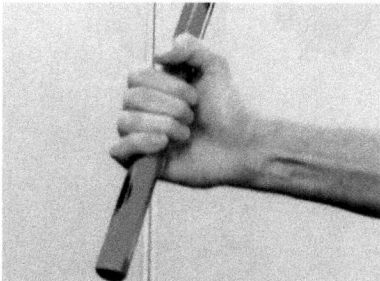

If you are going for this second, fast hit, keep as many fingers on the grip as possible. Smart, Filipino stick masters tell you to keep at least half your pinky hooked on your stick. You will never make the path of a complete, flat circle. It will be a cone. Experts are able to pull their elbows in a bit to make for a flatter cone and a faster second hit.

Keep part of the pinky engaged.

Sample Solution 3: Avoid the thumb up grip on the baton.

There is a naive, ignorant, negligence for people, especially security and law enforcement, to hold their batons in this manner. Without the thumb, ball of the thumb wrap, this grip is not maximized. Plus, as we see in the *Force Necessary: Hand* chapter, this thumb can be caught in a grip and locked in for a lot pain, and a loss of the stick. Look at the lower right. The man is even worse, with two fingers way off the stick, as though his three fingers could bend a fighting man over.

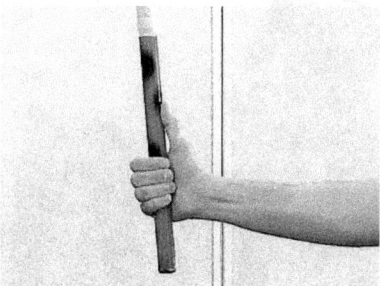

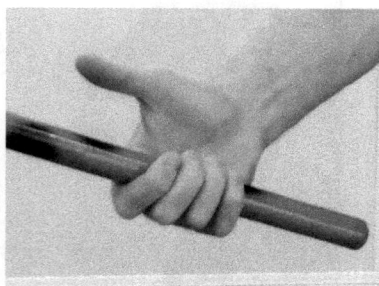

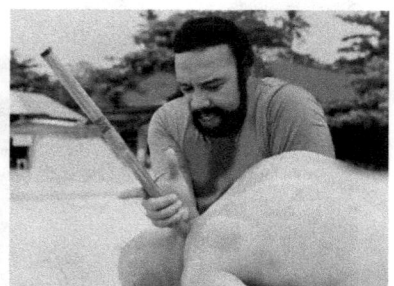

Thumb up on the stick.   *But this artsy thing is far worse.*   *More artsy, unreal crap.*

Sample Solution 4: The rowing motion. This is a pretty universal move against any middle-stick-area grab with single-hand, or a double-hand grab. The steps to remember for both are:

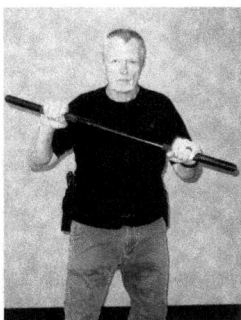

1: grab your stick with two hands, and pull. This may work? Maybe hit and/or low kick him.

2: with two hands, turn your stick to the right or the left, depending on his right or left-handed grab.

3: Go to the "outside" of his arms, so as to avoid being inside and punched easily.

4: Make your stick, virtually vertical.

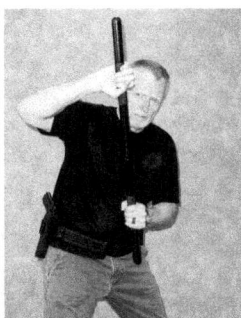

5: Outside of his grabbing arm, make a rowing circle to get a release. This puts him in a bit of a center lock.

6: Hit his forearm with your forearm. Hard.

7: If he gets the stick with 2 hands, do the same as above. And maybe hit or kick him in the shin but:

* you may crash his upper arm into his lower arm with lots of force and an accompanying "body drop," or-

* you may have to "double unlock" this, by rowing one arm and then the other. Two rows!

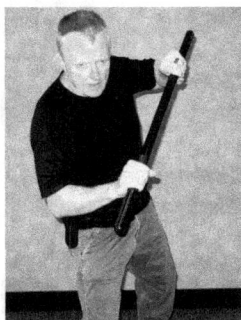

8: If you are caught "inside" his arms, you can still make a rowing motion to the outside. It will take a longer row, and you will be subject to an easy strike from the opponent. You will also lose the center wrist lock advantage. Outside the arms is better.

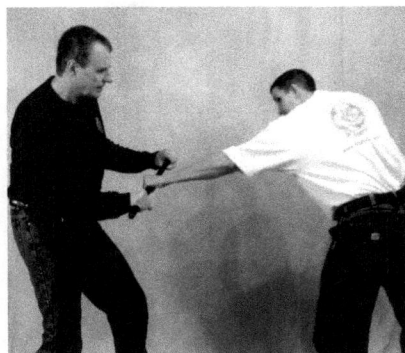

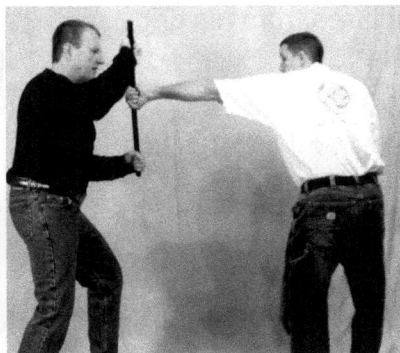

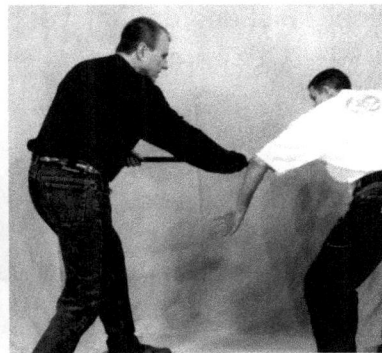

He grabs. You grab your stick with your free hand. Get it vertical. Row and smash forward.

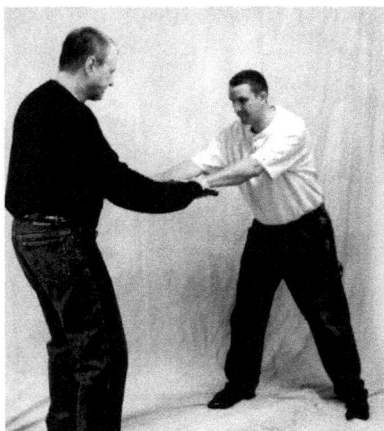

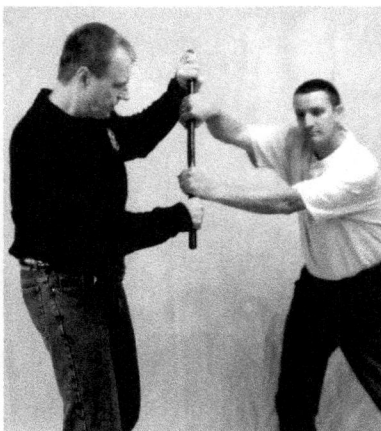

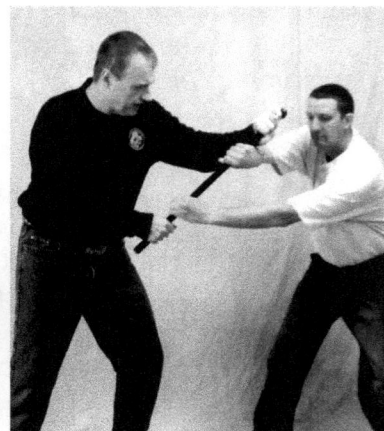

He gets a two-hand grab. You strike him and/or low kick him. You also get a two-hand grab.
Turn that stick as vertical as possible and slam down in a rowing motion. Try to hit both his forearms.

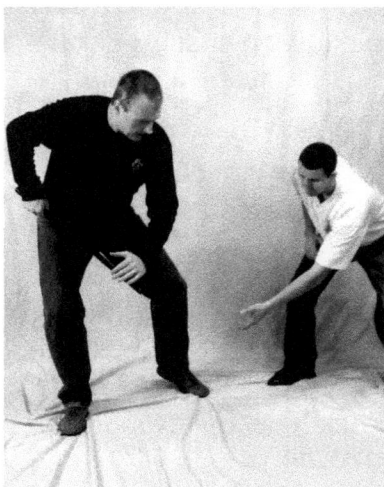

Power through both arms.

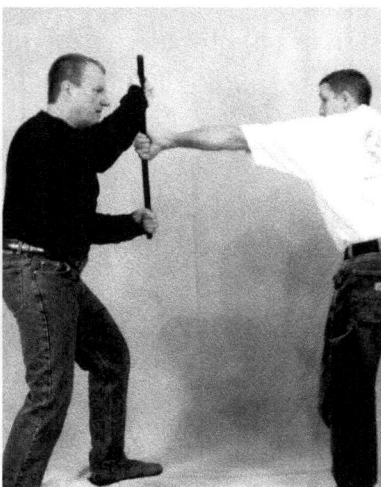

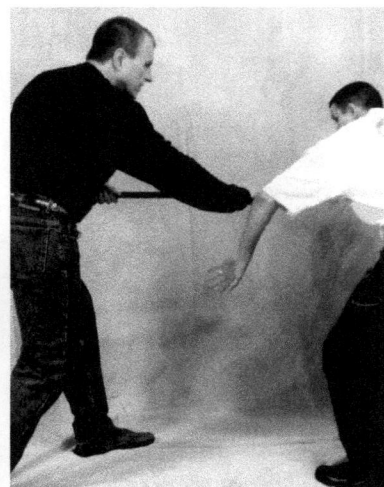

If you can't power through both forearms, you've at least got the top one. Switch sides quickly and make the second, rowing circle for a "double unlocking."

You can row forward or backward, but it seems the forward row is more successful. Will he grab your long flashlight or short stick? Use the same rowing concepts. Two handed grip. Try to get his wrist in an awkward position. Twist and/or yank your tool free from his grip.

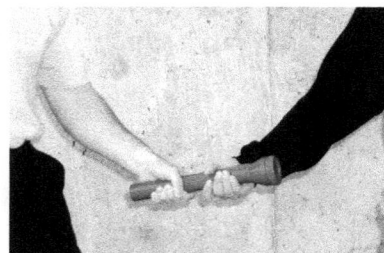

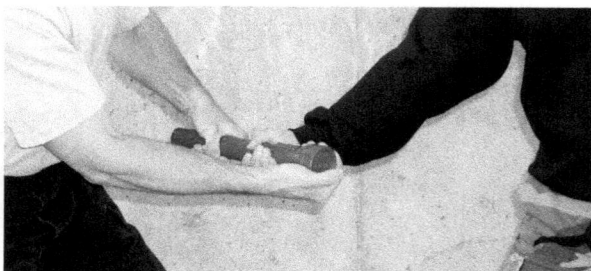

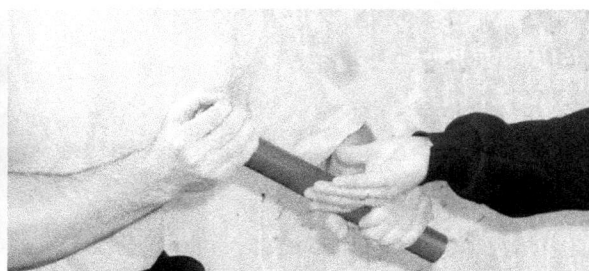

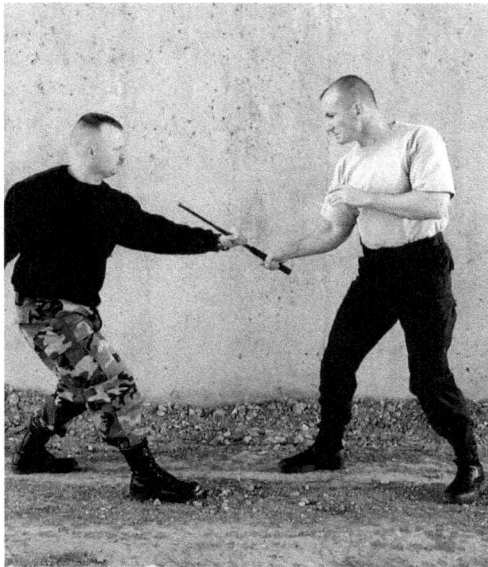

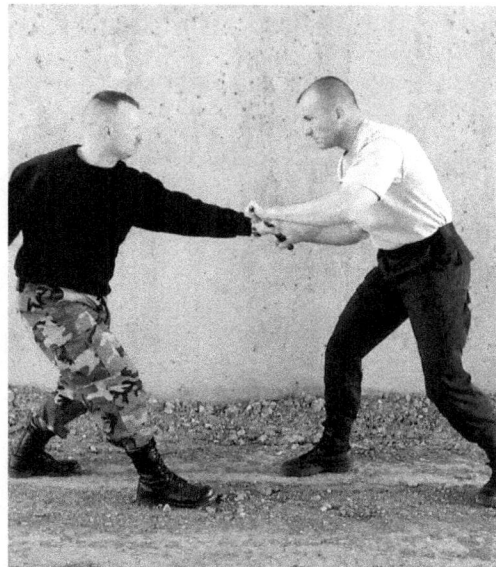

He's grabbed Mike Gillette's baton! Gillette gets a two-handed grip and pulls...

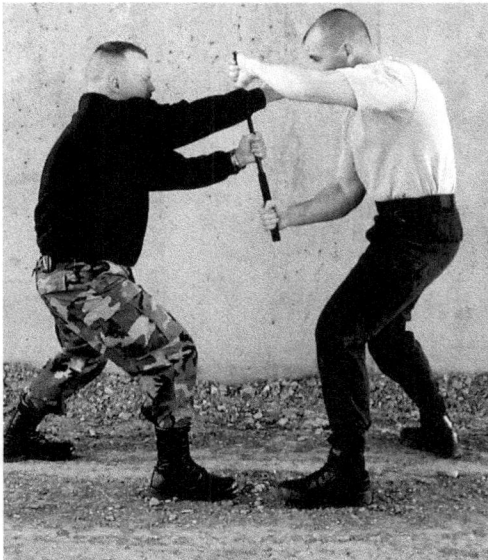

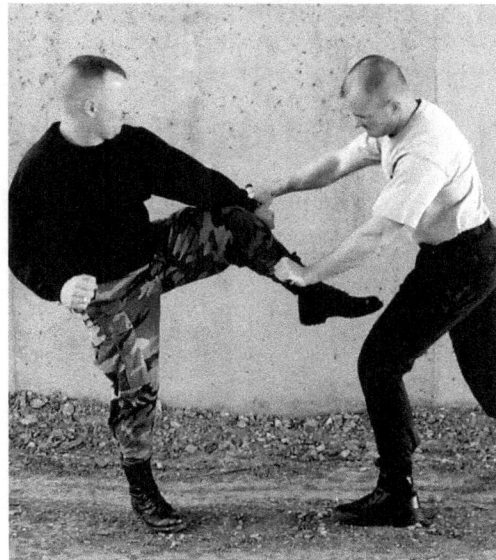

...it does not come free. He punches. Gillette blocks. He kicks. Gillette blocks.

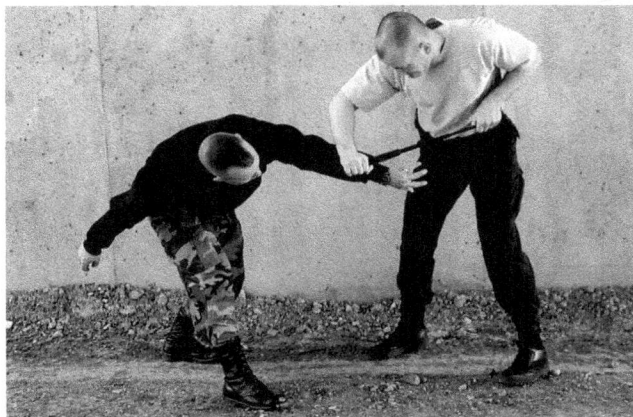

Gillette executes the "stick roll-over/row-over" move for the release.

Sample Solution 5: He grabs the end of your stick (or long gun) with one or two hands.
1: you grab your stick with two hands.
2: you make a tight circle around his hand or hands, causing locking situation. Then drive the weapon down in the best line.

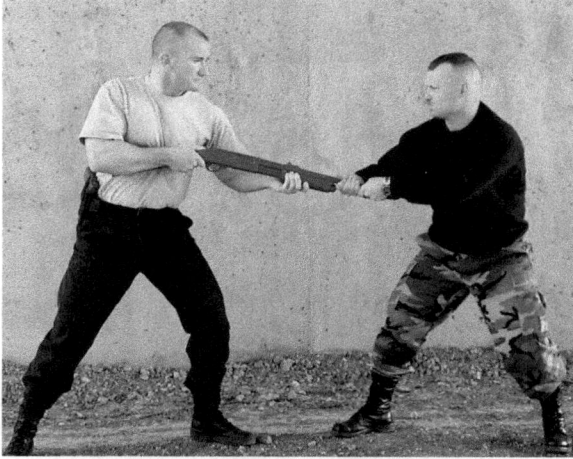
He grabs, and you don't want to shoot.

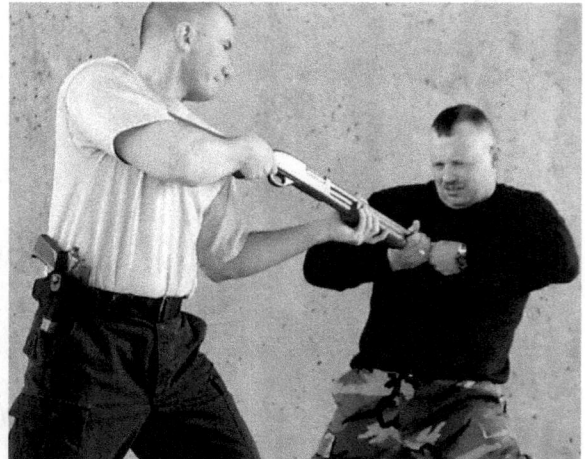
One solution - ram barrel into his chest.

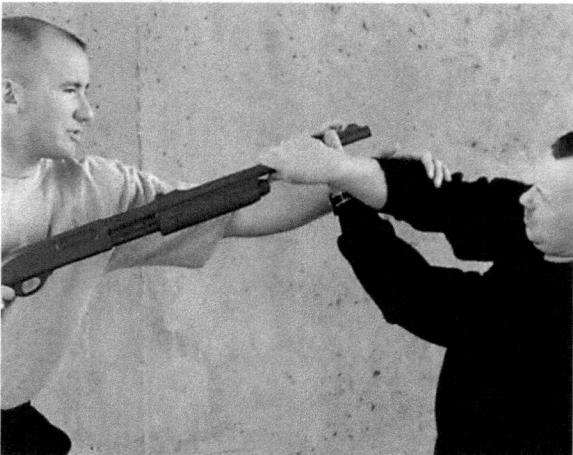
One solution - try to slap release the grab.

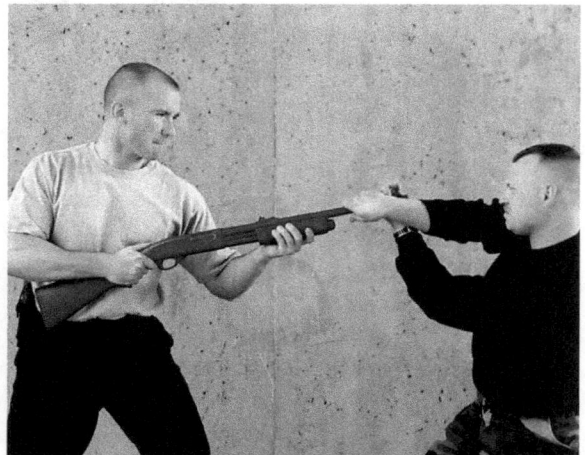
Popular solution, a circular release.

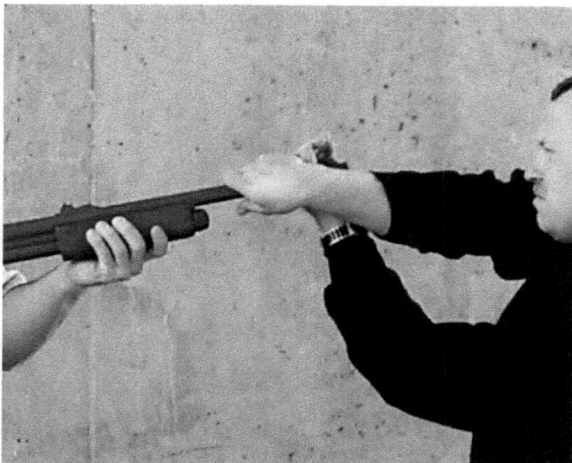
Clockwise or counter-clockwise.

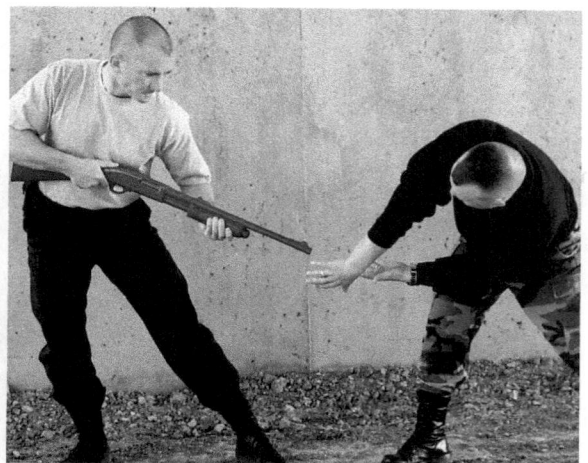
Get wrists in weak position, and push downward.

Sample Solution 6: Lose your stick? Take it back immediately. Then it seems the roles are reversed. It's you grabbing a stick now. And the beat goes on... (It's called "weapon recovery.")

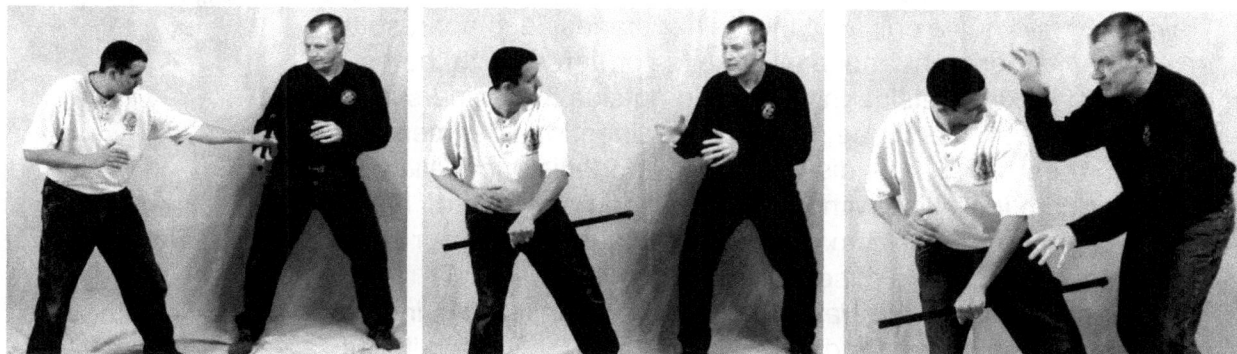

In the Clutches Of - Stick

This module of events fit perfectly into the *Stop 2* problem area. The various and common *Stop 2 Clutches Of Stick* positions are:

    1: Any configuration on the top-side, 3 to 9 o'clock, upper high-half of the clock.
    2: Any configuration on the bottom-side, 3 to 9 o'clock, lower-half of the clock.
    3: Mixed grips as in hands both high & low.
    4: Mixed grips as in left-hand versus right-hand, cross-grabs.
    5: The "accordion." Given the in-and-out motion of a fight, sometimes chests "bump."
    6: Your stick versus his unarmed, versus his stick, versus his knife, versus his pistol.

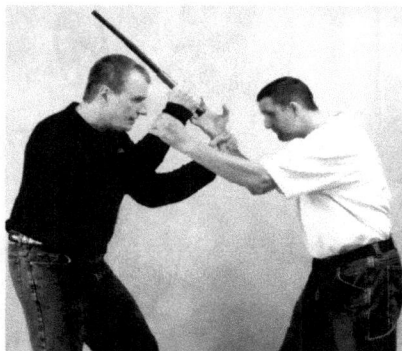

High end clutches.

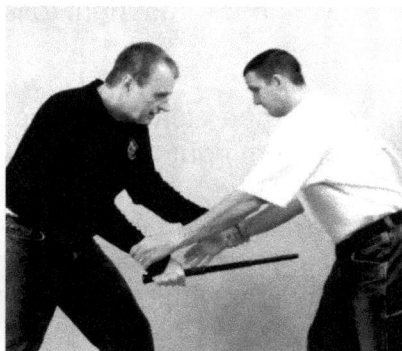

Low end clutches.

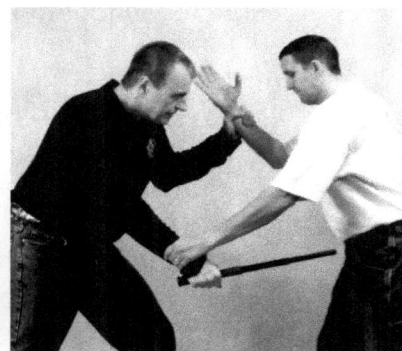

Mixed high and low.

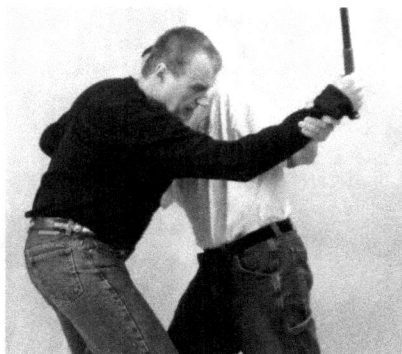

The accordion.

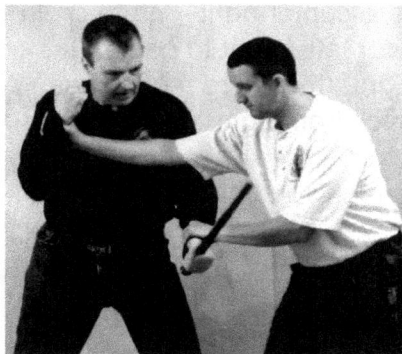

Righty versus lefty.

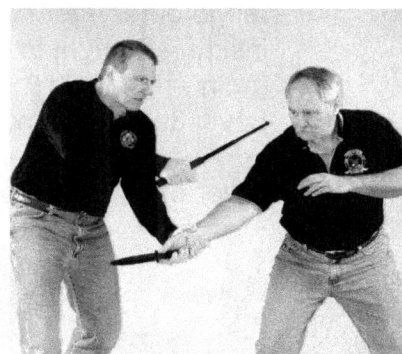

Stick versus unarmed and "other."

The In the Clutches Of, Stick! Statue Kick Drill
You can get caught in the "Clutches Of" situations, usually mixed weapon or high grips, you might get a quick kick in. To introduce this, to practice this, we use the statue drill as explained in *Stop 1 Training Mission One* drill, and the trainer stands, legs apart so the trainee can experiment and familiarize his or herself with the progression of kicking outside-inside-inside-outside the trainers legs. The trainer, being the statue, allows the trainee to experiment.

The nature of the arms distance, the *Stop 2* distance, allows for some freedom in kicking without being pushed or pulled off balance, as one might be with an arm wrap or bear hugs. Using your arms like the "accordion," can offset a push or a pull.

The *Force Necessary: Hand* course covers these kicks in its progression. Look there for detailed instruction if you need it. But here, do your best, as none of these kicks are "rocket science."

This statue drill kicking exercise emphasizes the:

* Frontal snap kick with shoes and/or shin.
    - left kick to shin - left to groin - right to groin - right to shin.

Next work back from right to left.

* Stomp kick.
    - left to right foot top - right to left foot top - left to left foot
    - right to left foot top. Next work back from right to left.

* Thrust kick.
    - left to right knee - right to left knee - left to left knee - right to left knee. Next work back from right to left.

* Low round kick.
    - left to right leg - right to left leg - left to left leg - right to left leg. Next work back from right to left.

* Knees (and there are many options.)
    - left to outer right - left to center right - left to groin - left to inside left - right to outer left - right to center left - right to groin - right to inner right. (there are more - see *FN: Hand* Level 3. Next, work back from right to left.

* Whatever other kicks you think you can get in.

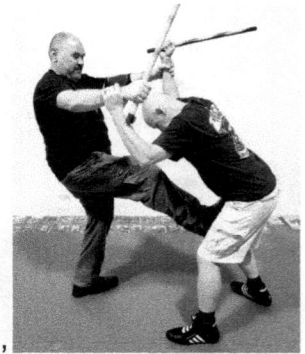
Frontal snaps.

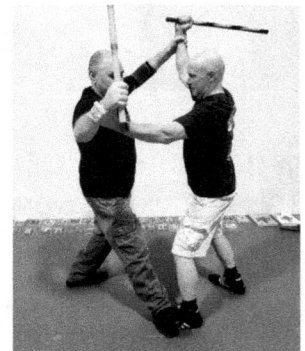
Stomps.

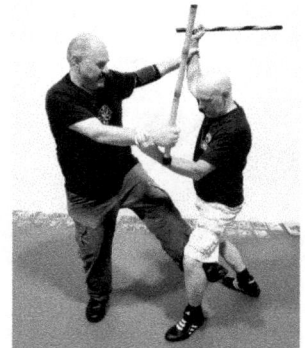
Low round kicks.

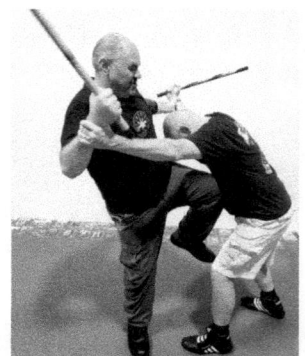
Knees.

Quick strikes examples once caught in the "stick clutches"

Depending upon his weapon, when caught in the clutches, you should use your stick immediately. Here are some options. Remember full on, combat scenarios with stick take-downs will be officially displayed in Training Missions levels 7, 8 and 9. Despite this official progression, I encourage schools, classes and seminar practitioners to work on stick take-downs at any time.

These quick hits will have to come from the variety of realistic catches that occur like high, low, mixed, right versus left, etc. What is the position of your caught hand? Can you really move his grab up and down? What is the length of your impact weapon? How much power can you generate from a grabbed strike?

Possible targets are:
- the head. This from a high grab position, or perhaps a low grab too, if reachable?
- the knees. This from a low grab position.
- the other caught limb as a possible impact disarm.
- maybe the stomach/torso? Depends.
- maybe the groin? This perhaps from a low grab position.

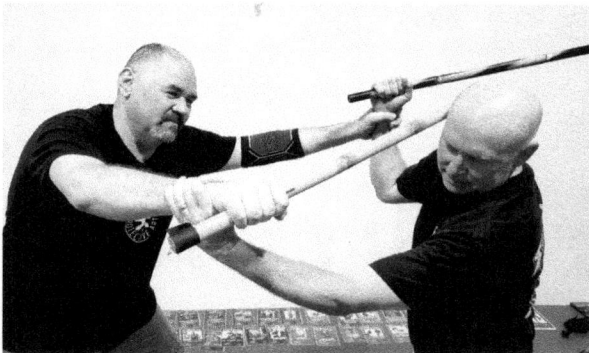

Quick fanning strike to the head.

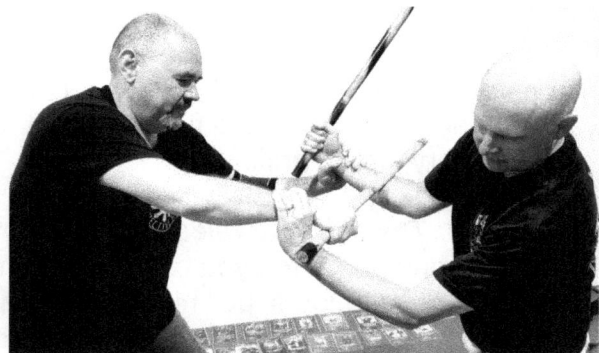

Quick Fanning strikes to his weapon-bearing limb.

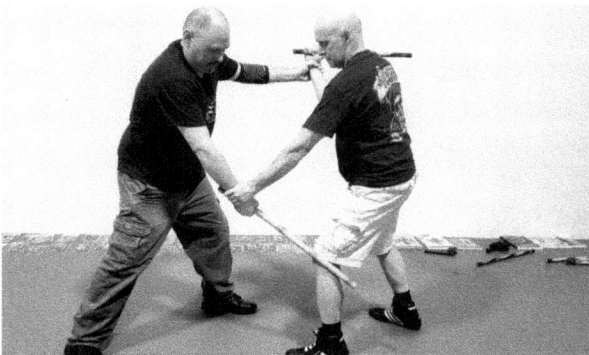

Low clutch catch? Quick strikes to his knee.

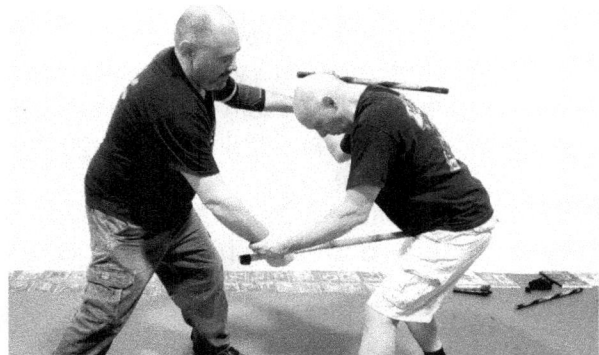

Low clutch catch? Quick strikes to the groin? Wherever...

A study of the major releases via the "stick clutches" format
Your stick limb/hand gets grabbed. High or low. These work versus one hand only grabs too and usually in Stop 2 to 6 also. This book only covers *Stop 2*, but you will be asked to review this releasing foundation as the *Stop 6* and *Training Mission* books continue.

Sample 1: The yank-out. Like a hit and retract, use your arm and whole body if need be to get out of this *Stop 2* grab. Same on the low end.

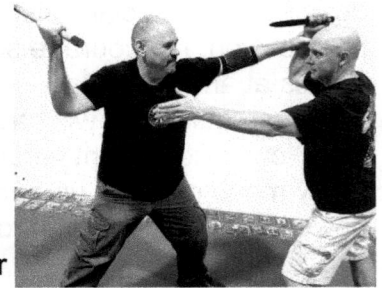
Yank-out release.

Sample 2: The circular release and the joint lock position releases. Rotating your stick hand clockwise or counter, clock wise can often get a release. It will depend on the grip, high or low. Sometimes a quarter-circle or a half-circle will allow you to use a quicker, joint lock release. At times, a second after the release, you can push the hand away with your saber or reverse grip, freeing a better path to your next attack, else the opponent will simply re-grab your limb. Look for this push-out opportunity in your practice.

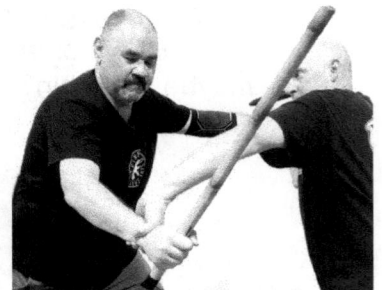
Circular releases.

Sample 3: The elbow rollover. This is really a joint lock release also, but it serves an honorable mention for its easy success. If you can, it's a) elbow up. b) elbow over his forearm. c) elbow down like a flapping motion. You can accompany that downward flap with a bit of a body drop against very strong grips.

Sample 4: The shoulder release. If you can't get a release from a strong grip? And you can judge from prior practice versus various heights, pull his gripping hand out from his body and get your upper torso under his arm, a bit sideways. Hammer your caught hand down as you stand up like a squat. This should get a release. Take care not to get caught in a head lock, by going a bit deeper in and a bit sideways.

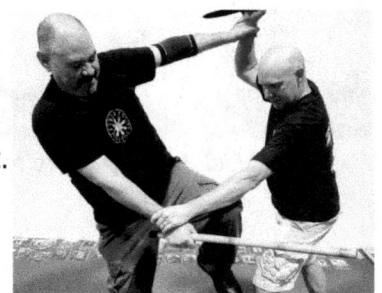
The knee release.

Sample 5: A knee release. On the low side of the clock, if you can't get a release, and you can judge from prior practice versus various heights, lift and drive you knee against his grabbing forearm, and pull your caught limb back and out.

Sample 6: A bite release. If you can't get a release, you can try stepping in and biting his arm, if his clothing makes this available.

Sample 7: Arm rams. Any cross arm catch, or when in a righty versus lefty jam-up, you could try to ram his arm up or down to get a release.

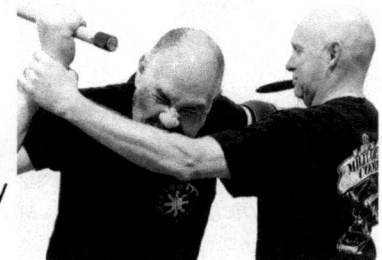
The bite release.

At the end of each of these sample events, the trainee should make some attempt to "finish the fight." with stick work and a takedown. But, this is only Level 2 and not the official time to mandate various, combat scenarios. Still, it is good classroom and seminar activity to get to work on these subjects.

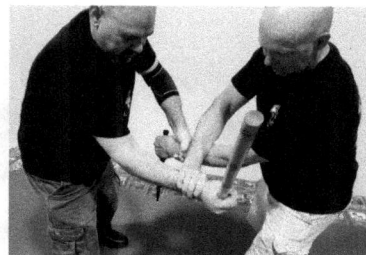

The arm ram release for righty versus lefty.

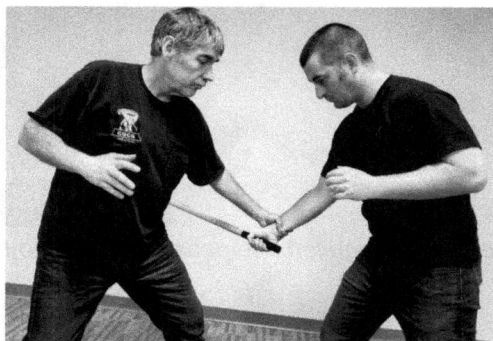

The 4 Corners Hand Switch exercise-drill - when releases fail
Using the hand switch method, work this drill in a four corner pattern. Trainee is armed with a stick (or a knife - see the knife chapter). He grabs your weapon limb with his free hand. The passed-off, freed stick should probably attack the weapon limb if armed, or head. I like to suggest that a weapon, hand switch may be done too, with the intensity of a relay race, baton hand-off at the Olympics.

Unarmed trainer grabs your right-handed, stick limb with his one hand:
> Event 1: Trainee is grabbed on his high right. He passes off stick to the left. Attack.
> Event 2: Trainee is grabbed on his high left. He passes off stick to the right. Attack.
> Event 3: Trainee is grabbed on his low right. He passes off stick to the left. Attack.
> Event 4: Trainee is grabbed on his low left. He passes off stick to the right. Attack.
> Next, switch to a left-handed stick grip and work these 4 events.
> Next, the trainer grabs and punches. Trainee blocks and hand switches.
> Next, the trainer grabs and stick attacks. The trainee blocks and hand switches.
> Next, the trainer grabs and knife attacks. The trainee blocks and hand switches.

Unarmed trainer grabs your right-handed, stick limb with his two hands:
> Event 5: Grabbed on the high right. Trainee passes off stick to left hand, and strikes.
> Event 6: Grabbed on the high left. Trainee passes off stick to right hand, and strikes.
> Event 7: Grabbed on the low right. Trainee passes off stick to left hand, and strikes.
> Event 8: Grabbed on the high left. Trainee passes off stick to right hand, and strikes.

At the end of each of these sample events, the trainee should make some attempt to "finish the fight." with stick work and a takedown. But, this is only Level 2 and not the official time to mandate various, combat scenarios. Still, it is good classroom and seminar activity to get to work on these subjects.

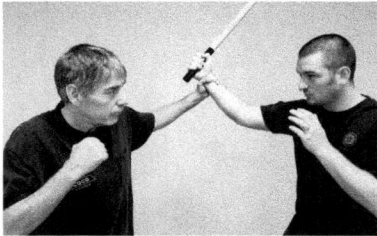

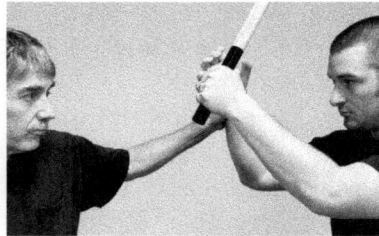

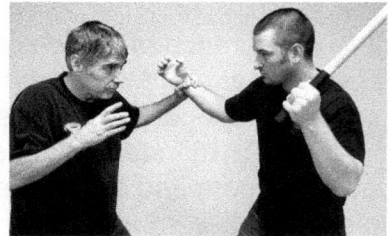

Switch event 1: Trainee is grabbed on his high right. He passes off stick to left hand and attacks.

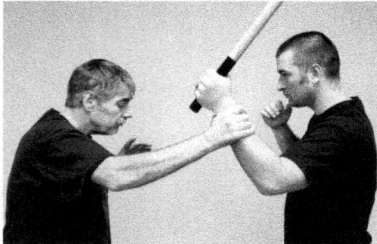

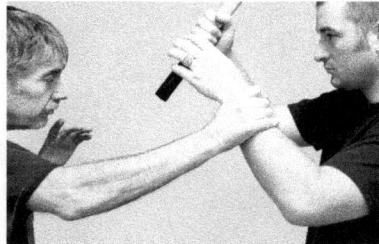

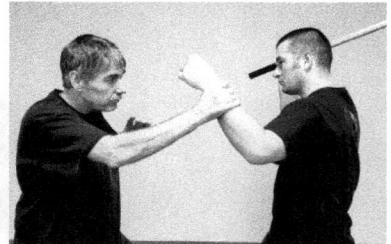

Switch event 2: Trainee is grabbed on his high left. He passes off stick to his right hand and attacks.

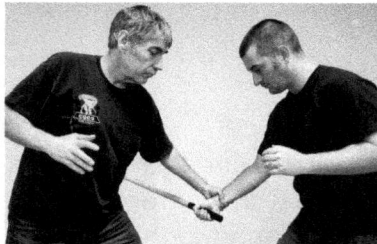

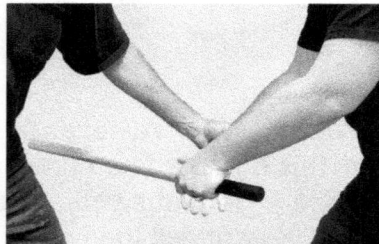

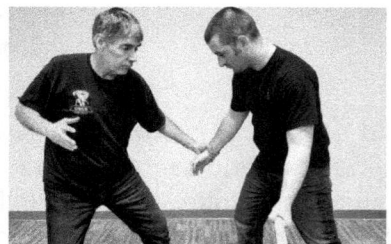

Switch event 3: Trainee is grabbed on his low right. He passes off stick to left hand and attacks.

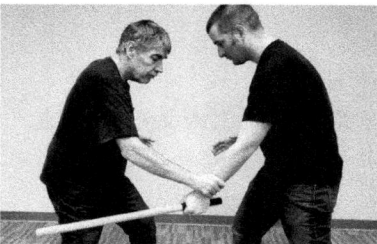

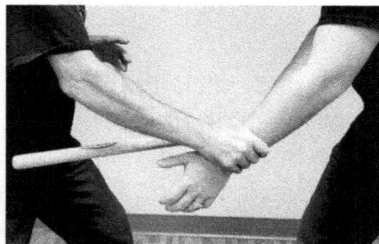

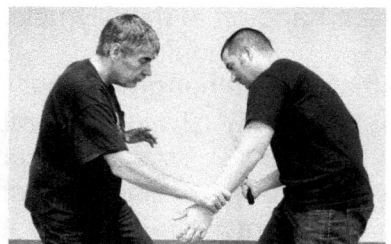

Switch event 4: Trainee is grabbed on his low left. He passes off stick to right hand and attacks.

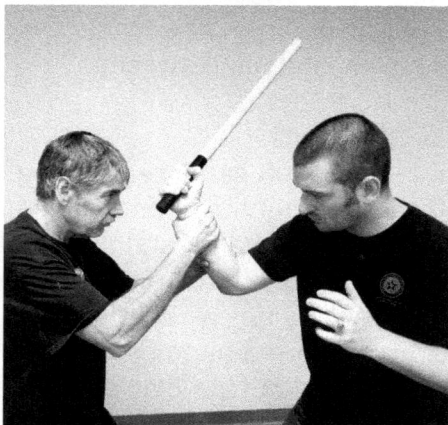

Work these same 4 corners versus a double hand grab.

This pass-off, hand switch must be done with the same fervor as a Olympic baton pass in a relay race. There are opportunities to do this successfully, but if you never do one once, it will not be in your "muscle memory." The pass off will be, like within all fighting, very situational.

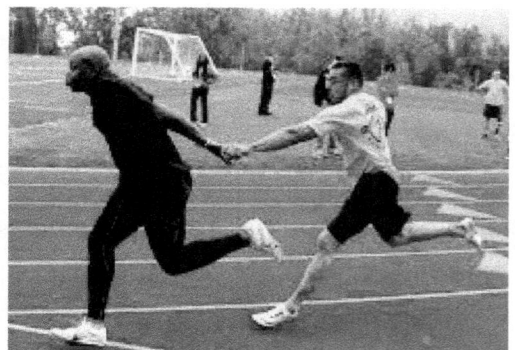

Can you block and hand switch your baton? Experiment with these situations and recognize the pros and cons, and the danger levels.

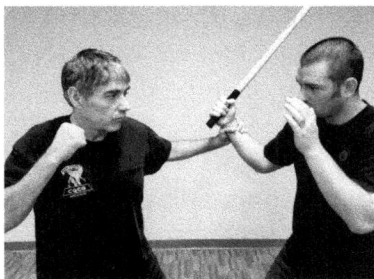

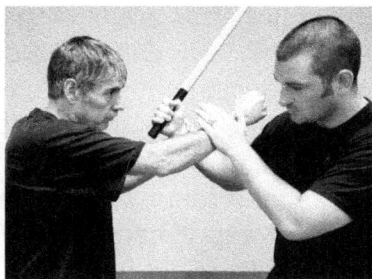

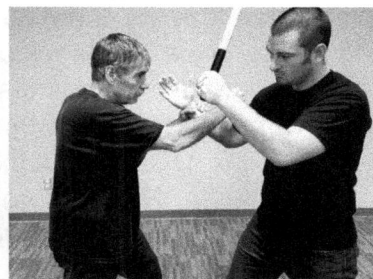

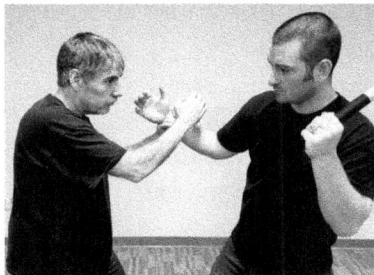

The suspect grabs your weapon limb and throws a punch at your face before you can attempt a releases. You block, and your block get very near your grabbed limb and stick. Try a hand switch.

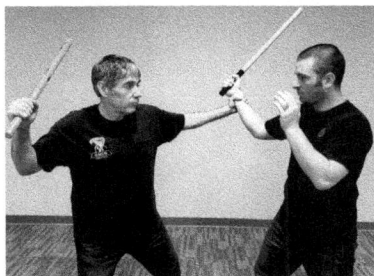

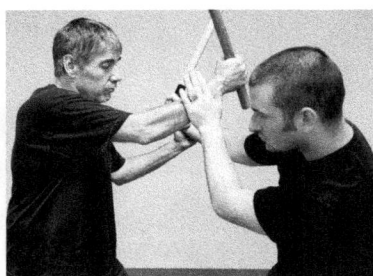

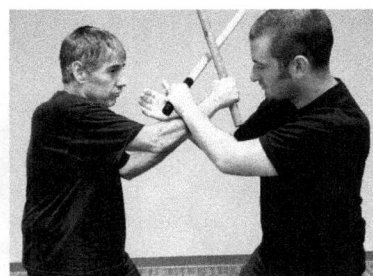

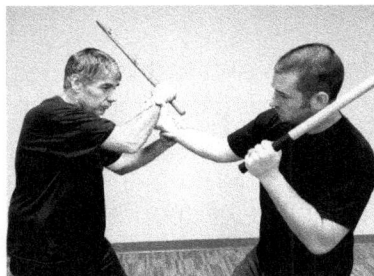

The suspect grabs your weapon limb and swings a stick at your head before you can attempt a releases. You block, and your block gets very near your grabbed limb and stick. Try a hand switch.

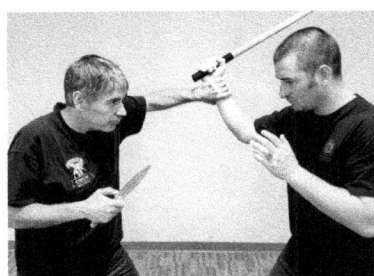

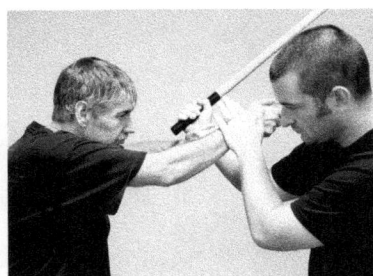

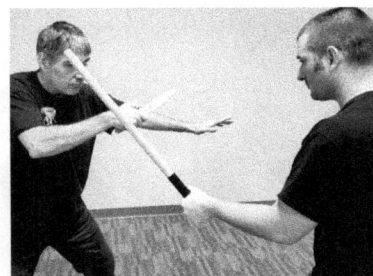

And lastly, the grab and knife attack. You block in desperation with no time to get a release, Should you try a hand switch? A quick withdrawal of his knife cuts your arm, but does he know to do that? Experiment with this.

Stress Stick Quick Draw Within the Tangler

He's rushed, your hands are "tied up" with each other. You see the need to draw your stick/baton from its carry site. But your hands are entangled. Now that we have covered the strikes while tangled, kicks while tangled, and the releases from tangles, we need to look at some of the particulars of enhancing your freedom to complete an impact weapon draw.Of note here, some 9 out of 10 people are right-handed.

Example 1: Just work the releases.

Now that you worked the releases, can you do them again and pull your stick? Where is your weapon carry site? Which hand is best to release?

An added step to this, might be this level's in and out footwork pattern. Can you move the carry site side (hip?) back for a more secure and safe draw? Then, can you twist the site away?

An collapsible, expandable baton needs a little time, space and momentum to open. Perhaps using it as a "palm stick," at first is smart. Palm stick, style strikes will be officially covered in later *Training Mission* books, but they are not rocket science and can be practiced now.

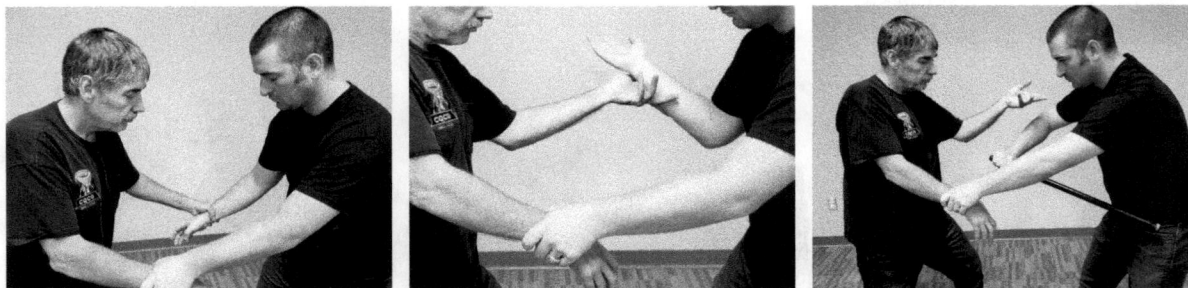

The trainer stalks, mad rushes in, stops at a tangle. Trainee releases and draws stick.

Example 2: The center lock delay

Working these for decades, teaching these for decades and watching thousands do them, I have learned that a handy distraction/delay is, when fingers entwined, the center lock, wristlock as shown in the unarmed chapter if this book. A twist of the hand and wrist and jar-lid-turning inward, has a stalling reaction. If done to his right hand or visible weapon-side hand, it confounds *his* quick draw.

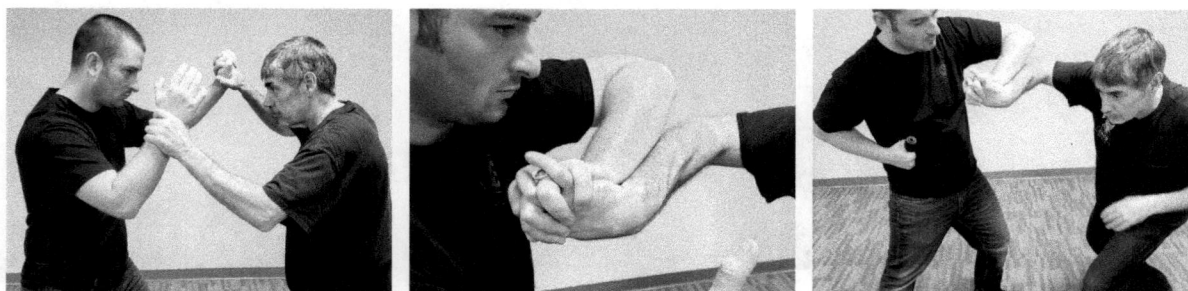

The trainer stalks, mad rushes in, and stops at a tangle. The non weapon hand is tangled by fingers.The center lock can distract, delay and puts the opponent in a poor position while the trainee get any release and draws a closed baton.

Example 3: Feeling for his draw - stick

When entangled you should be aware that he might draw a stick, a knife or a gun. Why is he suddenly letting go of your limb? Why is his hand dropping to a common weapon carry site? With that release, you may have to charge in and interrupt his weapon quick draw. This interruption can be done many grappling ways, such as a rear arm bar hammerlock. See the chapter in the first part of this book for details.

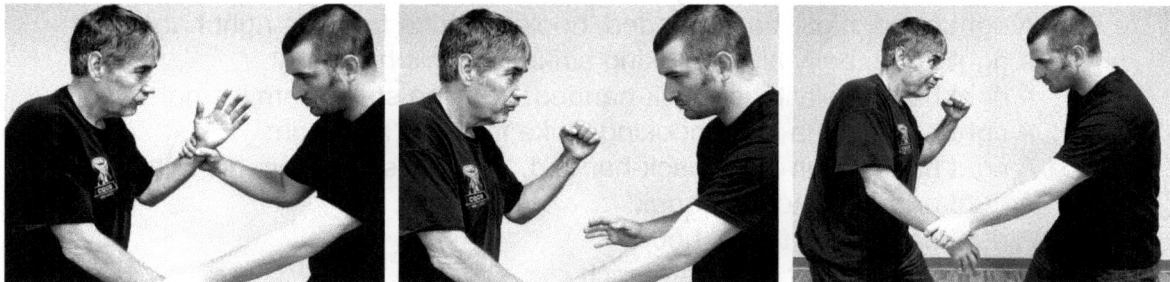

He's got you! He's letting go? His hand drops to a common weapon carry site. Hit him and carry on...

Example 4: He's drawing! Hitting the Pistol and or Knife Draw

Stop 2 is about also interfering with his weapon draws and this scenario falls into this category. If completely untangle yourself and you see a suspect reaching down to those carry sites we list in *Training Mission* books and films, you hit the hand going for the weapon.

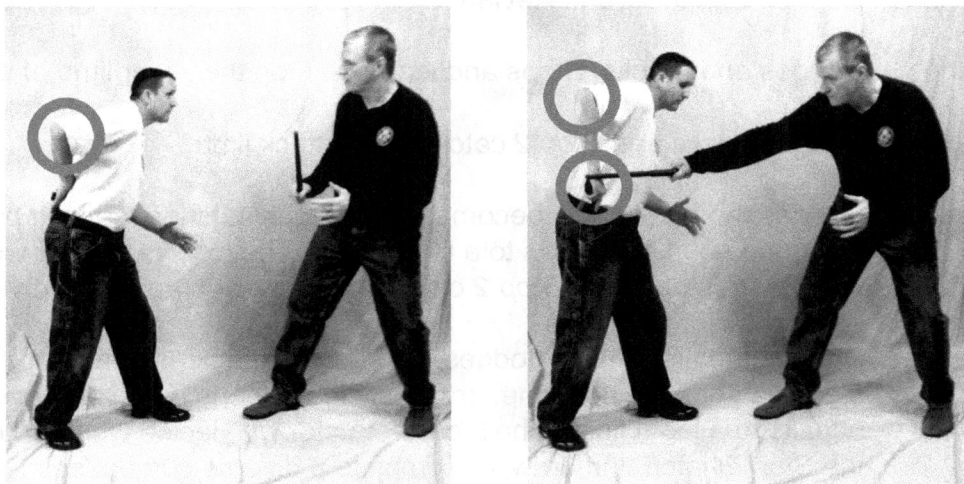

Shatter the elbow, or bash the hand.

The Stop 2 Ambush, Dodge, Evasion and Grab Stick Drill

As I warned in *Training Mission One*, you will see the Ambush Drill re-appear in various forms as the *Training Missions* continue. Here in *Stop 2* the trainee now grabs the arm attacks. Versus the leg shots, just dodge them with Level 2 "In and out" footwork. The weapon attack is a deadly force situation, causing a weapon response. A trainer stands before you. Close, but not too close. See the steps below. Review the Big 10 hand, stick or knife attacks:

    1: A right hand, high, hooking strike from his high right.
    2: A right hand, high, back-handed, hooking strike from his right hand.
    3: A right hand, belly high, hooking strike from his high right.
    4: A right hand, belly high, back-handed, hooking strike from his right hand.
    5: A right hand, thigh high, hooking strike from his high right.
    6: A right hand, thigh high, back-handed, hooking strike from his right hand.
    7: A right hand, low to high hook.
    8: A right hand, high to low hook.
    9: A right hand thrust to the stomach.
    10. A right hand thrust to the face.
    * Reset, and attack with the left hand.
    * Attack with hand, stick and knife.

Note and remember - each swing is an individual ambush attack. This represents 10 ambush attacks.

    The trainee

    Series 1: Dodges *without* footwork, just body elasticity. Review *Training Mission One*.

    Series 2: Dodges *with* footwork. Review *Training Mission One*.

    Series 3: Dodges and Blocks. Stops and learns to stop the lower limb of the attack.

    Series 4: Dodge, blocks and *Stop 2* catches the attack limb.

    Series 5: Dodges the first attack, becomes alert, stops/catches the next one. Draws knife and counter-attacks to a legal finish. The local instructor will decide whether to stop at the *Stop 2* catch and draw, or complete a diverse combat scenario.
    Dodges the first attack, dodges the second attack as one becomes alert, stops/catches the next one, draws stick, or opens baton and counter attacks to a legal finish. The local instructor will decide whether to stop at the *Stop 2* catch and draw, or complete a diverse combat scenario.

Note: This Ambush exercise might best be passed on to you with personal hands-on, instruction, as true, step-by step analysis, might take hundreds and hundreds of photos and a thousand words to document here. I hope what is presented here will inspire you and develops the skills of you and yours in *Stop 2* problems.

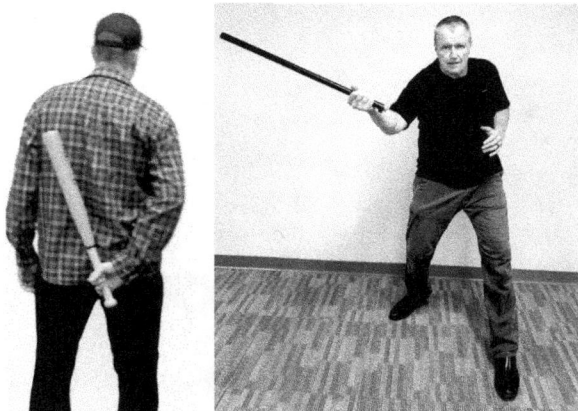

Ambush attack 1: Head shot from trainer's right. An inward strike.

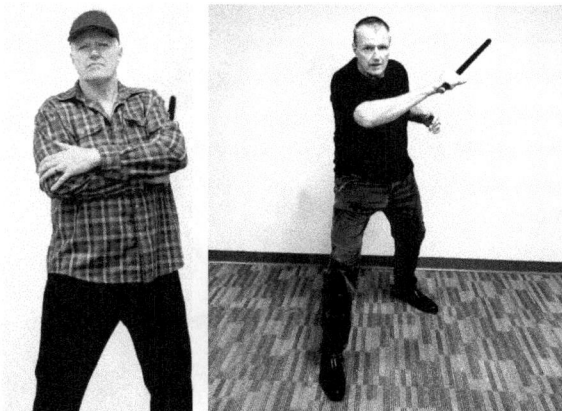

Ambush attack 2: Head shot from trainer's left. A backhand strike.

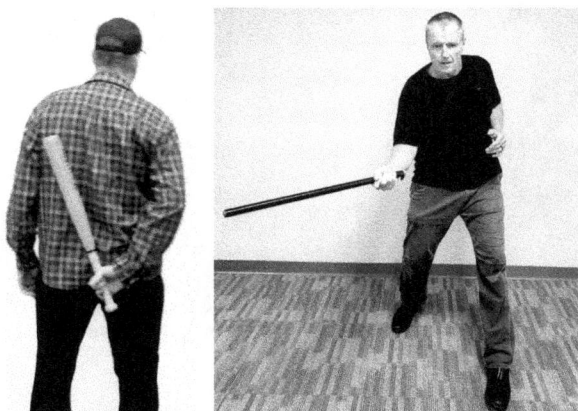

Ambush attack 3: Belly shot from trainer's right. An inward strike.

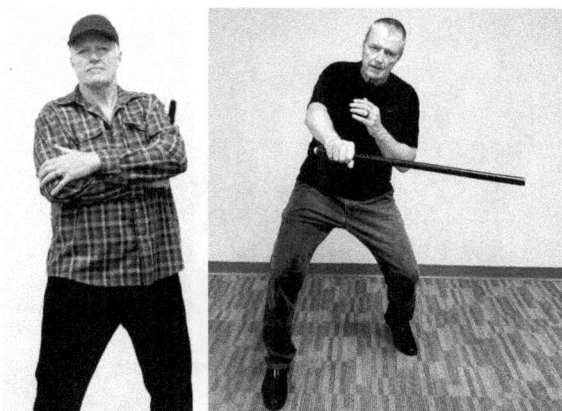

Ambush attack 4: Belly shot from trainer's left. A backhand strike.

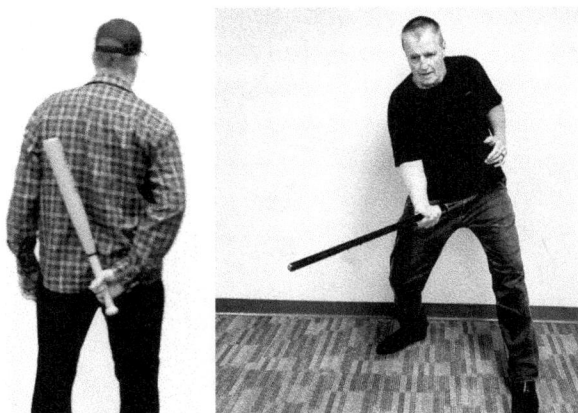

Ambush attack 5: Knee shot from trainer's right. An inward strike.

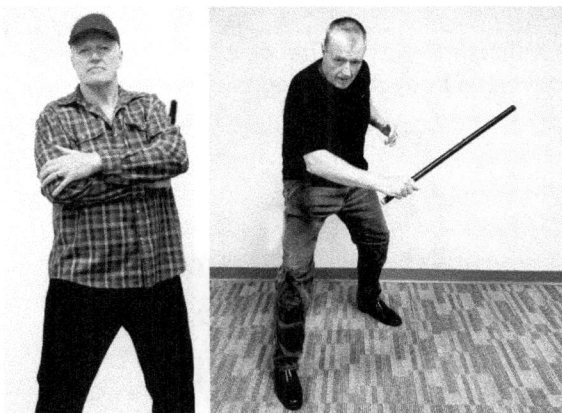

Ambush attack 6: Knee shot from trainer's left. A backhand strike.

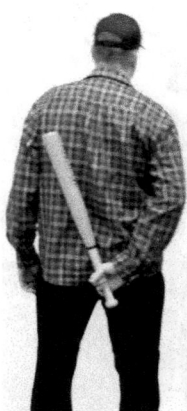

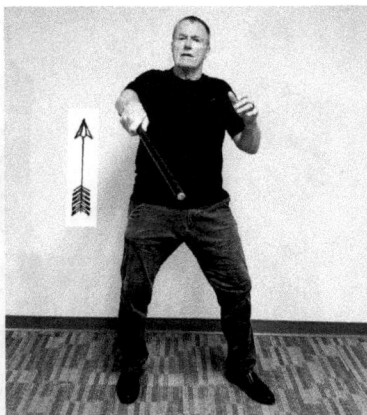

Ambush attack 7: Shot from trainer's low. Groin target? An upward strike.

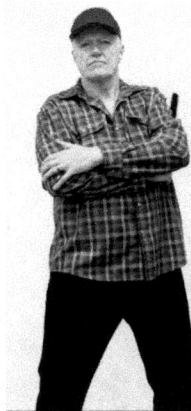

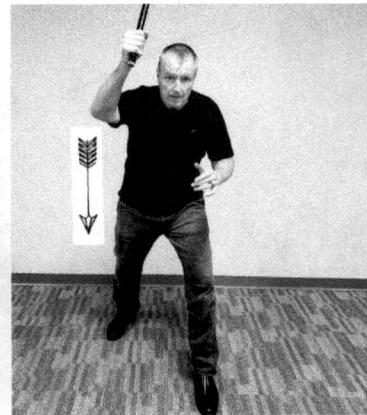

Ambush attack 8: Head or clavicle shot from trainer's high. A downward strike.

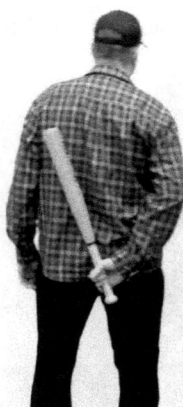

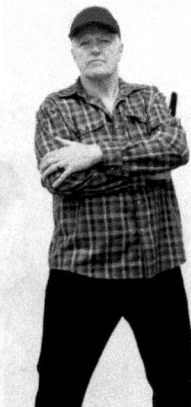

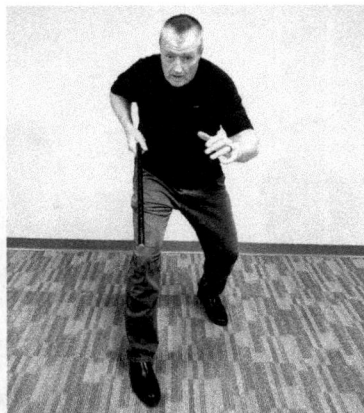

Ambush attack 9: Belly stab.

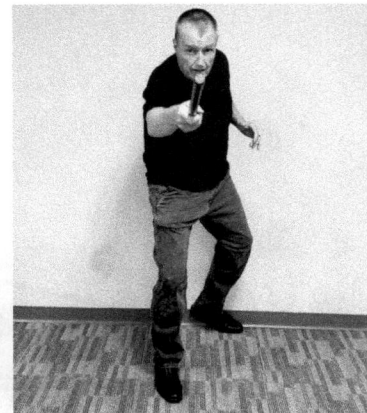

Ambush attack 10: Face stab.

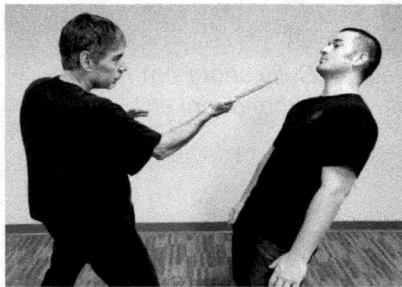

Ambush Series 1: Trainee only develops body elasticity dodging.

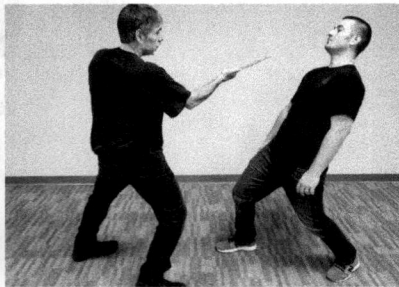

Ambush Series 2: Trainee develops dodging with footwork.

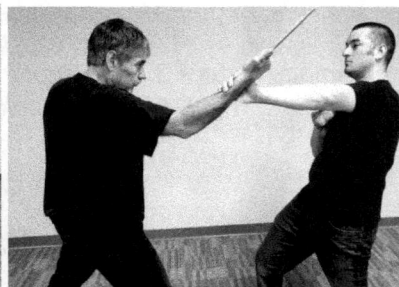

Ambush Series 3: Trainee only dodges and blocks.

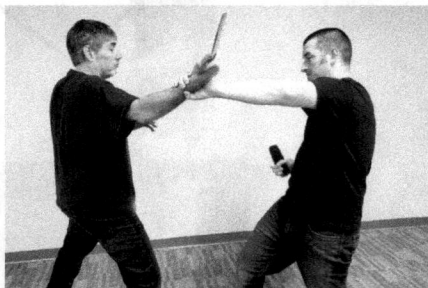

Ambush Series 4: Trainee dodges, blocks, catches and draws expandable baton.

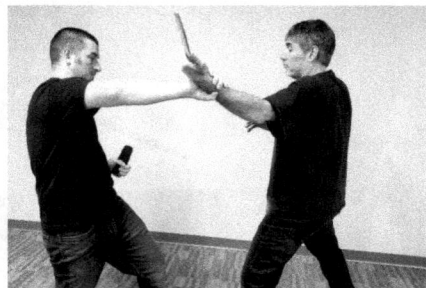

Ambush Series 5: Trainer attacks with multiples. Trainee combines responses.

Series 6: Trainee is alert to a very dangerous problem and has drawn out a stick. Trainer attacks while pulling a pistol and charges in to control the trainee's stick hand and fights. The trainee is "*Stop 2* grabbed." The trainee gets a release and fights back to any legal finish.

Tangler to Drawn Stick Series

Set 1: Trainee is alert to a very dangerous problem and has drawn out a baton. Trainer attacks unarmed and charges in to control the trainee's stick hand and fights. The trainee is "*Stop 2* grabbed." The trainee gets a release and fights back to any legal finish.

Set 2: Trainee is alert to a very dangerous problem and has drawn out a baton. Trainer attacks with a stick and charges in to control the trainee's stick hand and fights. The trainee is "*Stop 2* grabbed." The trainee gets a release and fights back to any legal finish.

Set 3: Trainee is alert to a very dangerous problem and has drawn out a stick. Trainer attacks with a knife and charges in to control the trainee's stick hand and fights. The trainee is "*Stop 2* grabbed." The trainee gets a release and fights back to any legal finish.

Set 4: Trainee is alert to a very dangerous problem and has drawn out a stick. Trainer attacks while pulling a pistol and charges in to control the trainee's stick hand and fights. The trainee is "*Stop 2* grabbed." The trainee gets a release and fights back to any legal finish.

Note: These 8 Tangler situations are great training grounds for a host of exercising and experimentation.

Suggested activities...

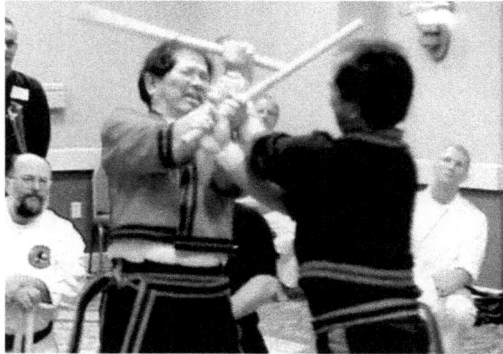

The world famous Remy Presas and Chris Chiu.

Modern Arnis is the name Remy Presas calls his Filipino art. He had popularized "Tapi-Tapi" as one of the studies within the system. Tapi-Tapi is a very close distance 1 versus1 drills, that involve the Stop 2 subject of hand, lower limb and weapon grabbing and releases. Its purpose is to teach you proper defense and reflexes. One of the partners delivers random attack, the other blocks it and retaliates.

Balintawak is another foundational Filipino system that spends a lot of time in this close zone and like Tapi-Tapi, it mostly covering stick on stick, live hand on opponent's weapon hand and stick.

The basic list of skills for these, the nuts and bolts of this process are listed here in this book, but anyone seeking more advanced, more challenging exercises can seek out these Filipino methods.

Suggested reading and viewing...

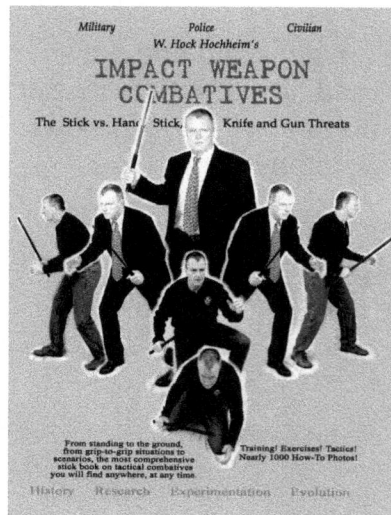

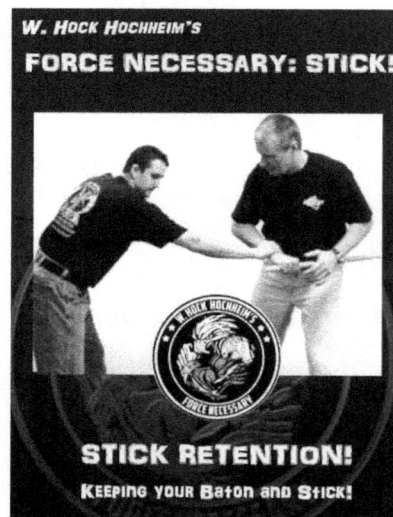

The Level 2 Stick Tangler drill

In *Training Mission One*, we pulled our weapon while the armed attacker stalked us. Now in *Stop 2* we explore when he stalks and mad rushes in. The trainer stalks, rushes in and only grabs the trainee's hands, wrists or lower forearms. Or both grab each others hands, wrists and lower forearms. The trainee solves the problem. Instructors should be aware of how well trained and experienced they are when managing scenarios, so as to decide how far into a combat scenario they should proceed. Participants should have safe training weapons and safety gear.

These may include two releases. The first release to get a hand free, a second one after the baton is drawn and that limb is re-grabbed. Use all the skills and tactics developed in this book.

Tangler to a Stress Quick Draw Series

1: This is a special scenario for those who feel as though an unarmed attacker, due to the totality of circumstances is a serious or deadly threat. This must be legally articulated later. Trainer mad rushes in and the empty-handed trainee is "Stop 2 grabbed." Trainee gets a grip release and draws a baton and uses it. Also, rehearses a threatening surrender.
* one rehearsal of a trainer surrender.
* several examples of impacts and takedowns.
    - some with a closed baton.
    - some with a fixed stick.

2: Trainer is armed with a knife. The trainer mad rushes in and the trainee is "*Stop 2* grabbed." Trainee gets a release and draws a baton and uses it.
* one rehearsal of a trainer surrender.
* several examples of impacts and takedowns.
    - some with a closed baton.
    - some with a fixed stick.

3: Trainer is armed with a stick. The trainer mad rushes in and the trainee is "*Stop 2* grabbed." Trainee gets a release and draws a baton and uses it.
* several examples of impacts and takedowns.
    - some with a closed baton.
    - some with a fixed stick.

4: The trainer mad rushes in while pulling a pistol, and the trainee is "*Stop 2* grabbed" with the trainee catching the pistol itself, the hands, wrist or forearm. Trainee gets a release and draws a baton and uses it.
* several examples of impacts and takedowns.
    - some with a closed baton.
    - some with a fixed stick.

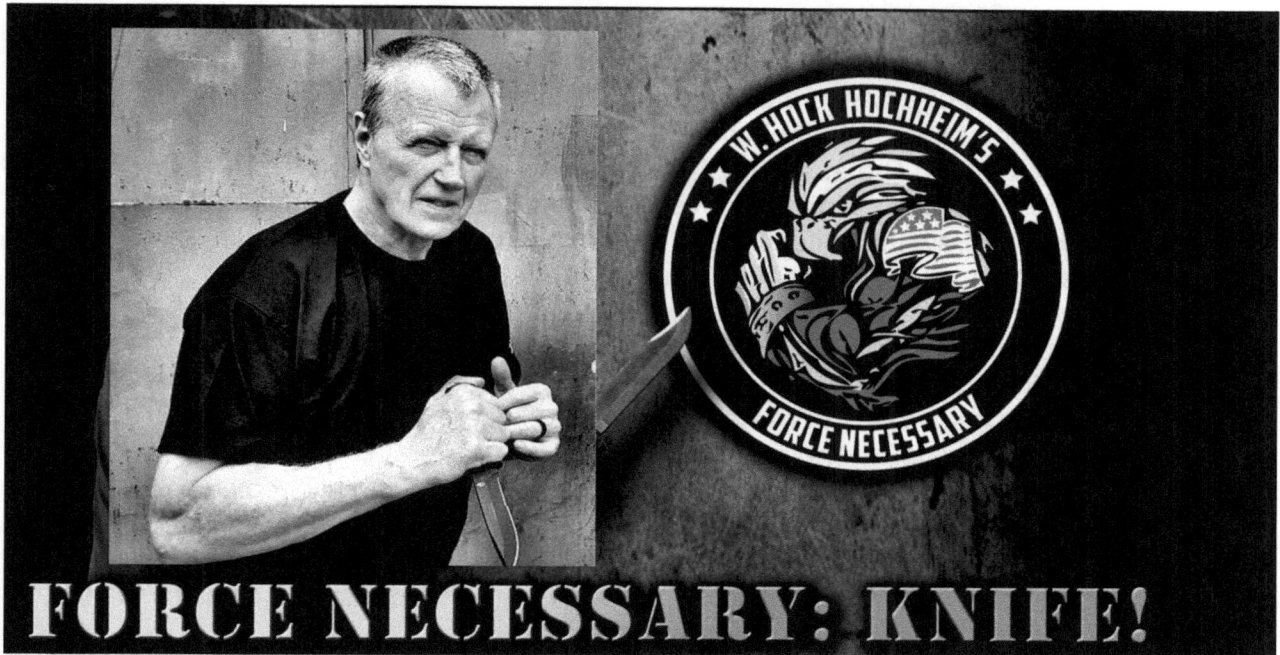

FORCE NECESSARY: KNIFE!

CHAPTER 21: FORCE NECESSARY KNIFE LEVEL 2

Review Training Mission One, Knife Level 1

Commonalities
    Examine *Stop 2* as explored within the Knife 2 context.
    Examine the "What" question as explored within the Knife Level 2 context.
    Examine the Footwork Drill #2: The In and Out Drill "while holding" a knife.
    Examine the grip releases from Part One of this book.
    Continue studying your local self defense laws.

Physical Performance Requirements
    Knife retention.
            - protecting the belt and "pocket."
            - protecting the drawn knife.

    Problem-solving firearm retention.
            - protecting the belt and sheath.
            - protecting the drawn knife when presented or be used.

    Problem-solving the Stop 2 version of the Ambush, Dodge, Evasion, Counter Exercise

    Problem-solving the Tangler Exercise.

    Hitting, grabbing and interfering with the enemy quick draw.

Stop 2 of the Stop 6: Grabs on Fingers, Hands, Wrist and Weapons

In Knife Level 1 we drew the knife under various stressors, under the *Stop 1* parameters of a hands-off, somewhat distant showdown.

The main thrust here in Knife Level 2 is solving the *Stop 2* problems with a knife. The essence of the study is the *Death Grip of the Knife* Drills. Familiarization of that covers a lot of problem-solving. You are about to draw the knife, or have drawn the knife and the enemy grabs your weapon-side limb. You may grab his weapon-bearing limb too, or not. You are holding a knife. The enemy might be:

- empty-handed.
- holding a stick, or sheathed stick.
- holding a knife or a pocketed or sheathed knife.
- holding a pistol or one holstered or tucked.
- holding a long gun, or has a long gun slung/attached to his body.

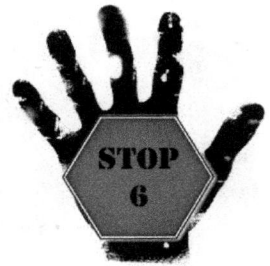

What-Knife of the Ws and H Questions?

Look at the beginning of this book to study the overall what questions. Specific to the knife, here are some "what-knife" to consider:

What knife will you buy and/or carry? Folder? Fixed blade? Small? Big? Double edge? Single?

What knife training course will you take?

What is your mission? What if any mission do you have?

What will you be wearing that either covers or conceals your knife?

What are your the local laws about knives? Carrying? Brandishing? Using?

What do you expect to accomplish with your knife?

What is your "weapons continuum" Are you also carrying other weapons too?

What is the weapons disparity? Disparity is defined as, lack of similarity or equality; inequality; difference: a disparity in age; disparity in rank. And a disparity of weapons, such as knife versus a pistol.

What happens next? After you used that knife, what happens next? Redemption? Jail? Law suit?

What will this cost me?

Continue to try and collect, and answer the "what-knife" questions.

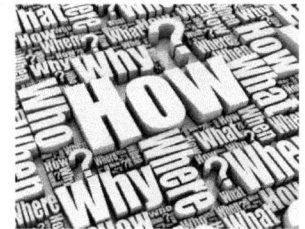

Footwork #2: The In and Out ,"While Holding Knife" Footwork
As previously covered in the first part of this book, practice the in and out footwork pattern while holding a knife, saber grip and reverse grip. You should add strikes on each step.

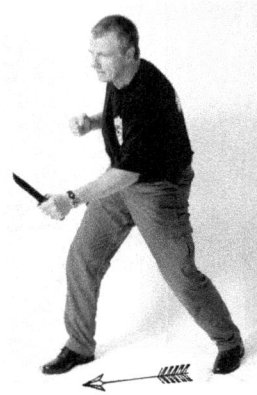

> *Series 1*: Left foot is anchored in the axis. Right foot works in and out at about 2 and 4 or 5 o'clock. Hold and work the knife saber and reverse grips

> *Series 2*: Right foot is anchored in the axis. Left foot works in and out at about 10 and 7 or 8 o'clock. Hold and work the knife saber and reverse grips

> *Series 3:* Quick review of *Stop 1*: Step and draw the knife.

> *Series 4*: Slash and stab
> - step in and out and slash with a saber grip.
> - step in and out and stab with a saber grip.
> - step in and out and slash with a reverse grip.
> - step in and out and stab with a reverse grip.
> - step in and out and saber block.
> - step in and out and reverse grip block.
> - step in and out and block, and any strike combination.

>< * right-handed.
* left-handed.

Combinations:
> - step in and out and any saber stab or slash.
> - step in and out and any saber stab or slash.

Freestyle:
> - freestyle blocks and strikes while moving in and out.

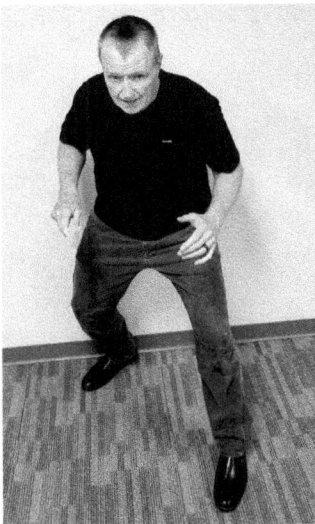

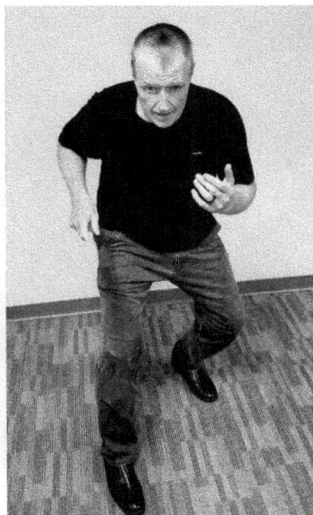

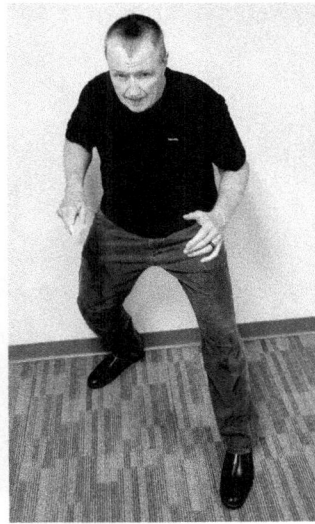

Sample: Right foot steps up, steps in, the right foot steps back, steps out.

Protecting the belt, or pocket

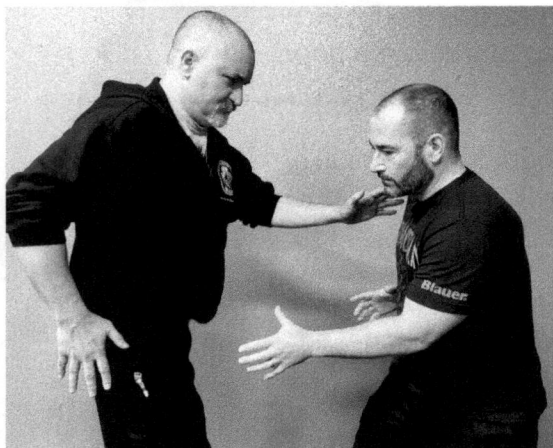

He sees you are dropping your hand to get a weapon. He sees the knife clip on your pocket.

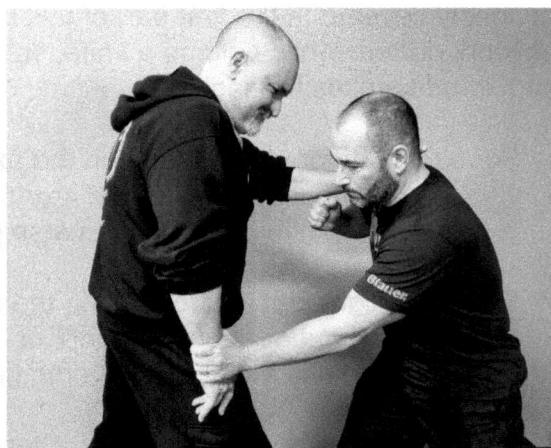

He grabs only your hand. Not getting to the knife. Total retention madness next? No.

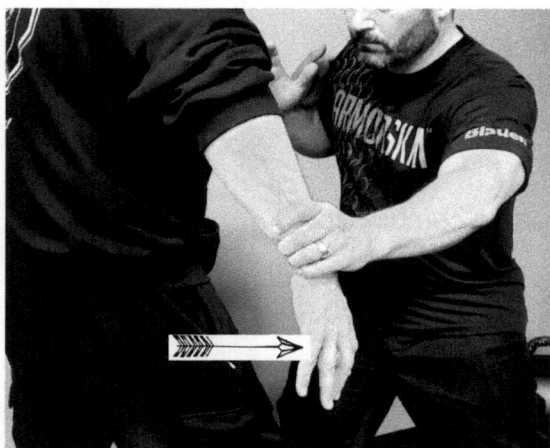

You remove your hand from your weapon. The weapon is not involved!

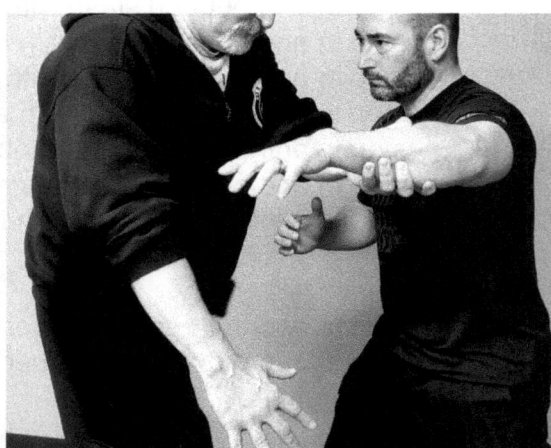

You push-pull, slap-release his grip on your hand. Step away from the grip.

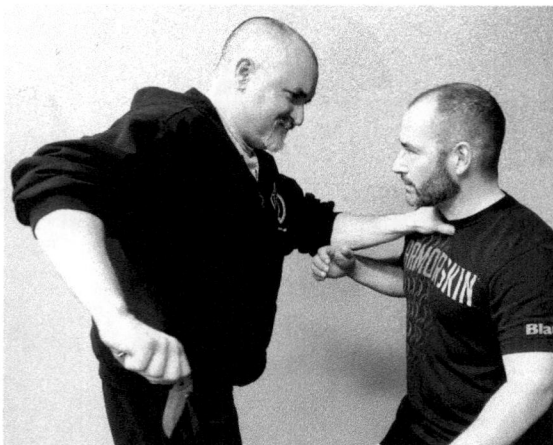

Draw if still needed.

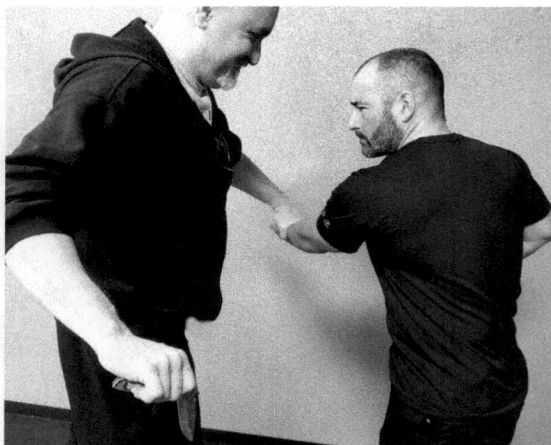

Or release his grip, or hang on, arm drag to the side for a clearer path to draw.

Protecting the Drawn Knife

Knife disarming is dangerous, situational and difficult. But disarms occur everyday, all over the world, even by totally untrained people. Remaining ignorant about them, because you have been told they are impossible, is not a solution. *Stop 2* is more about retention than disarming, and a deeper delve into the aspects of knife disarming with begin in later *Training Missions.*

Suffice to say that a solid grip on your drawn knife is important. One of the things I've written extensively about since the 1990s is what I call the *Cancer Grip.* This very, very silly thing any citizen, soldier, or even a small child would look at and know would not cut a baloney sandwich on soft white bread. The thumb and the ball of the thumb simply MUST be on the knife to stab or slash and keep hold of the knife. Normal people look and say, "Why of course!" But you would be surprised. Not all people agree.

You might receive some knife training from some of these groups, so beware. Usually they are Filipino or Silat based, groups which are automatically presumed to be knife experts. Do not blindly follow everyone and everything.

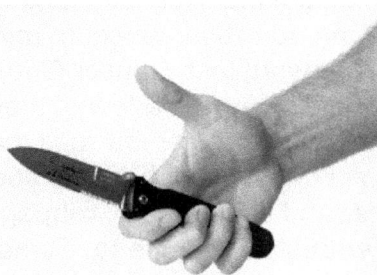

The cancer grip.

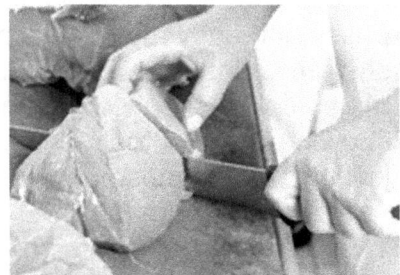

Butchers use their thumbs and ball of their thumb to cut meat.

Probably the most trouble I have gotten into in the established martial arts world was over this very silly knife grip. Worldwide, I was accused of defaming and disrespecting famous Filipino "Godheads." They called me rude, disrespectful and wrong. Some martial supply companies refused to sell me gear. A Kali group in Germany, declared that:

> "... what Hock doesn't know is that, yes, we hold the knife that way, but when we stab or slash, we grab down on the handle completely during the stab or slash."

So, we are then to presume that if one is unlucky enough to be in a knife duel, or face someone unarmed, or face someone with a stick, you are to half-hold a knife in a ridiculous, useless, unsolid manner while dueling? Then you predict an accidental, incidental contact in the chaos of a duel, and...squeeze the knife handle. Then open your hand up again to an incomplete grip? That's your plan? If you see an instantaneous opening from an attack, you quickly squeeze the handle, cut or slash, then retract back to a worthless grip?

There would seem to be no sensible excuse for this. It is more than obvious that any contact with the knife, accidental, incidental or on purpose would cause an easy disarm from that worthless grip.

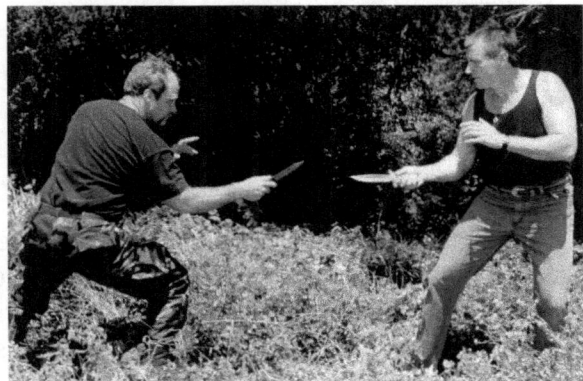

Keep a solid grip to retain your knife.

But, there is more,
"Well Hock, that high thumb is used to hook and catch the knife bearing wrist."

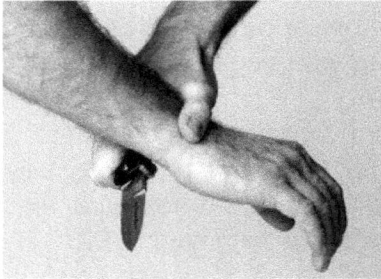

So this one hard-to-do, low probability trick is offered as sole reason we must over-use, over train, fight with a terrible grip? A grip with high probability, knife loss upon any contact?

Even just phasing in and out of this lame, artsy, Cancer Grip, as famous instructors mindlessly do when teaching, is thoughtless and dangerous.

I am told that to this day, you will still see some of the very big FMA names demonstrating and teaching knife drills and slipping mindlessly off into the lame Cancer Grip. It's prissy and artsy and looks cool? It's an addictive dance. In my travels, I too still see students mindlessly practicing with the worthless Cancer Grip. They are all FMA vets. I began collecting photos of them. I will display just a few of them here, but hope I am not showing much of their faces, as I do not want to embarrass them as people. I want you to know not to do these mindless, stupid grips, lest it become your muscle memory. These photos are from magazines, seminar and course ads, webpages and even book covers. These are all instructors you have entrusted your life to. Some are quite famous. Challenge their ideas.

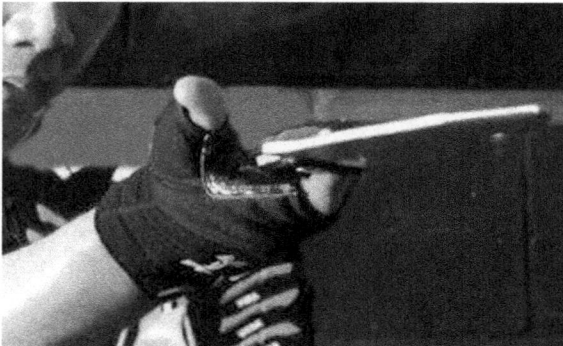

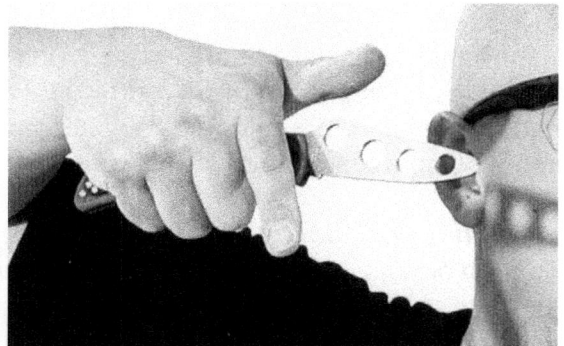

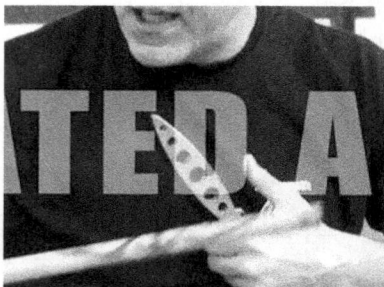

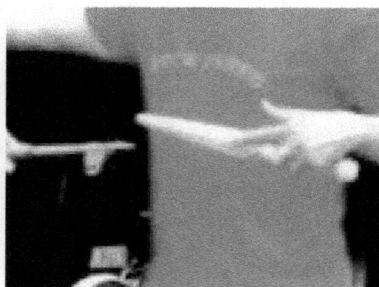

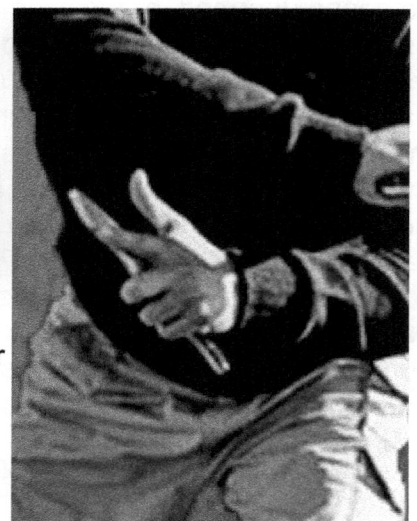

You should not put your finger out on the blade. It will hamper your stab, as the stab will only penetrate up to your finger, limiting your success. Military and crime forensics report that stabs are more successful than slashes. Why limit your success by limiting the penetration of the stab with your finger?

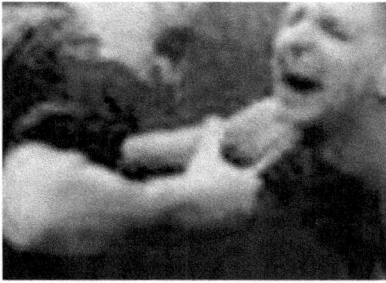

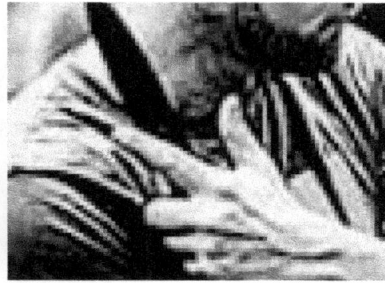

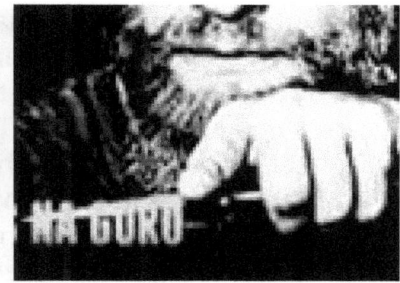

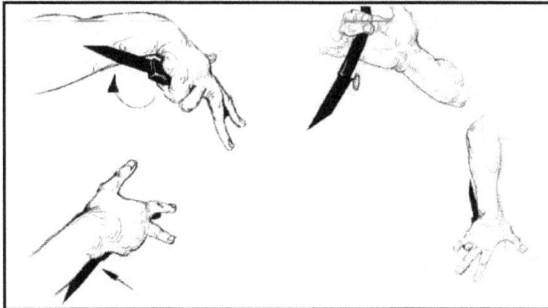

This is some instructional artwork for knife manipulation. I will not embarrass the system head or the system by naming them. It is all open-finger handicapped, stupid, artsy junk.

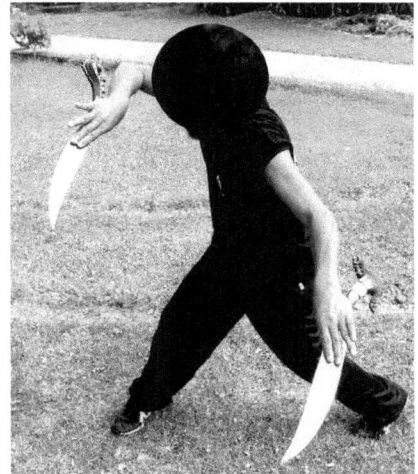

WTF?

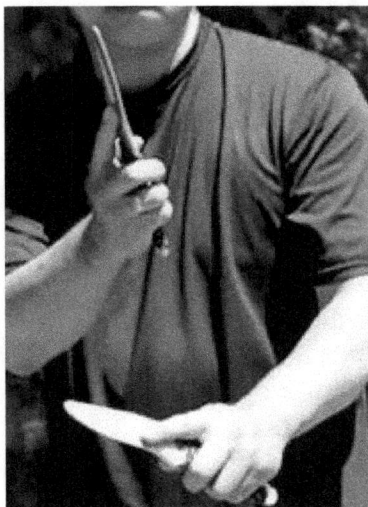

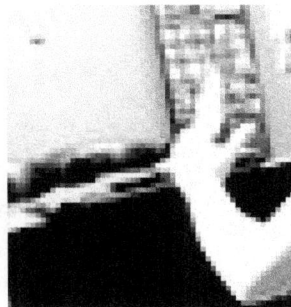

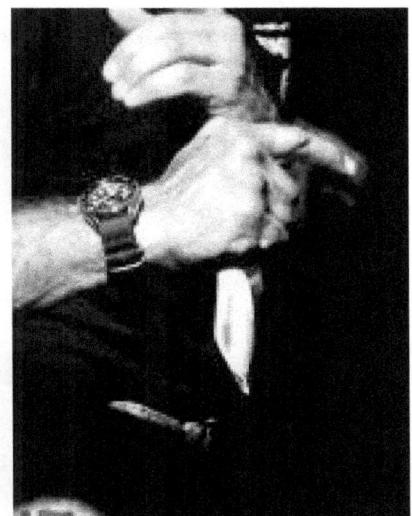

The knife is a great equalizer, but not God's gift to equalization. But, you can do a lot of stupid stuff and maybe get away it. If you want to maximize your chances for survival, stop this infection. Use your hand and all your fingers to hold your knife, to retain your knife, whether presented or slashing or stabbing. Military veterans laugh at such artsy nonsense.

The Death Grip of the Knife Exercise (The "Catch" Sets)
The exercise creates a foundation for solving *Stop 2* problems. The various and common *Stop 2* Death Grip positions are:

1: Any configuration on the top-side, 3 to 9 o'clock, upper high-half of the clock.
2: Any configuration on the bottom-side, 3 to 9 o'clock, lower-half of the clock.
3: Mixed grips as in hands both high & low.
4: Mixed grips as in left-hand versus right-hand, cross-grabs.
5: The "accordion." Given the in-and-out motion of a fight, sometimes chests "bump."
6: Your knife versus his unarmed, versus his stick, versus his knife, versus his pistol.

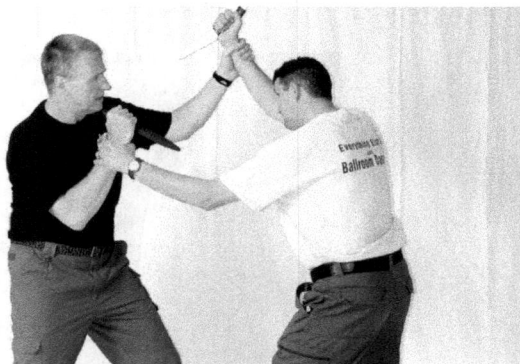

Any configuration on the top-side, upper high-half of the clock. 3 to 9 p.m.

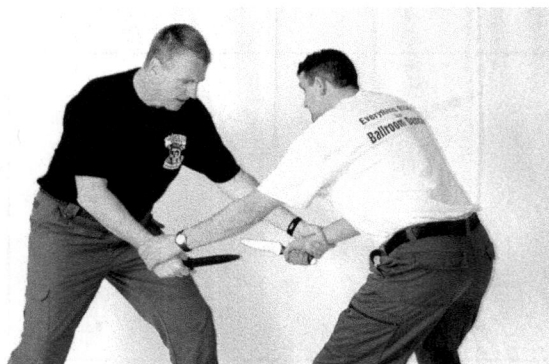

Any configuration on the low-side, low-half of the clock. 3 to 9 p.m.

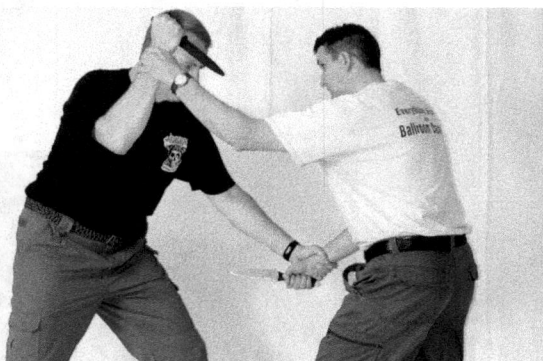

Mixed grips as in hands high & low.

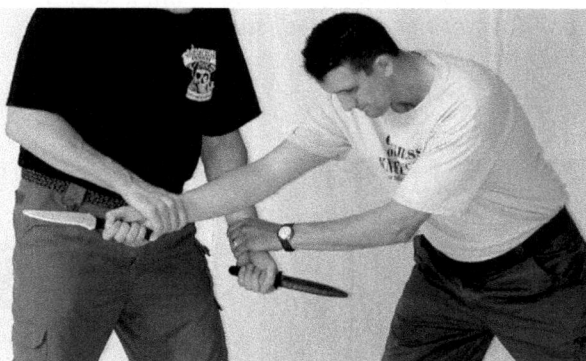

Mixed grips as in righty versus lefty.

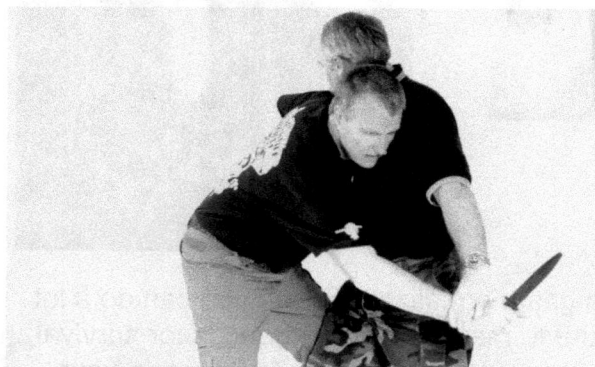

The "accordion." Given the in-and-out motion of a fight, sometimes chests "bump."

These are *Stop 2* common samples of problems. Being "caught red handed" can occur in the following Stops too, way closer in, all the way to the ground. We will cover those problems in later books.

Saber and knife grips many vary. There have been some law enforcement studies that suggest high or higher stab attacks often involve the reverse grip and mid-to-lower stab attacks often are saber grips. These are natural. However there are a few newer knife courses that are making practitioners pick one or the other grip for everything, which can be limiting, and a big mistake.

The Knife Death Grip, Statue Kick Drill

You can get in the Death Grip situations, usually mixed or high grips, you might get a quick kick in. To practice this, we use the statue drill, and the trainer stands, legs apart so the trainee can experiment and fabularize his or herself with the progression of outside-inside-inside-outside the trainers legs. The trainer, being the statue, allows the trainee to experiment.

The nature of the arms distance, the *Stop 2* distance, allows for some freedom in kicking without being so easily pushed off balance, as one might with an arm wrap.

The fact that the enemy's hands/forearms are being held, hinders the opponent's ability to stab your kicks. If the hands are low? This availability might lead to a kicking leg slash or stab.

The *Force Necessary: Hand* course covers these kicks one by one in its progression. Look there for detailed instruction if you need it. But here, do your best, as none of these kicks are "rocket science." This Statue Drill exercise emphasizes the:

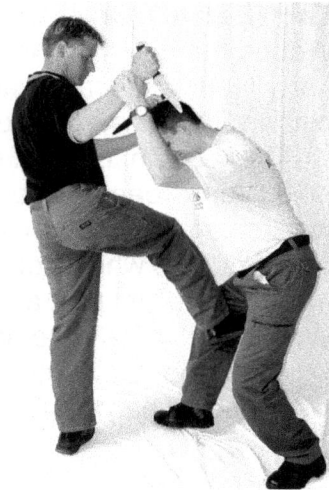

Frontal snapping kick to shin and groin.

* Frontal snap kick
    - hitting with the shoe tip, sides, instep, shin.
    - left kick to shin - left to groin - right to groin - right to shin. Next work back from right to left.

* Stomp kick
    - left to right foot top - right to left foot top - left to left foot - right to right foot top. Next work back from right to left.

* Thrust kick
    - left to right knee - right to left knee - left to left knee - right to right knee. Next work back from right to left.

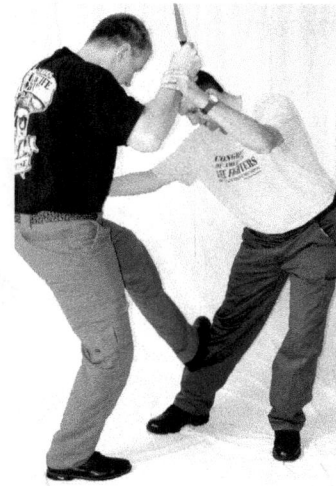

Thrust kick to knee.

* Round kick
    - left to right leg - right to left leg - left to left leg - right to right leg. Next work back from right to left.

* Knees (and there are many options.)
    - left to outer right - left to center right - left to groin - left to inside left - right to outer left - right to center left - right to groin - right to inner right. (there are more - see *FN: Hand* Level 3). Next work back from right to left.

* Whatever other kicks you think you can get in.

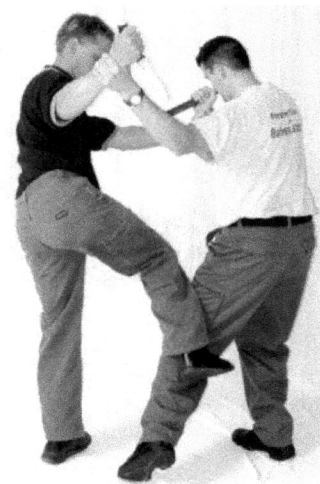

Round kick to legs.

The 12 Death Grip Forearm Woundings

Wound the defense, wound the offense. These were first shown to me by JKD instructor Larry Hartsell decades ago. I vaguely remember him saying the method came from a certain Filipino system, but I do not recall which one.

The 12? On the high side, which we think will be a reverse grip, 3 stabs to forearm that holds your weapon limb. Weakening this. Then 3 stabs crossing over to his weapon side, weakening his weapon side. "Wound his defense, then wound his offense." That's 6 stabbing wounds, which could be a slash too. Why 3 and 3? Well, its better than 1 and less than 16. We just pick a decent number to do the job. More than enough. Not too many. Wounding his defense arm, weakens it and should allow you to attack his other arm.

The other 6? Same ones on the low line, which we think will be a saber grip. Three to his grabbing hand limb. Three to his weapon side limb. Six high. Six low.

Mixed? Those 12 would be basic training. But what if the grips weren't just like these? Perfect high and perfect low? Like a saber grip high and not a reverse grip when the tip is not near his forearm? What if when low and with a reverse grip, and that tip isn't near the forearm? What if one grip was high? The other low? Mix up the responses.

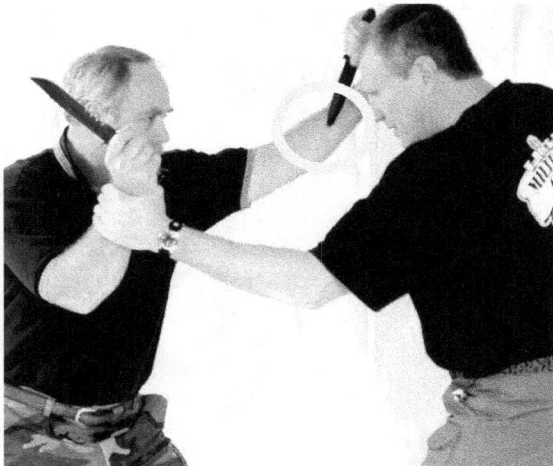

3 stabs/cuts to his defense.

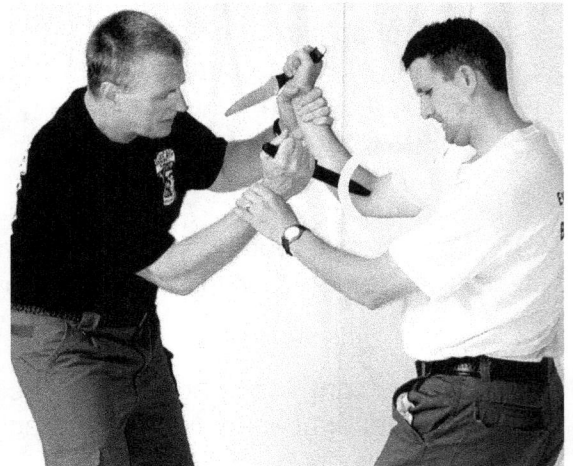

Defense weakened and 3 to his offense.

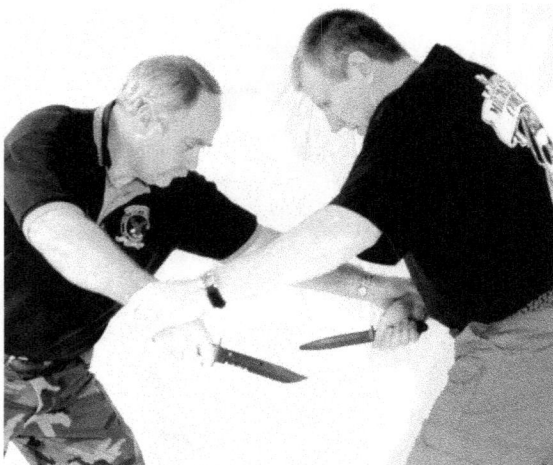

The same for the low line catches.
Three and 3. For a total of 12.

Mixed catches? Mix these basic moves and experiment. For example, you might kick the opponent, spit in his eye and attack the other limb, wounding his offense.

High catch basics.
- 3 to the catching limb (his defense)
- 3 to the weapon limb (his offense)

Low catch basics.
- 3 to the catching limb (his defense)
- 3 to the weapon limb (his offense)

A Study of the Major Releases via the Death Grip

Your knife lower limb/hand gets grabbed. High or low. These work versus one hand only grabs too and also usually in Stop 2 to 6. This book covers *Stop 2* only, but you will be asked to review this releasing foundation as the *Stop 6* and *Training Mission* books continue.

Sample 1: The yank-out. Like a hit and retract, use your arm and whole body if need be to get out of this *Stop 2* grab. Same on the low end.

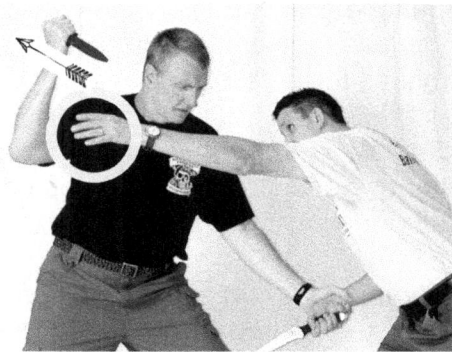
The yank-out release.

Sample 2: The circular release and the joint lock position releases. Rotating your knife hand clockwise or counter-clockwise can often get a release. It will depend on the grip, high or low. Sometimes a quarter-circle or a half-circle will allow you to use a quicker, joint lock release. At times, a second after the release, you can push the hand away with your saber or reverse grip, freeing a better path to your next attack, else the opponent will simply re-grab your limb. Look for this push-out opportunity in your practice.

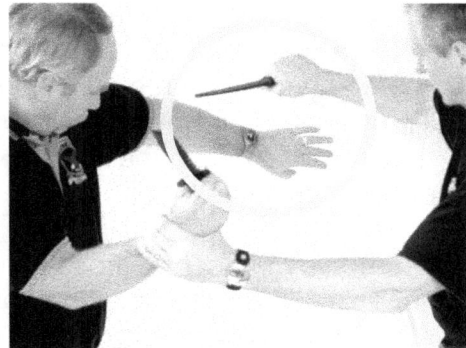
A circular release. This one counter-clockwise.

Sample 3: The elbow rollover. This is really a joint lock release also, but it serves an honorable mention for its easy success. If you can, it's 1) elbow up; 2) elbow over his forearm; 3) elbow down like a flapping motion. You can accompany that downward flap with a bit of a body drop against very strong grips.

Sample 4: The shoulder release. If you can't get a release from a strong grip? And you can judge from prior practice versus various heights, pull his gripping hand out from his body and get your upper torso under his arm, a bit sideways. Hammer your caught hand down as you stand up like from a squat. This should get a release. Take care not to get caught in a head lock, by going a bit deeper in and a bit sideways.

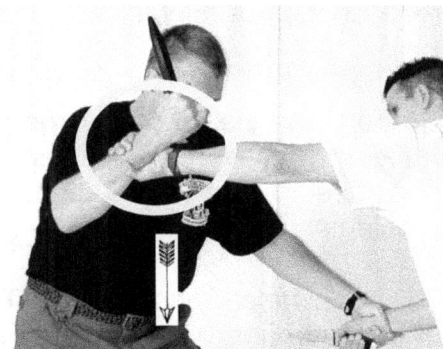
A joint lock release. He's in a center lock position. Jam knife down.

Sample 5: A knee release. On the low side of the clock, if you can't get a release, and you can judge from prior practice versus various heights, lift and drive you knee against his grabbing forearm, and pull your caught limb back and out.

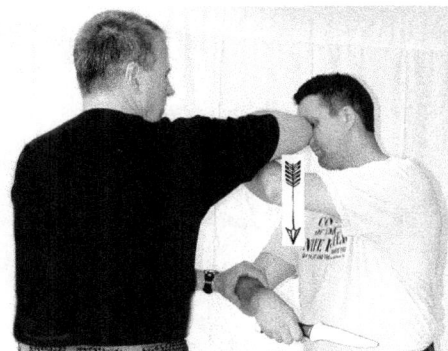
An elbow rollover.

Sample 6: A bite release. If you can't get a release, you can try stepping in and biting his arm, if his clothing makes this available.

Sample 7: Arm rams. Any cross arm catch, or when in a righty versus lefty jam-up, you could try to ram his arm up or down to get a release.

Sample 8: A arm stab to his defense grab that shocks him back. When we execute the forearm woundings, he may jerk back freeing your knife hand from his grip.

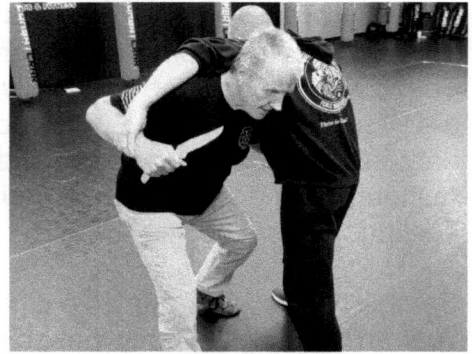
A shoulder squat release.

Sample 9: He accidently grabs the knife itself. Whether you are saber or reverse grips, high or low, the enemy may accidentally grab your knife trying to catch your limb. Practice twisting the blade to destroy his hand, then yank the knife back.

At the end of each of these sample exercises, the trainee should make some attempt to "finish the fight." with knife work and a takedown. This is only Level 2 and not the official time to mandate combat scenarios. But it is good classroom and seminar activity to get to work on these subjects.

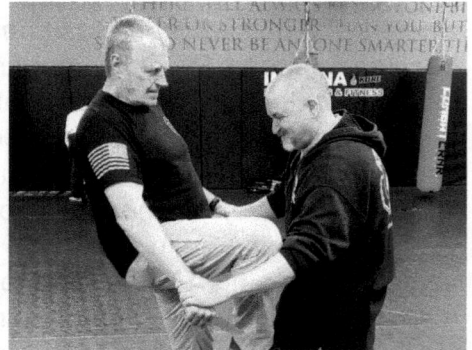
A knee release, "on the low."

Some Other Death Grip Type Solutions/Responses
Here are some other solutions you should know, that don't directly lead to a release. One and two-hand grip problems.

1: The Pommel Chest Charge. The hand grips are high or low, saber or reverse. Can't get a release? He's too strong? Can you bring the pommel of your knife to your chest, lean in and run in? Take care not just to strike his sternum, and work around the chest bone structure.

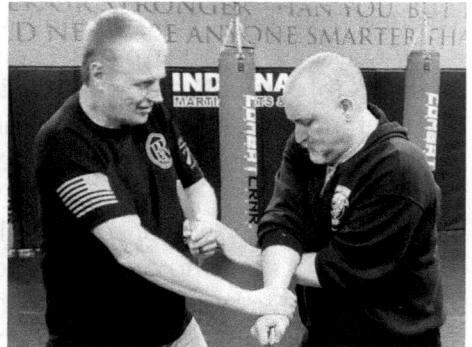
Arm rams, when crossed.

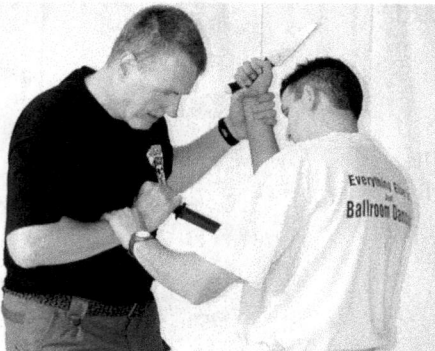
The pommel chest charge.

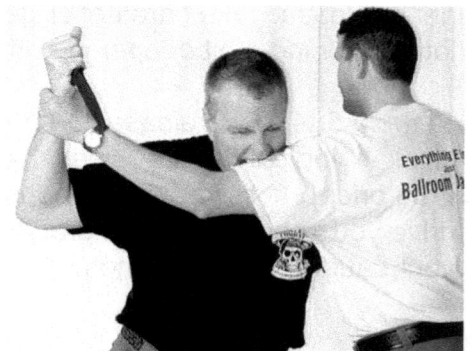
A bite release.

2: Arm swing to thigh attack. Low death grip. Having trouble getting that release? Can't even seem to get an arm bend? Using your captured knife limb, lift or pull the capture so that he might resist by pulling down. Take his pulling down momentum and sweep down to a serious stab or slash on his inner thigh, thinking about the hitting the location of the femoral artery.

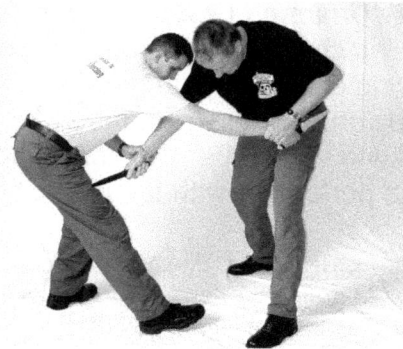

Arm swing to thigh attack.

3: The Knife Disarms as Studied through the Knife Death Grip Format: Push-pulls, strips and carving out the disarm of his knife. You catch. He catches. You do the 3 and 3 woundings. Maybe a kick. Then take on the knife disarms for experience.

High Catch Push-Pull-Strip - Reverse Grip (learn now to protect your thumb).

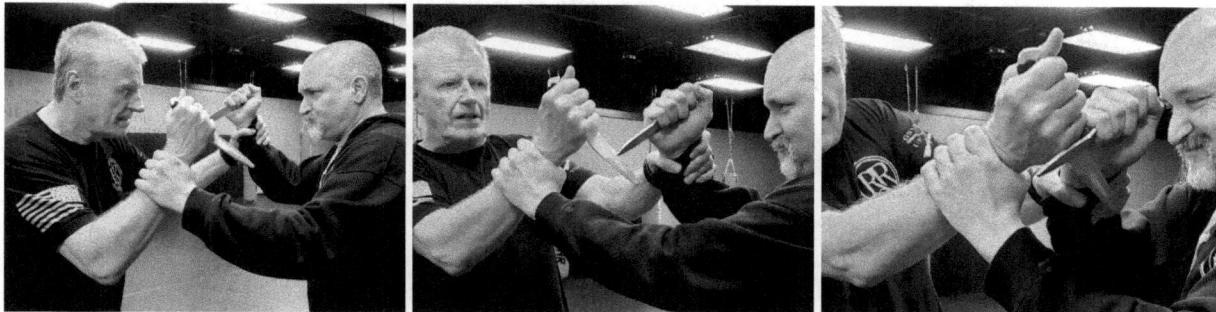

High catch. 3 and 3. Bring his wounded arm in. Take your knife and in and around his knife and shove/cut his knife out of his hand, shooting it away.

Low Catch Push-Pull-Strip - Saber Grip (learn now to protect your thumb).

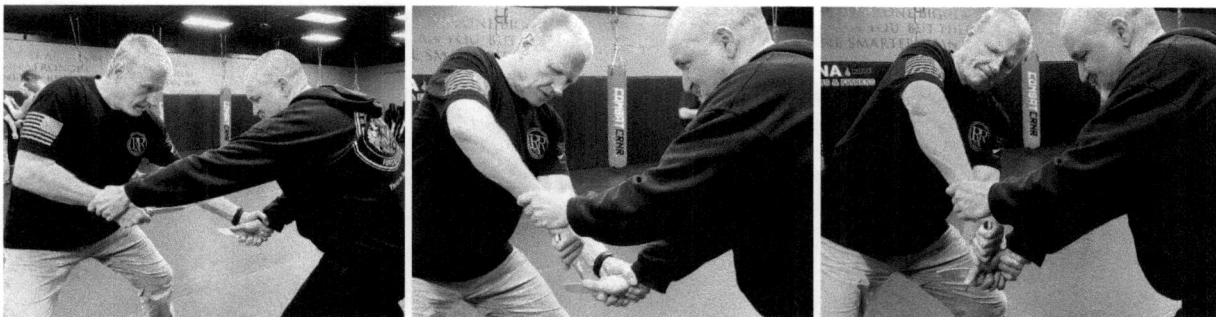

Low catch. 3 and 3. Bring his wounded arm in. Take your knife and in and around his knife and shove/cut his knife out of his hand, shooting it away.

Optional Death Grip Disarm Skill Drill
Do this standing, kneeling, topside, backside, right side ground, left side ground. Try to roll into these positions. You can start the "push" to simulate the strip," them flow into the next position. This circumstance may happen in all 6 of the *Stop 6* collisions.

4: Unarmed Grabs on Your Knife Limb: The Knife Hand Switch Drill Series

The circumstances warrant you to draw a knife. You might be searching a suspicious area and discover a dangerous, unarmed suspect. You might be circumstantially overwhelmed by one or more unarmed bad guys. You've drawn your knife, or just barely drawn your knife. He grabs your knife limb to interrupt you. I like to suggest that a weapon, hand switch is performed with the intensity of a relay race, baton hand-off at the Olympics.

One hand. High grip. You switch hands and stab if needed.

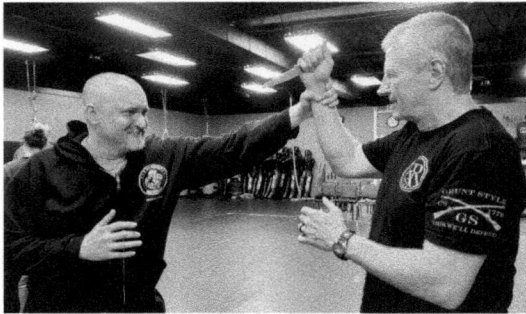

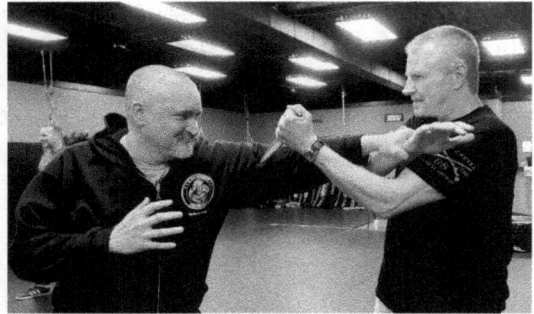

He single-hand grabs. High. You pass the knife off to the other hand. Attack if need be.

One hand. Low grip. You hand switch and stab if needed.

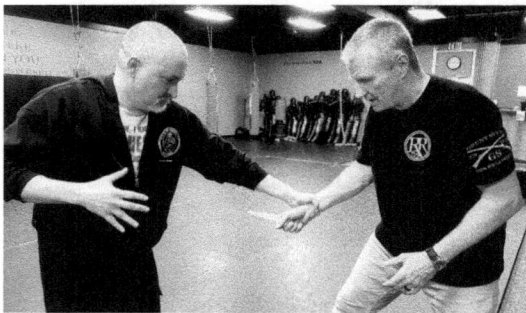

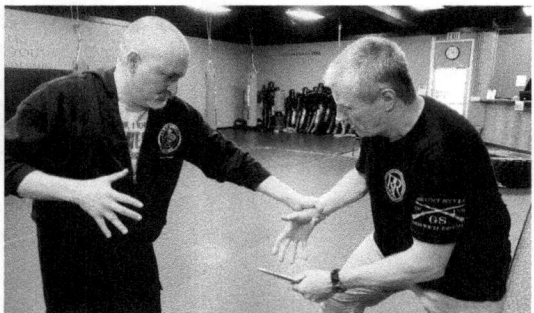

He single-hand grabs. Low. You pass the knife off to the other hand. Attack, if need be.

Two hands. High grip. You hand switch, and stab if needed.

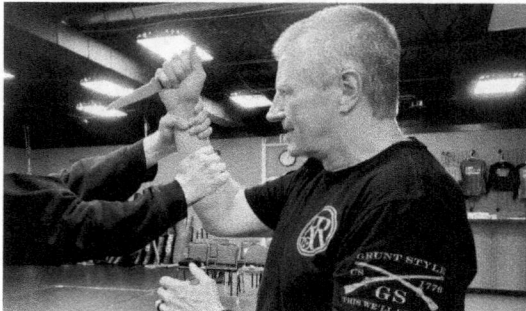

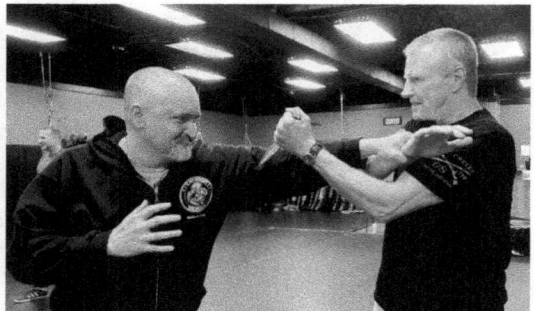

He double-hand grabs. High. You pass the knife off to the other hand. Attack, if need be.

Two hands. Low grip. You hand switch, and stab if needed.

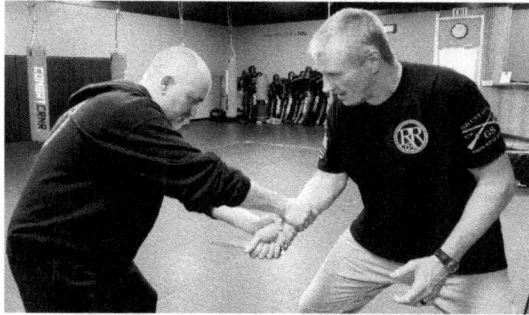

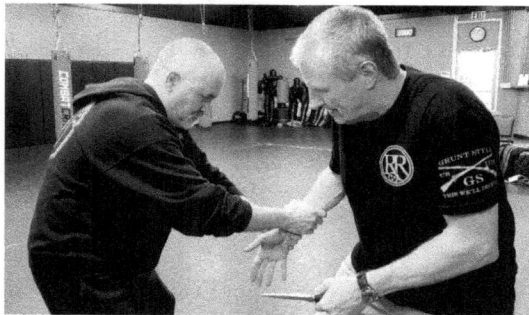

He double-hand grabs. Low. You pass the knife off to the other hand. Attack, if need be.

Center area grip. Versus a right or left hand single grip, hand switch, and stab if needed.

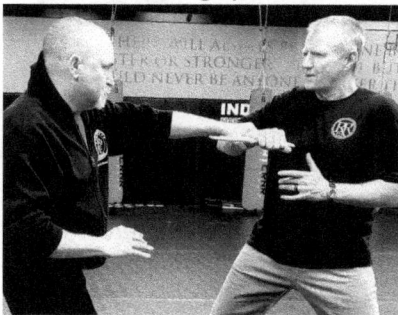

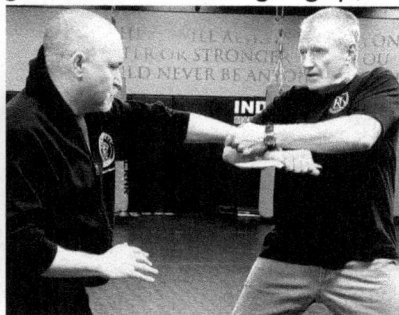

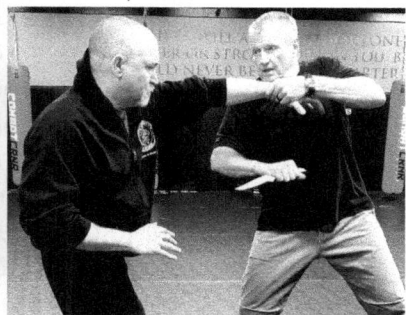

Common single hand, cross-over grab in your center-line area. No pass-off on this. The push-pull release in the best direction. Stab if still needed. This is a pretty universal move.

Using the hand switch method, work this drill in a four corner pattern. Trainer is unarmed, or armed with a stick or knife. He grabs your weapon limb with his free hand. The passed-off, freed knife should probably attack the weapon limb if armed, throat or face/head. I like to suggest that a weapon, hand switch is done with the intensity of a relay race, baton hand-off at the Olympics.

Unarmed trainer grabs your right-handed, stick limb with his one hand:
 Event 1: Trainee is grabbed on his high right. He passes off knife to the left. Attack.
 Event 2: Trainee is grabbed on his high left. He passes off knife to the right. Attack.
 Event 3: Trainee is grabbed on his low right. He passes off knife to the left. Attack.
 Event 4: Trainee is grabbed on his low left. He passes off knife to the right. Attack.
 Next, switch to a left-handed stick grip and work these 4 events.
 Next, the trainer grabs and punches. Trainee blocks and hand switches.
 Next, the trainer grabs and stick attacks. The Trainee blocks and hand switches.
 Next, the trainer grabs and knife attacks. The Trainee blocks and hand switches.

Unarmed trainer grabs your right-handed, stick limb with his two hands:
 Event 5: Grabbed on the high right. Trainee passes off knife to left hand, and strikes.
 Event 6: Grabbed on the high left. Trainee passes off knife to right hand, and strikes.
 Event 7: Grabbed on the low right. Trainee passes off knife to left hand, and strikes.
 Event 8: Grabbed on the high left. Trainee passes off knife to right hand, and strikes.
 activity to get to work on these subjects whenever possible.

At the end of each of these sample events, the trainee should make some attempt to "finish the fight." with legal knife work and a takedown. But, this is only Level 2 and not the official time to mandate various, combat scenarios. Still, it is good classroom and seminar activity to get to work on these subjects.

Stop 2 Knife Tip: Weapon Retention versus the Interrupted Knife Quick Draw

We have taken a hard look at the releases. Knowing them, we must cover this problem. This is a hands-on, Stop 2 problem. Citizens, military and police often carry knives in spots that are visible to the enemy and criminals. This is especially true of the fad in recent years of carrying a small, easily accessible knife on ones belt in the pelvis area. These knives are easily snatched by opponents, especially when in *Stop 4, 5, and 6* close quarter problems.

One way to solve that problem is don't wear one there. It is ironic that many pistol carriers worry and work out to prepare for snatched guns by having various levels of retention holsters for their handguns, yet think nothing of having a

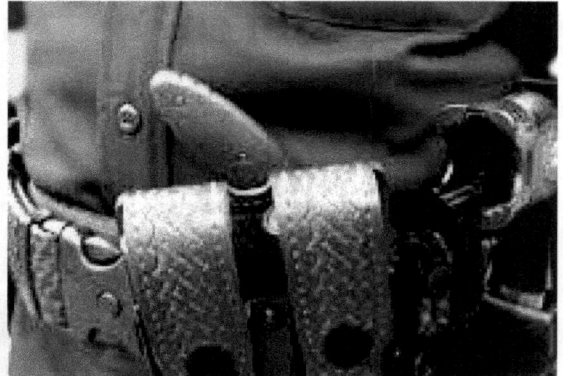

Retaining these knives in close quarters grappling can be difficult. They are easily seen by an enemy and easily removed from your belt and used back on you.

small, visible, so easily, snatchable knife up front near their belt buckles. Some think the knife will be used to interrupt a pistol snatch. Maybe. Maybe not. Small knife stabs are often initially felt as punches and slashes can be ignored.

An opponent sees your hand drop to another very common carry site on your body for a knife, such as the pocket or hip, belt line area. Your knife could be in a sheath or clipped to a pocket or belt line. He may strike you or grab you first! So, for starters you may want to block those attempts. Think about the math on this. Who is righty and who maybe a lefty? Same side grab or cross grab? Which hand may strike? Which hand may grab? Will both hands grab and there is no strike? Work on all of these in class.

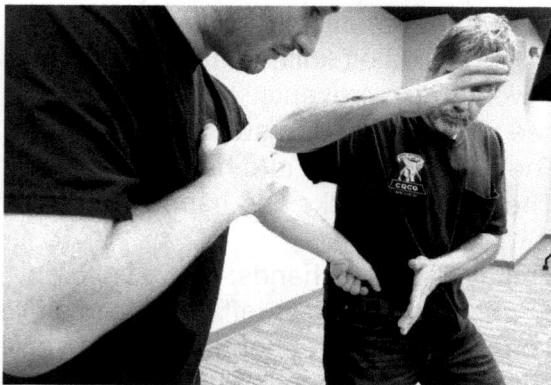

Train to slap attempted grabs at your weapons away.

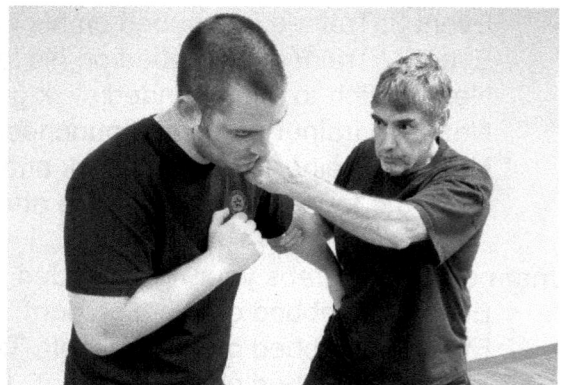

Train to capture the hand on your carry site weapon and to strike the throat and eyes of the enemy.

Stop 2 Knife Tip: Remember The Center Lock Delay

Working these for decades, teaching these for decades and watching thousands do them, I have learned that a handy distraction/delay is, when fingers entertained, the center lock, wristlock as shown in the unarmed chapter of this book. A twist of the hand and wrist and jar-lid-turning inward, has a stalling reaction. If done to his right hand or visible weapon-side hand, it confounds *his* quick draw.

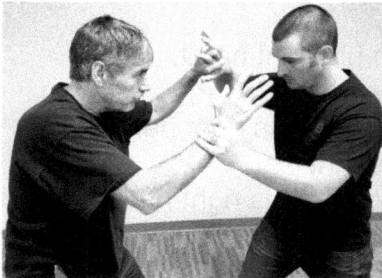

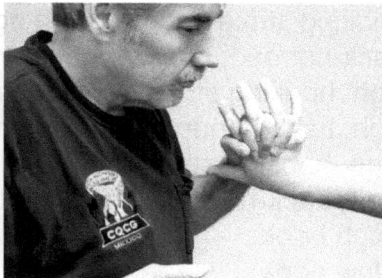

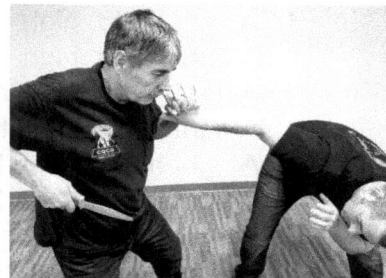

Stop 2 Knife Tip: Remember Feeling for His Draw

When entangled you should be aware that he might draw a stick, a knife or a gun. Why is he suddenly letting go of your limb? Why is his hand dropping to a common weapon carry site? With that release, you may have to charge in and interrupt his weapon quick draw. This interruption can be done many grappling ways, such as a rear arm bar hammerlock. See the chapter in the first part of this book for details.

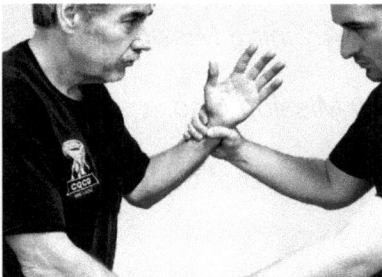

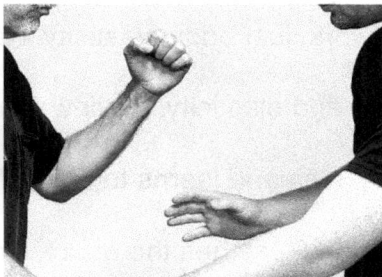

He's got you, yet...   *...he let go? Why the hand drop to common carry sites...*   *He's going for a weapon. Hit him, and carry on...*

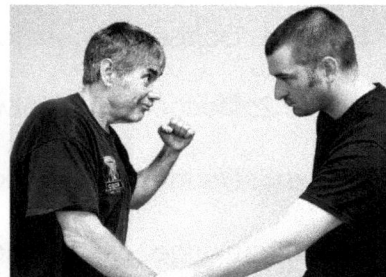

Stop 2 Knife Tip: Hitting the Pistol and or Knife Draw

Stop 2 is about also interfering with his weapon draws and this scenario falls into this category. If you completely untangle yourself and you see a suspect reaching down to those carry sites we list in *Training Mission* books and films, you hit the hand going for the weapon.

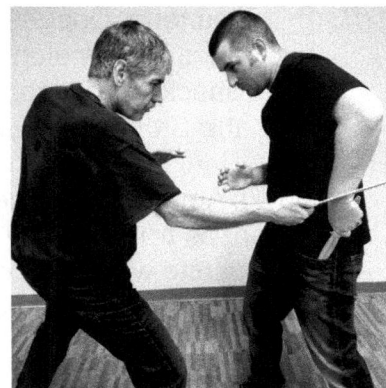

The Stop 2 Ambush, Dodge, Evasion and Grab Drill

As I warned in *Training Mission One*, you will see the Ambush Drill re-appear in various forms as the *Training Missions* continue. Here in *Stop 2* the trainee now grabs the arm attacks. Versus the leg shots, just dodge them with Level 2 "In and out" footwork. The weapon attack is a deadly force situation, causing a weapon response. A trainer stands before you. Close, but not too close. See the steps below. Review the Big 10 hand, stick or knife attacks:

       1: A right hand, high, hooking strike from his high right.
       2: A right hand, high, back-handed, hooking strike from his right hand.
       3: A right hand, belly high, hooking strike from his high right.
       4: A right hand, belly high, back-handed, hooking strike from his right hand.
       5: A right hand, thigh high, hooking strike from his high right.
       6: A right hand, thigh high, back-handed, hooking strike from his right hand.
       7: A right hand, low to high hook.
       8: A right hand, high to low hook.
       9: A right hand thrust to the stomach.
      10: A right hand thrust to the face.
      * Reset, and attack with the left hand.
      * Attack with hand, stick and knife.

     Note and remember - each stab and slash is an individual ambush attack. This represents 10 separate ambush attacks.

The trainee
Series 1: Dodges *without* footwork, just body elasticity. Review *Training Mission One*.

Series 2: Dodges *with* footwork and elasticity. Review *Training Mission One*.

Series 3: Dodges and blocks. Stops and learns to block the lower limb of the attack.

Series 4: Dodge, blocks and *Stop 2* catches the attack limb.

Series 5: Dodges the first attack, becomes alert, stops/catches the next one. Draws knife and counter-attacks to a legal finish. The local instructor will decide whether to stop at the *Stop 2* catch and draw, or complete a diverse combat scenario. Dodges the first attack, dodges the second attack as one becomes alert, stops/catches the next one, draws knife, or opens folder and counter attacks to a legal finish. The local instructor will decide whether to stop at the *Stop 2* catch and draw, or complete a diverse combat scenario.

Note: This Ambush exercise might best be passed on to you with personal hands-on, instruction, as true, step-by step analysis, might take hundreds and hundreds of photos and a thousand words to document here. I hope what is presented here will inspire you and develops the skills of you and yours in *Stop 2* problems.

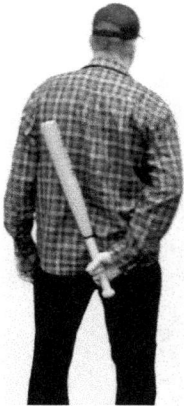

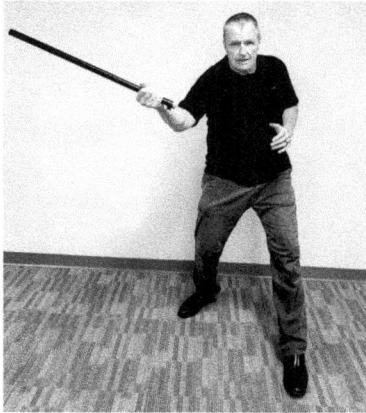

Ambush attack 1: Head shot from trainer's right. An inward strike.

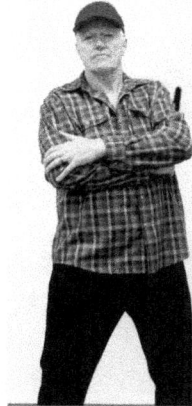

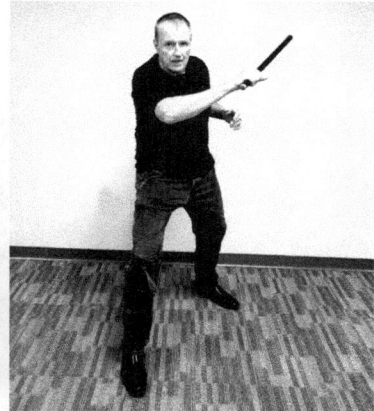

Ambush attack 2: Head shot from trainer's left. A backhand strike.

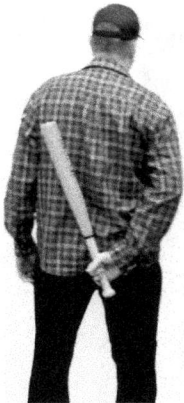

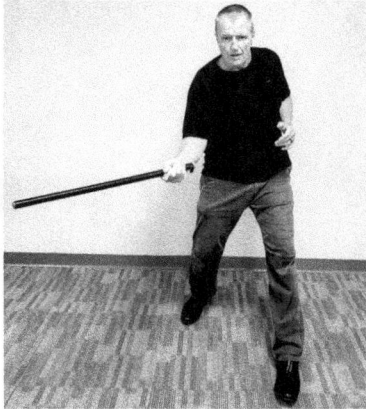

Ambush attack 3: Belly shot from trainer's right. An inward strike.

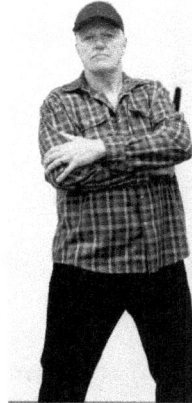

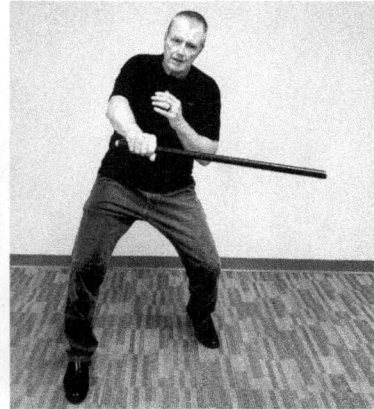

Ambush attack 4: Belly shot from trainer's left. A backhand strike.

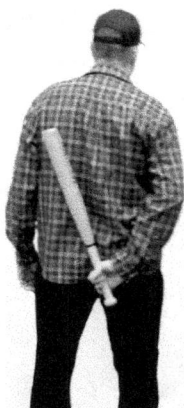

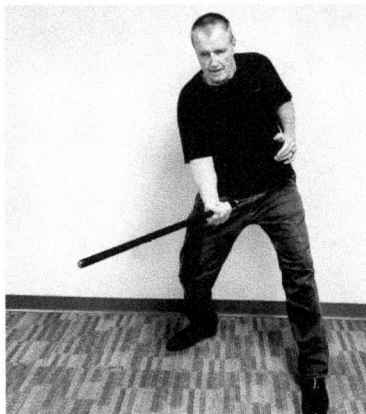

Ambush attack 5: Knee shot from trainer's right. An inward strike.

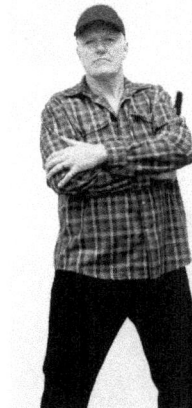

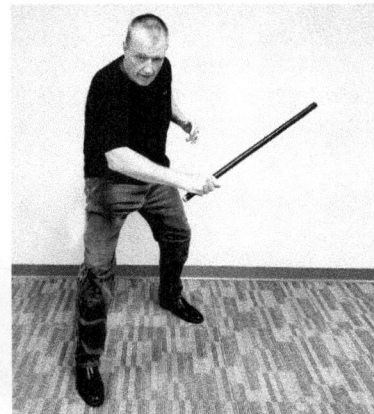

Ambush attack 6: Knee shot from trainer's left. A backhand strike.

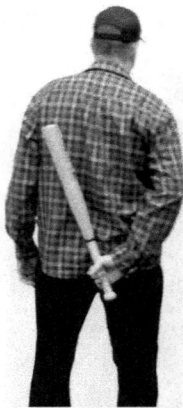

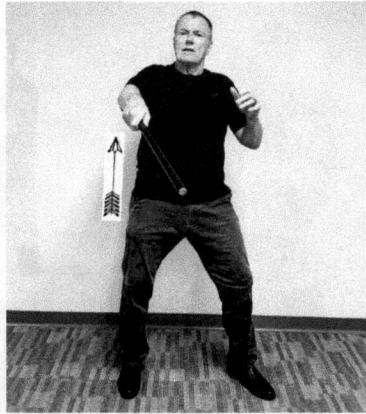

Ambush attack 7: Shot up from trainer's low. Groin target? An upward strike.

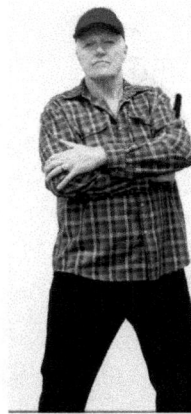

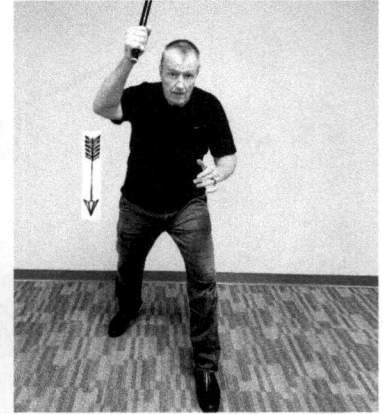

Ambush attack 8: Head or clavicle shot from trainer's high. A downward strike.

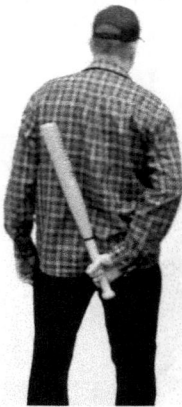

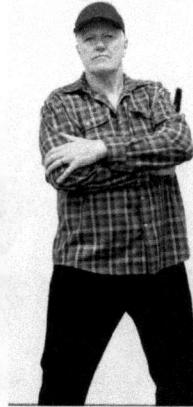

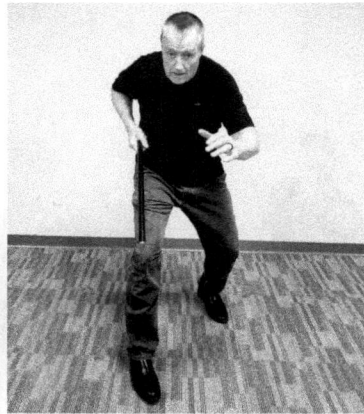

Ambush attack 9: Belly stab.

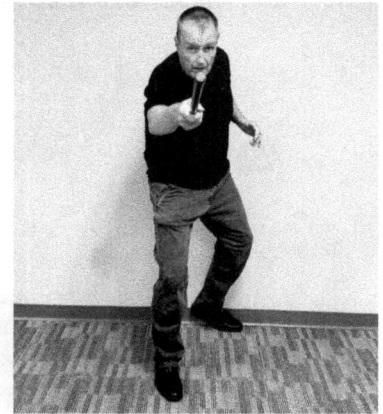

Ambush attack 10: Face stab.

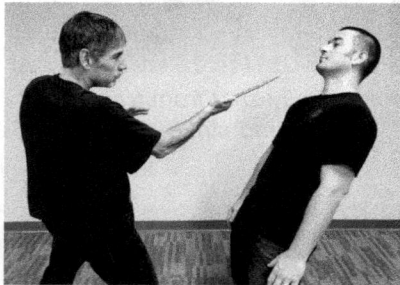

Ambush series 1: Trainee only develops body elasticity dodging.

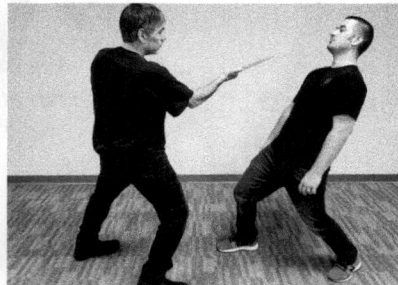

Ambush series 2: Trainee develops dodging with footwork.

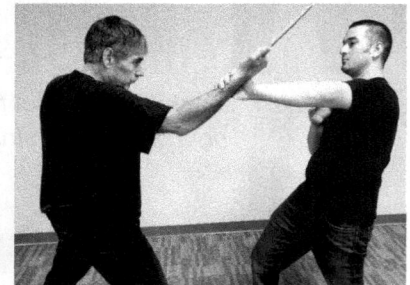

Ambush series 3: Trainee only dodges and blocks.

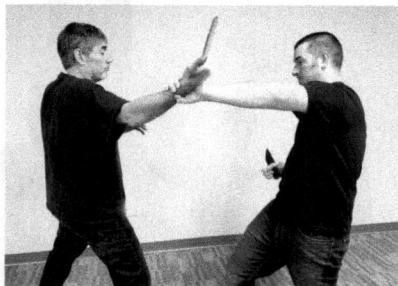

Ambush series 4: Trainee dodges, blocks, catches and draws knife.Uses knife.

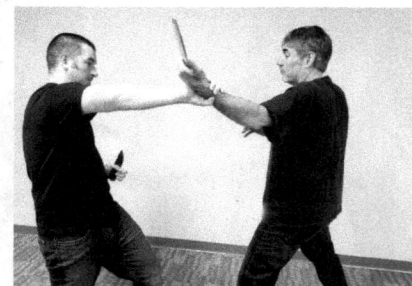

Ambush series 5: Trainer attacks with multiples. Trainee combines responses.

The Level 2 Knife Tangler Exercise Drill

In *Training Mission One*, we pulled our weapon while the armed attacker stalked us. Now in *Stop 2* we explore when he stalks and mad rushes in. The trainer stalks, rushes in and only grabs the trainee's hands, wrists or forearms. Or both grab each hands or wrists. Trainee solves the problem. Instructors should be aware of how well trained and experienced trainees are when managing scenarios, so as to decide how far into a combat scenario they should proceed. Participants must have safe training knives and protective gear conducive to the level of safe ammo.

   These may include two releases. The first release to get a hand free, a second one after the knife is drawn and that limb is re-grabbed. Use all the skills and tactics developed in this book.

Tangler to a Stress. Quick Draw Series

   1: This is a special scenario for those who feel as though an unarmed attacker, due to the totality of circumstances is a deadly threat. This must be legally articulated later. Trainer mad rushes in and the empty-handed trainee is "Stop 2 grabbed." Trainee gets a grip release and draws a knife and uses it. Also, rehearses a threatening surrender.
      * one rehearsal of a trainer surrender.
      * several examples of knife use.
            - with a closed folder, strikes and takedowns.
            - with an open folder, strikes and takedowns.

   2: Trainer is armed with a knife. The trainer mad rushes in and the trainee is "*Stop 2* grabbed." Trainee gets a release and draws a knife and uses it.
      * one rehearsal of a trainer surrender.
      * several examples of use.
            - with a closed folder, strikes and takedowns.
            - with an open folder, strikes and takedowns.

   3: Trainer is armed with a stick. The trainer mad rushes in and the trainee is "*Stop 2* grabbed." Trainee gets a release and draws a knife and uses it.
      * one rehearsal of a trainer surrender.
      * several examples of use.
            - with a closed folder, strikes and takedowns.
            - with an open folder, strikes and takedowns.

   4: The trainer mad rushes in while pulling a pistol, and the trainee is "*Stop 2* grabbed" with the trainee catching the pistol itself, the hands, wrist or forearm. Trainee gets a release and draws a knife and uses it.
      * several examples of use.
            - with a closed folder, strikes and takedowns.
            - with an open folder, strikes and takedowns.

5: Trainee is alert to a very dangerous problem and has drawn out a knife. Trainer attacks while pulling a pistol and charges in to control the trainee's knife hand and fight. The trainee is "*Stop 2* grabbed." The trainee gets a release and fights back to any legal finish.
* several examples of strikes and takedowns.

Tangler to Drawn Knife Series

1: Trainee is alert to a very dangerous problem and has drawn out a knife. Trainer attacks unarmed and charges in to control the trainee's knife hand and fight. The trainee is "*Stop 2* grabbed." The trainee gets a release and fights back to any legal finish.
* one rehearsal surrender threat.
* several examples of strikes and takedowns.

2: Trainee is alert to a very dangerous problem and has drawn out a knife. Trainer attacks a stick and charges in to control the trainee's knife hand and fight. The trainee is "*Stop 2* grabbed." The trainee gets a release and fights back to any legal finish.
* one rehearsal surrender threat.
* several examples of strikes and takedowns.

3: Trainee is alert to a very dangerous problem and has drawn out a knife. Trainer attacks a knife and charges in to control the trainee's knife hand and fight. The trainee is "*Stop 2* grabbed." The trainee gets a release and fights back to any legal finish.
* several examples of strikes and takedowns.

4: Trainee is alert to a very dangerous problem and has drawn out a knife. Trainer attacks while pulling a pistol and charges in to control the trainee's knife hand and fight. The trainee is "*Stop 2* grabbed." The trainee gets a release and fights back to any legal finish.
* several examples of strikes and takedowns.

Note: These 8 Tangler situations are great training grounds for a host of exercising and experimentation.

Suggested reading and viewing...

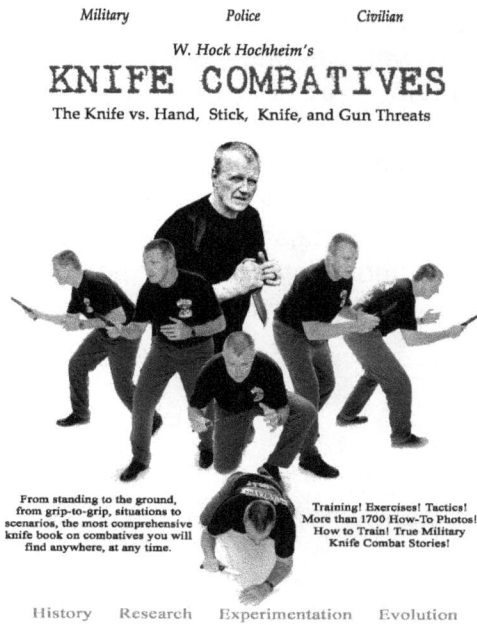

Military   Police   Civilian

W. Hock Hochheim's

KNIFE COMBATIVES

The Knife vs. Hand, Stick, Knife, and Gun Threats

From standing to the ground, from grip-to-grip, situations to scenarios, the most comprehensive knife book on combatives you will find anywhere, at any time.

Training! Exercises! Tactics! More than 1700 How-To Photos! How to Train! True Military Knife Combat Stories!

History   Research   Experimentation   Evolution

The book!

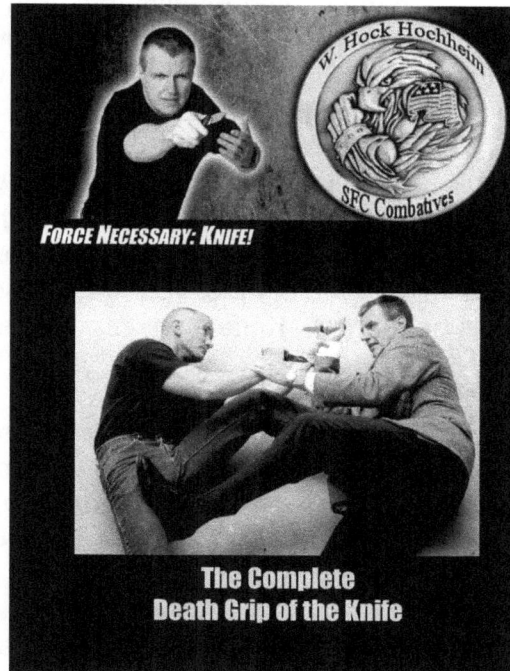

FORCE NECESSARY: KNIFE!

The Complete Death Grip of the Knife

A film for this topic!

FN Knife Addendum 1: Should I Even Dare to Use a Knife to Defend Myself?

A motto for my Force Necessary: Knife course is "Use your knife to save your life!" It's also for desperate times and situations. Mine is a politically correct slogan that sets the stage for the carry-and-use doctrine.

The knife can be used for less-than-lethal purposes and lethal purposes. Yes, less-than-lethal despite its reputation. The edged weapon is not well looked upon in the legal systems of the civilized world. I must warn you that if you use one to defend yourself you usually will be harshly regarded and will be working under an emotional and costly deficit to clear yourself of legal trouble.

Carrying alone can be a problem. Most pocket and belt carry knives are illegal in many countries and in some cities and states in the United States, unless you have a very common sense reason to do so, such as your job. If you run across the street to grab a cup of coffee, from your factory job, you may be grilled by authorities about your pocket knife. (This has happened.) Knife who, what, where, when, how and why?

Who are you to carry a knife?
What do you do that requires a knife?
Where do you do this knife-as-tool work?
When do you need a knife on your job or work?
How will you use this knife on your job or work?
Why such a knife?

These are some of the legal questions authorities will consider, investigate and ask about your knife-carry in these knife-restricted areas.

There is also a citizen-based, "never-knife" and "anti-knife" knife movement, if you will, in certain self defense and combatives programs. Many of these groups are in countries where knife carry is illegal. I get the message from several Krav Maga schools also, which is a bit surprising. I hear –

"I'll never have a knife!"
"I'll never need a knife, I have my unarmed skills."
"Even if I disarm a knife, I'll just throw it off."
"Carrying knives are illegal where I live. I won't have one."
"I don't need knife training. Everyone already knows instinctively how to use a knife."
"People who like and use knives are crazy, like criminals."
"There are no self defense knife-use incidents where I live. Why bother with a knife?"
"Have you seen the kinds of people that carry and train with knives? They're a cult. A crazy, wacky cult!"
    …and so on.

Knives are quite ubiquitous. They are in the kitchens and probably the garages of every home in the world. They are in every restaurant in the world, and every business in the world that requires a minimal amount of handy work. There was a stabbing the other day in a Walmart. A man got a for-sale knife off a shelf and used it on another customer. This ubiquity renders some of the above quotes moot. And I might address the "There are no self defense knife use statistics where I live. Why bother then?" comment. I usually hear it from people/instructors/school owners who live in countries where knife-carry is illegal. There are consistent numbers of knife and gun crime but not knife self defense. Could that be that knives are just not allowed on the streets for the normal law abiding citizen? The no-knife mentality bleeds over to forgetting the knife, like Judo people forget to punch.

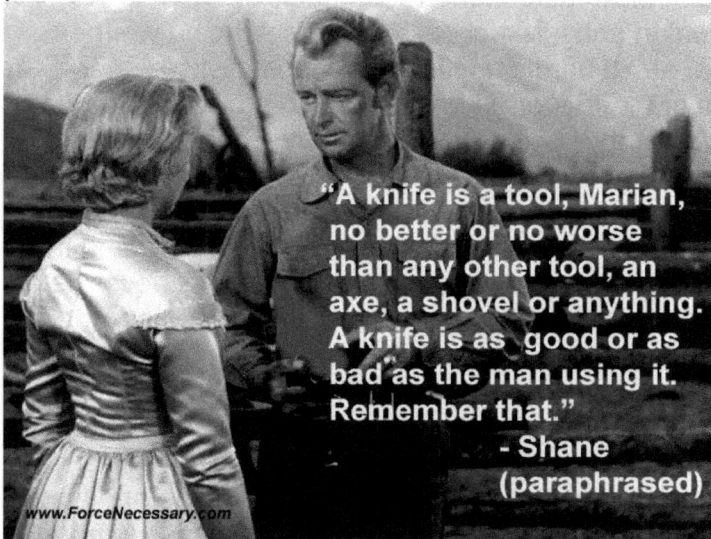

"A knife is a tool, Marian, no better or no worse than any other tool, an axe, a shovel or anything. A knife is as good or as bad as the man using it. Remember that."
- Shane
(paraphrased)

www.ForceNecessary.com

Still, despite the stigma, I carry on with my own knife course, the *Force Necessary: Knife*. Here's why; and, perhaps - should you ever need them - you can use some of my talking points to justify your own legal positions. The following is how and why I justify a "nasty, violent" knife course.

First off, I understand your anti-knife concerns. I really do. I have wrangled with these issues. I have no particular fascination with knives themselves. I feel the same way about guns and sticks. I do not collect them, in the same way I wouldn't collect wrenches or hammers, or all tools in general. These things to me are tools. Some folks do collect knives and of course that's a fine hobby. But since I feel this way, this detachment, I might offer a very practical viewpoint on the subject, along with, needless to add, my decades of investigating knife crimes might add some value too.

We live in a mixed weapon world and therefore I accept the challenge of trying to examine this…hand, stick, knife, gun world. Carry, possession and use laws aside, it's still a hand, stick, knife, gun world. It's a world of war and crime that includes weapons. We fight criminals and/or worse, we fight enemy soldiers.Sometimes we escape them. Sometimes we capture them. Sometimes we have to injure them. And, sometimes we have to kill them.

A person (who lives anywhere) should know how to use a stick, a knife or a gun, despite the laws possessing them. I am not talking about legal or illegal possessing here, as in walking around with an illegal weapon in your pocket. I am just talking about use. Using it. Knowing. Messing with it. Familiarization.

The Big Picture.
Martial instructors with statistics of things that almost never happening? A whole lot of things hardly ever happen in some areas. There are 330 million people in the United States. Millions in other countries. And the odds of being a victim of any hand, stick, knife or gun crime is quite small in comparison. Keep this in mind when we discuss one hand-fighting-only instructor in the USA who declared it was a waste of time to bother learning long gun disarming. "Long gun attacks never happen," he said. "You would be smarter to get on a treadmill than learn long gun disarming." He said these very things the same week a guy walked into a church with an AR-15 and killed people. Annually, consistently, people use long guns like hunting rifles and shotguns in crimes.The problem exists. Since it exists, the problem requires solutions and one movement is in the available, existence of long gun disarming training.

Stats also that say that knife defense hardly ever happens too? That beatings with impact weapons "never happen." That fistfights and unarmed beatings hardly ever happen. I agree in the big picture. I think you would discover though that even simple, unarmed fights are also extremely rare when compared to population size and the billions of personal interactions people have every day.

So then, if an actual, unarmed fight, or an actual unarmed attack/crime is so very, very rare in comparison to the population and interactions numbers, why do we then bother to practice any self-defense at all? If hardly anything happens? Why bother with your unarmed Krav Maga? I ask this of the "never-knife," people, the "never long-gun" person, the unarmed-only trainer. Why bother doing anything then? Does your "no-knife" logic carry over to "no-hand," "no-stick, "no-gun?" None of it happens a lot anyway. Why bother?

Crime rates are small compared to the over-all population. Most of you reading this now will never be in an unarmed fight, never a knife fight, never be shot, or never be a victim of crime. Still we work on these problems because on some level we know, it has happened, will happen and could happen to you and yours.

A study of the FBI crime records disclosed that through the years, 40 percent to 90 percent of the people the police must fight, are armed in some fashion. That's a lot of weapons out there in the civilian world. But, of course, in the history of crime and war, a knife (and sharp, knife-like things) has been used, dare I say, countless times in combat. Since this "no-knife-no-matter-what" essay aired on social media back in 2016, Brits, Europeans and Australians have presented examples when desperate people have used knives to save lives and have been acquitted, even within their strict laws. Even guns have been used in self defense and shooters were acquitted in ""no gun" worlds. In the end, the "totality of circumstances" (a legal term) and common sense should usually win out. We hope! Should you ever, even dare to use a knife to save your life? It will certainly be ugly. There will be ramifications.

I do get a kick out of the knife simpletons who say, "just stick the pointy end in someone." Well, there are mental and physical and situational and legal issues to work on and work out. I also find it interesting that many of these same folks spend thousands and thousands of dollars to own and learn how to stick the…"pointy end of a bullet," into someone. A simpleton might say back to them, "What? Just point the barrel and pull the trigger. Stick the pointy end of a bullet into someone." I would never say that about shooting and I won't say that about the knife either.

Mental. Physical, Situational. Legal. I hope I don't have to mention a long list of examples here. Training with a knife creates a desensitization of its use, something most people need. They need the speed, strength and coordination to overcome an opponent and their reflexive arms. What are the positions and situations of use. And the legal issues! One could write a textbook about these vital legal things.

And I would be remiss not to comment here on the subject listed above on "lost," dropped or disarmed knives in this essay. You might not have a knife, but he does! And in your unarmed combatives class, your Krav Maga class in "no-knife" countries still practice knife disarms ad nauseam. You break the guy's nose and execute Disarm #22. It worked!

Two things then happen to the knife :
        - The knife either hits the floor, or,
        - The knife is now in your trained or untrained hand.

What happens next? One naysayer mentioned above says he will just "throw that knife away" and continue to fight on versus one, (two or more) bad men unarmed. What size room are you in, anyway? And just because the knife (or gun) is on the floor doesn't mean the bad guy can't lunge down in a second's flash and get it back. The lethal threat is not over because the knife has hit the floor at your feet. It's still within lunge and reach and the deadly intent has been established with his assault.

Knives! Look…hey…they exist. They are everywhere. To save your life and the lives of others, use them when and where you got them. It's a hand, stick, knife, gun, world. If you call yourself a self defense, combatives, survivalist, you must have a working knowledge of hand, stick, knife, gun world.

Warning though, if you use a knife, even legally, you will still be rung through the legal ringer. First the knife carry-and-use stigma. Then your background, your comments on social media, your "unusual" (they will call it) interest in weapons. Your knife brand name and your knife social group. Your tattoos. Everything will be used against you. And you will spend a lot of money on lawyers. I have written about these obstacles extensively elsewhere. Violence sucks in general, but this will suck a bit worse.

So, despite all the negativity, I still maintain the *Force Necessary: Knife* course as a storehouse of information and research on the subject. Somebody has to do it. Knife versus hand. Knife versus stick. Knife versus knife. Knife versus gun threats. Standing on down to floor/ground. Legal issues. Use of Force. Rules of engagement. Psychology. History. (Certainly not just knife dueling.)

I will leave you "never-ever-knife" folks with this thought. This question. It's 4 a.m. and you hear two thugs breaking in your back door. Your spouse and kids are asleep. Presuming you are unfortunate enough, deprived enough, not to have a gun handy, do you reach for the biggest kitchen knife you can get your hands on? Or, will they get to your big kitchen knife first instead, as so many home invaders and rapists like to use *your* kitchen knives, so they aren't caught with a knife in transit. If you don't even think about getting a kitchen knife in that very dark moment? You are a very poorly trained, self defense, survivalist. If you do realize you need to get the biggest knife you can find? You may have just joined that crazy knife cult you so quickly dismiss!

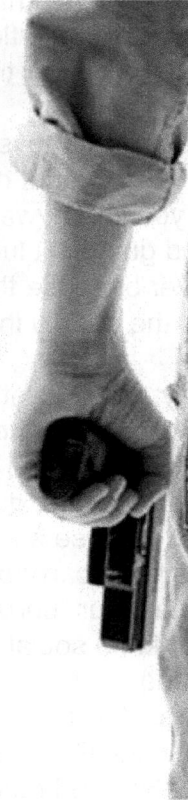

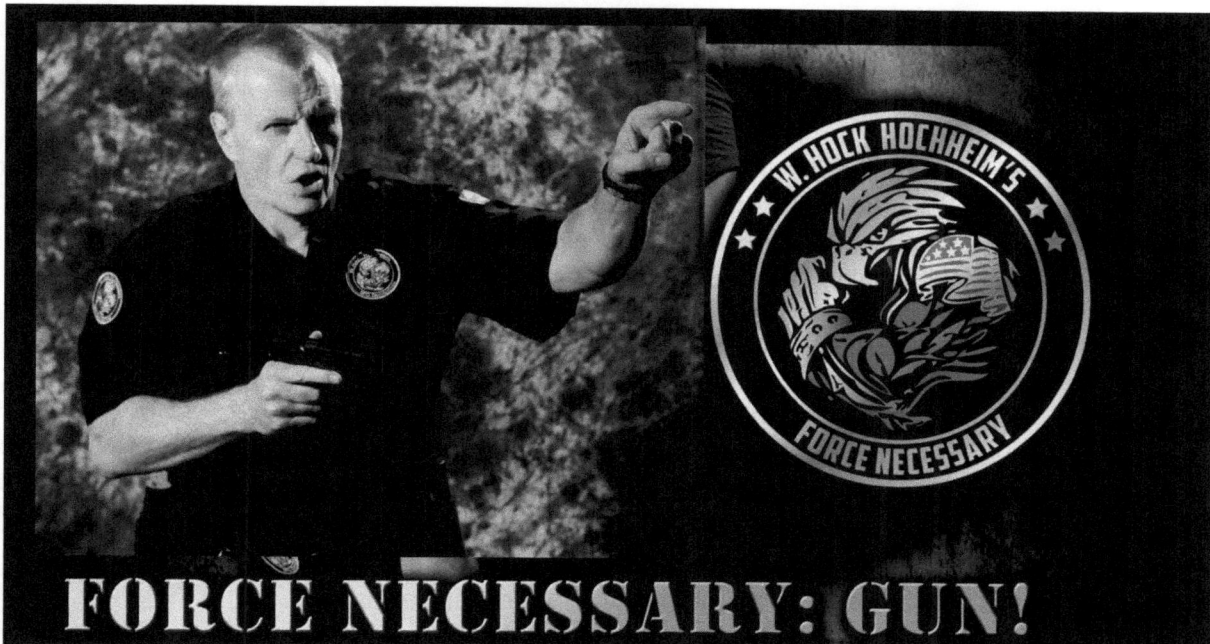

FORCE NECESSARY: GUN!

CHAPTER 22: FORCE NECESSARY: GUN "EXTERNAL FOCUS" LEVEL 2

Review Training Mission One and Gun Level 1

Review Commonalities

Examine *Stop 2* as explored within the Gun Level 2 context.
Examine the "What" question as explored within the Gun Level 2 context.
Examine the Footwork Drill #2: The In and Out Drill "while holding" a gun.
Examine the universal grip releases from Part One of this book.
Continue studying your local self defense laws.

Physical Performance Requirements

Problem-solving firearm retention.
- protecting the belt and holster, lanyard or shoulder carry long gun.
- protecting the drawn pistol or long gun while drawn, while presented, while being fired.

Problem-solving the *Stop 2* version of the Ambush, Dodge, Evasion, Counter Exercise

Problem-solving the Tangler Exercise.

First - A Note on Safety

Start training sessions with a safety briefing on live fire and levels of simulated ammo fire. While the classic 4 basic gun safety rules cover live fire, they cannot cover simulated ammo training in precisely the same way, because we will absolutely be pointing and shooting training weapons at each other. Constantly. Be constantly vigilant about your training weapons, and your fellow trainees and trainers. This creates a heavy burden of concern. And do not create casual bad habits with simulated ammo pistols that may play over to real firearms. Remember the course safety motto, *"We are each other's safety officers."*

Stop 2 of the Stop 6: Grabs on Fingers, Hands, Wrist and Weapons

In Gun Level 1 we drew the pistol and raised the rifle under various stressors, under the *Stop 1* parameters of a hands-off, somewhat distant showdown. The main thrust here in Gun Level 2 is solving the *Stop 2* problems. The essence of the study is the *"Death Grip of the"* Drill. Familiarization of that covers a lot of problem-solving. You are about to draw the pistol, drawing, or have drawn the pistol and the enemy grabs your weapon-side limb or your gun. You may grab his weapon-bearing limb too, or not. You are holding a weapon. The enemy might be:

- empty-handed.
- holding a stick, or sheathed stick.
- holding a knife or a pocketed or sheathed knife.
- holding a pistol or one holstered or tucked.
- holding a long gun, or has a long gun slung/attached to his body.

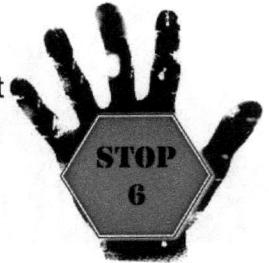

The "What-Gun," of the Ws and H Questions?

Look at the beginning of this book to study the overall what questions. Specific to the gun, here are some "what-gun" to consider:

What gun will you buy and/or carry?
What gun training course will you take?
What is your gun "mission?" What if any mission do you have?
What will you be wearing that either covers or conceals your
  weapon?
What are your the local laws about guns? Carrying? Brandishing? Using?
What do you expect to accomplish with your gun?
What is your "weapons continuum" Are you also carrying other weapons?
What happens when you become "adrenalized" with a gun?
What is the weapons disparity? Disparity is defined as, lack of similarity or equality;
  inequality; difference: a disparity in age; disparity in rank. And a disparity of
  weapons, such as knife versus a pistol.
"What happens next? After you use that gun, what happens next? Redemption?
  Jail? Law suit?

Continue to try and collect, and answer the "what-gun" questions.

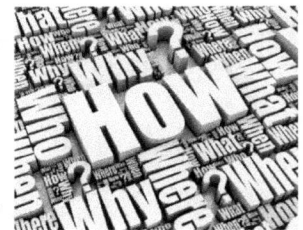

Footwork #2: The In and Out , "While Holding" a Firearm, Footwork
As previously covered in the first part of this book, practice the in and out footwork pattern while holding a pistol, one hand or two handed, and a long gun.

Series 1: Left foot is anchored in the axis. Right foot works in and out at about 2 and 4 or 5 o'clock.
- while holding a pistol.
- while holding a long gun.

Series 2: Right foot is anchored in the axis. Left foot works in and out at about 10 and 7 or 8 o'clock.
- while holding a pistol.
- while holding a long gun.

Series 3: Quick review of *Stop 1*:
- step and draw the pistol, and re-holster.
- step and raise the long gun.

Experiment with:
* barrel up.
* barrel down.
* extended grip.
* contracted grip.

Series 4: One hand grip:
- step while holding a pistol.

><

Series 5: Two hand grip:
- step while holding a pistol.
- step while holding a long gun.

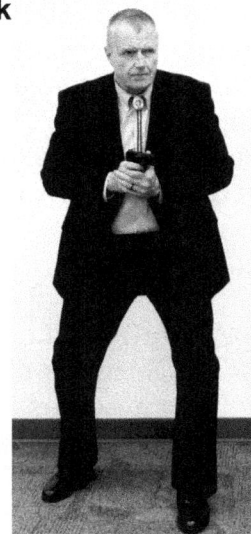

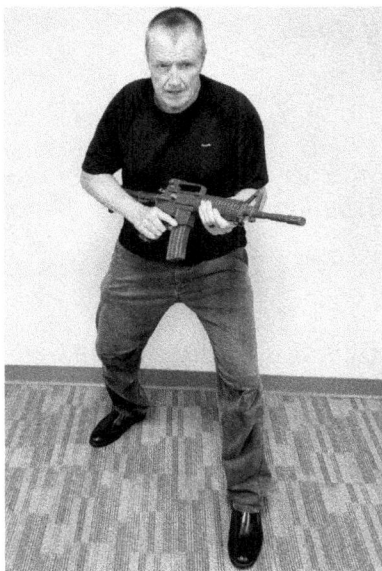

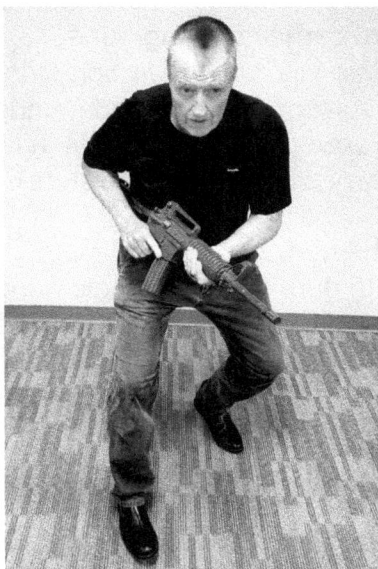

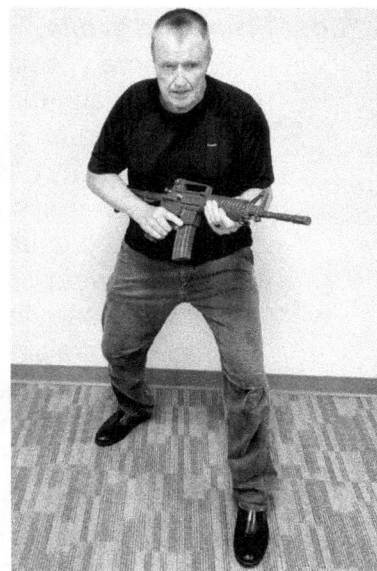

Sample: Right foot steps up and in, then right foot steps back and out, whole holding a long gun.

"Protecting the Belt" and "Protecting the Drawn Gun."
In Gun Level 1 we've drawn the pistol, "raised" or "dismounted" the long gun in stressful situations, within a no-contact, *Stop 1* range. Here in Level 2 we remain very much in the beginning draw events and will cover the challenge in the vitally important subject of grabs You grab. He grabs in general and handgun retention. Stress draws and retention are important in all *Stops* of the *Stop 6*, so lessons learned here are important. The mission of Level 2 and *Stop 2* is protecting the belt and protecting the drawn pistol, and "raised" long gun.

Where They Look?
Suspects often peek or stare at their goals. They size you up and also your gun carry sites. You might use the old police line, "Sir, do you mind looking at me when I talk to you, and not at my pistol?" This lets them know you are aware of this.

Overall retention, "who, what, where, when, how and why."
Who will try and take it, who is taking my gun?
What will be, what is, the situation?
Where will this happen? Locations? Where am I carrying my gun on my person?
When am I vulnerable for a gun loss?
How will I react? How will he? How good is your holster? Your carry system?
Why am I there? Why is he disarming me?

Gun experts report an annual "90 percent" police rate of serious injury and death from your own lost weapon, if your gun is taken. There are no such studies done concerning citizens. Still, it is a very serious incident to have your gun taken. It will be a legal, case-by-case situation.

"Lost From and While." Why we lose our pistols and long guns
- review primary, secondary and tertiary sites for handguns.
- review sling and lanyard carries for long guns.
- review the search chapter in *Training Mission One*.
- you gave it away? We surrender the weapon, under some sort of coercion. If I may suggest, never give up your gun. More on this in later *Training Missions*.
- taken from the usual carry sites (usually holsters).
- we lose the weapon -
    * while carrying the gun.
    * while drawing the gun, from our single hand and/or double hand grips.
    * while presenting the gun, from our single hand and/or double hand grips.
    * while firing the gun, from our single hand and/or double hand grips.
    * while moving with the drawn gun, from our single hand and/or double hand grips.
    * in doorways and cornering.
        - counter with slice the pie if you can.
        - counter with third eye" contracted two hand grip.
        - counter with one hand contracted grip.

Part 1: Protecting the "Belt and the Undrawn Weapon."

How will an opponent grab your pistol at its carry site? How will he lunge for your carry site? How close is too close? Enforcement experts suggest two giant steps and a lunge away is a safer distance, which still can be traversed in but a second.

- Grab 1: hits you first (once or multiple times) and then grabs for your gun.
- Grab 2: grabs your gun first and then hits you (once or multiple times).
- Grab 3: hits and grabs all at once.
- Grab 4: with a solo hand, right or left hand 12, 3, 6, and 9 o'clock.
- Grab 5: with two hands, 12, 3, 6, and 9 o'clock.
- Grab 6: possibly from above (Stairs? Or, you are downed?).
- Grab 7: possibly from below (Stairs? Or, he is downed and reaching up?).

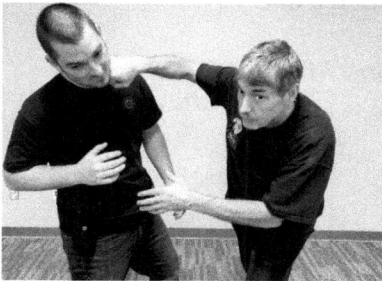
Hits you first, then grabs for your gun.

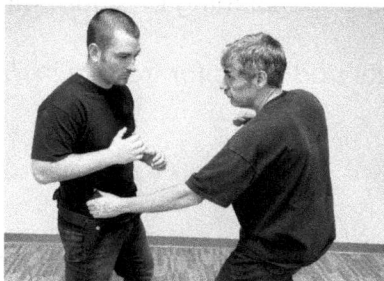
Grabs your gun first, then starts hitting.

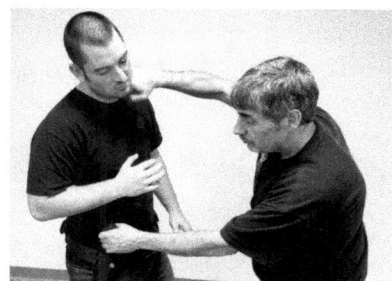
Hits and grabs at the same time.

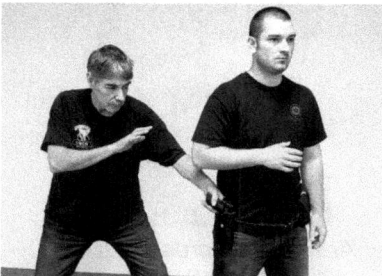
Solo hand grab from 12, 3, 6 and 9 o'clock.

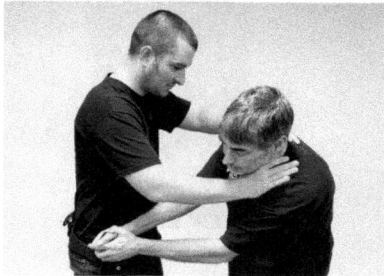

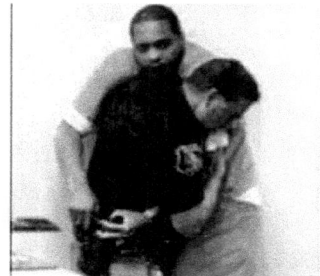
Both hands grab from 12, 3, 6 and 9 o'clock.

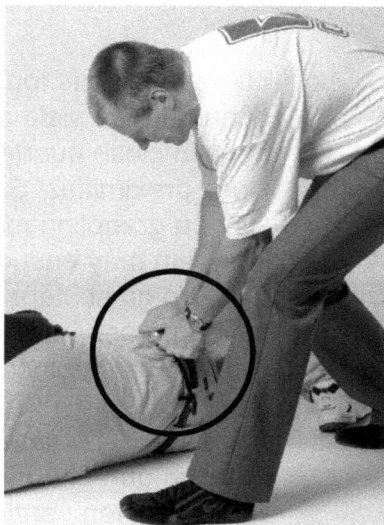
From above.

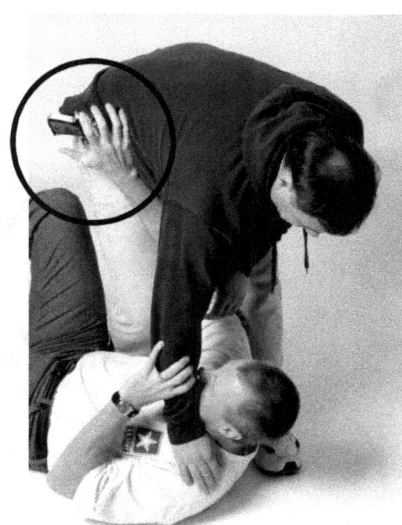
From below.

Protecting the belt: How is your interview stance in regard to weapon retention?
Given the list potential list of grabs, how do you stand in suspicious or dangerous situations? Consider...

> - your arm positions?
>> * lightly cross arms to protect shoulder holsters.
>> * arm tight against your hip carry.
>
> - gun back or gun forward?
>> * as in a stance with your legs. One foot forward or back.
>> * as in a stance with your torso.
>> * as in holster positioning on your belt, or carry site.
>
> - review the tip-offs and clues for trouble in _Training Mission One._

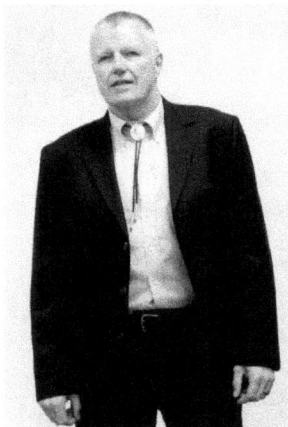

Arm tight against hip carry.

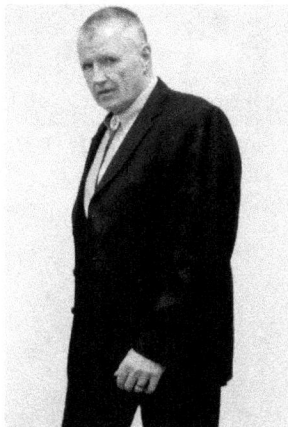

Weapon side back.

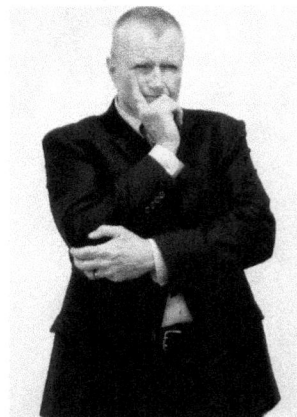

Arms lightly crossed for shoulder holsters, as well as configured for a jacket sweep and draw.

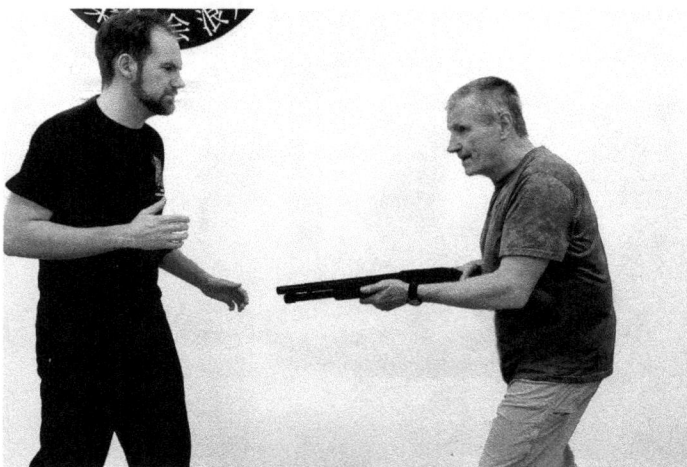

How close is too close?

How close is too close? It is often hard to wield around long guns in close quarters and in close proximities. Sling or no sling, a grappling match over a long gun may ensue. Remember the "two giant steps and a lunging reach," advice, and how fast such a distance can be leaped.

In my past, I have foregone the long gun and used a pistol instead, when I anticipated tight quarters. The choice is yours.

Protecting the Belt: Your holster and retention possibilities

As a reminder, most common criminals do not use holsters. They stick their pistols in their belt line or pockets. "Girlfriend holster," - gang members, thugs and terrorists around the world often have their girlfriends hold their weapons, so when searched by authorities they are unarmed. So, you might say, holsters come in "all shapes and sizes," and qualities.

We, the non-criminals, the "nice, good guys" worry over, contemplate, argue about and buy "nice, good" guns, and "nice, good" holsters. And we are still often killed by unskilled, thoughtless, holster-less, untrained, muggers, thugs, or nut-cases. Such is the importance of, nature of the interview and/or ambush studies. A review of the weapon carry sites:

- *Primary carry sites*, as in on the body in the "quick draw," location, such as pockets and belt line. Think "quick draw."

- *Secondary carry sites,* as in "back up," locations on the body. The clothing diggers, like boot/ankle weapons and neck knives, even pistols, places that require a few seconds to procure a weapon. Think "back-up."

- *Tertiary carry sites*, as in off the body. They are weapon sites just hidden somewhere, or are always hidden there, like. well, anywhere! A glove box in a car. Under a seat or chair. On a shelf, on a stone wall? Use your imagination. Think "lunge and reach."

Some things to consider about holster selection are:
- what, where is your carry site on your body?
- what threat level do you want?
- general durability and quality?
- will your holster "travel with the grab" on and around your belt in the space between belt loops or uniform keepers?
- do you have the $100 holster and the $5 belt? And is the holster solidly connected to the belt. You do not want to pull your gun and the holster come out with it.

"Yes, we have the $10 holster (or belt) for the $10 life." (Old saying.)

Protecting the belt: Retention holster mechanisms...

...are intended to prevent the gun from being drawn or obtained by anyone other than the intended user, or prevent the gun from coming easily loose from the holster. There are various "threat" levels and holsters developed into "safety systems" in the last decades. For the many holster companies, the level of retention on a holster directly corresponds to the number of retention mechanisms that keep the gun from coming out of the holster.

Military vet and firearms expert, Mike Woods described this history best, "Back in 1973, former FBI agent and police instructor Bill Rogers started designing and building some excellent duty holsters that incorporated improved retention capabilities. In an effort to quantify these improvements, Rogers created a testing protocol in 1975 that awarded retention "levels" to holsters.By the mid-2000s, Safariland had even introduced the first Level IV and V-designated holsters, indicating they were capable of resisting four or five Level I-style attacks (respectively) as their security devices were disabled step-by-step, in sequence."
I would like to relate four holster retention stories.

Retention story #1
Several years ago I taught at a major US city police academy, an in-service combat-ives course. Running there also was the rookie class.There was a woman in this rookie class that was consistently having her pistol taken during defensive tactics classes. Instructors told me she'd purchased a high level (many tricks to draw) retention holster. There were so many twists and turns, pushes and pulls, that she herself could not draw her own gun. Their final qualifications were coming up and she absolutely refused to give up her new safer holster, even though she literally could not pull the gun out on demand! I left before there was a conclusion. My best guess though, is she changed holsters.

Retention story #2
I was teaching a Chicago seminar once that was attended by a large group of area police officers. One of the scenarios I taught was drawing and shooting after your stong-side/gun-side arm had been incapacitated as in injured or shot. You cross-draw, pull your gun with your support hand, taking care not to accidentally insert your pinky into the trigger guard, a common discharge problem from this angle. We do this standing and on the ground with simulated ammo as the practitioner actually has to shoot a moving, thinking person closing in and/or shooting back. Next came a break and I saw all the officers over in one corner of the gym, their support arm stretching and reaching unsuccessfully around their backs to pull their pistol. Only the skinniest, most limber, police woman could do it. I asked them what they were doing, and they told me that their guns and holsters were department issue. The holster retention device would not allow for such a frontal, angle removal. That holster company feared that gun take-aways would usually occur from the front. In order to pull the pistol from that model holster, a shooter had to grab the gun pull/angle it back, and then out. This holster prohibited the easy, common sense draw I, and so many others, teach. (And, what about drawing while seated in a car?)

Retention story #3
In the 90s I was teaching an Air Force SWAT-style team and the San Antonio SWAT team. I was, once again doing simulated ammo scenarios and was doing one on the ground, on my back. I asked for a gun belt and an SAPD SWAT officer quickly gave me his. On my back, when time to draw and shoot, I could not remove the pistol from the holster. We all gathered around closely to inspect this. The SWAT officer's holster had several retention tricks built in. His holster company had decided that most pistols were removed from the front, requiring a pull backward first, then out. Since I was flat on my back, I could not pull the gun back. No one, all vets, in the class had thought of this, least of all this SWAT officer until this experiment. One would think that a holster company would put such news on the packaging label and advertisement.
      "WARNING! You cannot draw this weapon when down on your back!"

Retention story #4
Back in the day," as a detective, I was working with a fellow investigator on a case when we heard of a very nearby armed robbery on the police radio. We were so close, we actually saw the suspect run from the store. We drove as far as we could to chase

him, then had to bail from the car and follow on foot. A few fences were jumped and the robber got into a cement factory with a large, open gravel lot, and big trucks. We'd split up, but we both saw the robber stop by a truck as we could see his legs under the truck. We drew our guns as we closed in, and my partner pulled his .45 out on the run. He pulled the pistol AND paddle holster out and pointed it at the bad guy. He made a violent jerk and the holster flew off the pistol. The robber, facing our two guns, surrendered. We laughed about it later because we were a little crazy back then, but we also learned a lesson about holsters.

Retention story #5
The Sandpit Travesty. One of my officer friends once, lost his pistol and was shot and killed by a fugitive. Without revealing any personal details, this SWAT officer had a retention duty holster on regular duty, but when on a SWAT assignment had a "drop" holster as shown previously, a low, thigh, tactical holster, minus any retention. His pistol was taken in a ground fight, and he was shot in the head. Since sad events like this, retention devices started appearing on the most "tactical" of holsters, (even Taser holsters).

His agency went on a PR, press junket to prove how much they cared about the subject, suggesting that holster retention was so well trained. They filmed a news segment for TV with their officers training in a sandpit. A trainer grabbed a trainee's holstered pistol and tried to remove it. The trainee held on and basically the two engages in a stupid, standing wrestling match – four hands on a holstered rubber gun. Sometimes falling down in the ruckus.

Perhaps to an ignorant novice, this seemed like terrific, tough-guy, training? But it is not. No one threw a punch, kicked a nut, yanked head hair, popped an eye, or broke a bone. A bad guy wanting to kill you will do all these things. An officer, wanting to stay alive will do all these things. All the things that cannot happen full speed in training, but can be partially simulated, yet still are totally ignored. And like you learn to forget to punch in Judo, bad training makes you forget how to survival fight. This is not preparing an officer, or any one toting a gun, to respond properly to a disarm attack. And that is why, this sort of sandpit style training is a stupid travesty. And it doesn't have to be in a sandpit either, as you'll find stupid anywhere.

Retention stories summary
Mike Woods sums it up by saying, "Buyer Beware. So, if you're shopping for a holster - as an individual or as an agency buyer - you need to go beyond the ratings and advertising hype by fully understanding how the various security features work. You also need to ask hard questions about the specific tests and criteria that a manufacturer uses to rate their products. Until the industry unites around a single standard, it's not enough to assume that Brand X's Level III rating denotes a comparable level of security, durability and quality as Brand Y's Level III rating. Your choice of duty gear is too critical and your safety too important to be influenced by clever marketing. Ask tough questions, get the details, and make sure you're comparing apples-to-apples."

Protecting the Belt: Holsters

Holster retention comes in two "flavors": **passive retention** and **active retention**...

   Passive retention is retention force that's inherent to a holster by virtue of its design and construction. To put that a little better, the materials used and the shape of a holster make it hold a pistol to a certain degree. Any natural retentive properties a holster has without having to do anything to it is the passive retention.

   Active retention, on the other hand, is user-actuated in that an active retention device has to be engaged. Some holsters have one or the other, and some have both - it all depends on the design of the holster in question. Usually, a "retention holster" will have multiple retention devices, offering far more security than many standard carry holsters."

- AlienGearHolsters.com

Post Falls, Idaho

Protecting the Belt: Holster samples

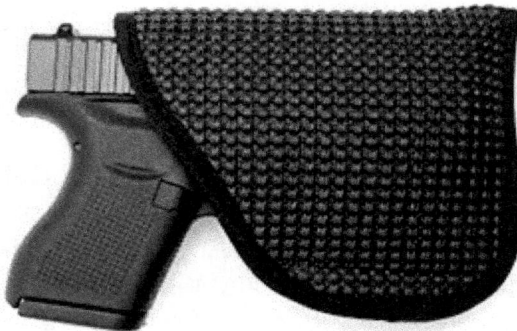

A friction holster.

Holster sample 1: Friction! Called "passive resistance" holsters
A passive resistance holster has no bells and whistle tricks. The holster is usually a tight, tight fit with your precise gun. That tight fit is all the resistance offered.
   There are "sticky" holsters. Friction on the inside and friction on the outside, too. As advertised - the "friction" holster is made from a black textured material that is lightweight, durable and sweat resistant. It is both comfortable and functional. The holster stays in place by using friction in the pocket and/or compression in the waistband. This unique combination allows the handgun to be easily and safely drawn, while leaving the holster securely in place. You have to see if you trust all that. Your choice.

Holster sample 2: Thumb "breaks"
The thumb break is usually made of the same material as the holster. A thumb break, or sometimes called a retaining strap, is a safety device installed on many holsters to prevent a weapon from being unintentionally drawn. The thumb break is held in place by a simple snap mechanism, usually metal, which may be disengaged by pushing the thumb upward against it.

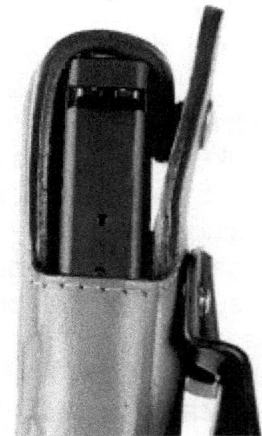

The simple thumb break. As you access the pistol, the process alone seems to pop open the snap.

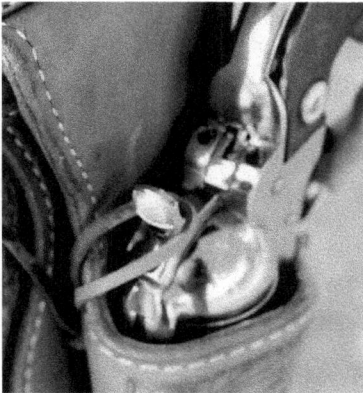

Even the old cowboy holsters had a retention "device." A simple leather loop. A "hammer loop."

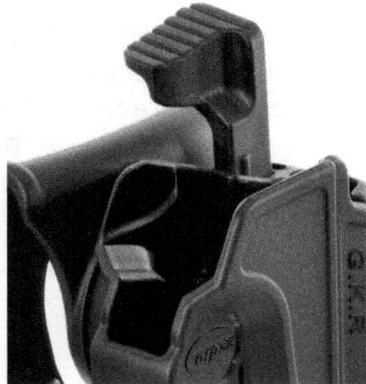

This is thumb "drive." Push down on that grooved "pump" and the pistol is released for a draw.

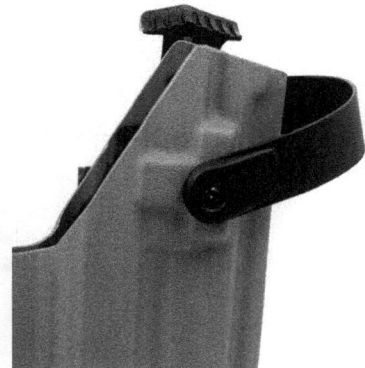

The "hood." This Centaurian model has a "humb-drive" release, that allows the hood to slip forward.

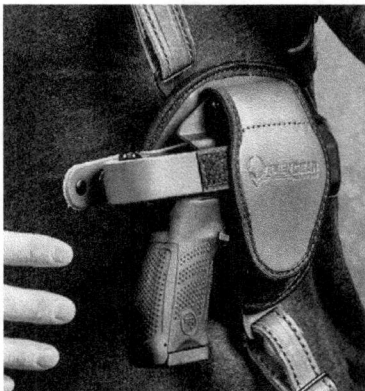

Thumb break on a shoulder holster.

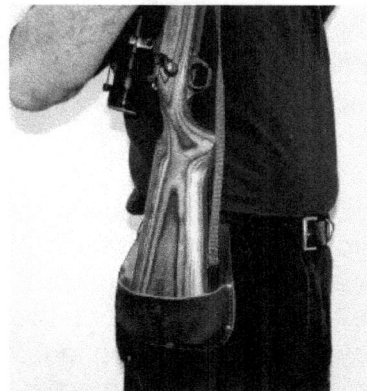

Ever see a..."rifle holster?"

One thing we have learned after wrestling around with replicas in thumb break holsters, is that the thumb break can be rather easily dislodged by an enemy too, just in the act of grabbing and wrestling over the gun.

Holster sample 3: Modified draw stroke retention
Drawing a gun from a common holster is simple. You just pull the pistol up and out of the holster. But, as I mentioned in the above stories, the directions of the pull has been restricted and /or modified. These holsters require the user to push or pull and/or twist the gun to facilitate its removal from the holster. You might have to push down first, or rock the gun back or forth, or pull and twist in or out to draw the weapon. Manufacturers always claim, the complications of a draw is simply a "training issue."

Holster sample 4: Retention screw options

In any application, screws are used to draw things more tightly and hold them together better. In this case, it's the same for holster tension screws. The more you tighten down on the screws, the better the fit and friction between holster and gun. Screws can line up the side of a holster, set for your choice of when the gun "breaks" from the holster.

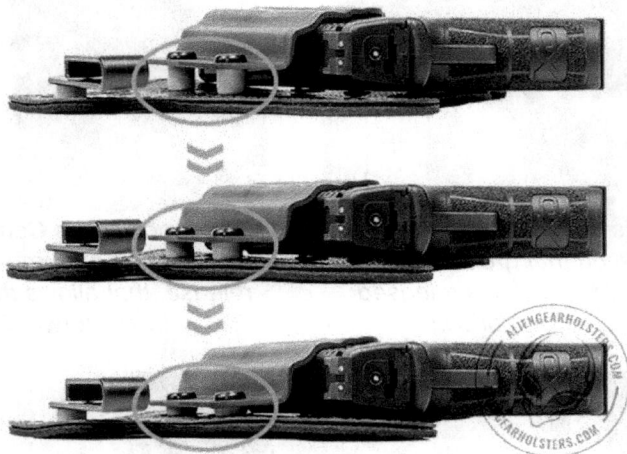

AlienGearHolsters.com demonstrates the retention screw concept.

Holster sample 5: How high or low do you go?

If you have a hip carry holster, the "height" on your holster affects your draw and retention strategies. You can select a high ride on the belt, medium ride on the belt, low on the belt, even a very low, tactical "drop leg." All these have retention considerations and "who, what, where, when, how and why" questions to pursue. For example, a high ride might be protected at times by a tight arm or tight elbow pressed against it. A medium or low-ride might be protected by your hand's easy access.

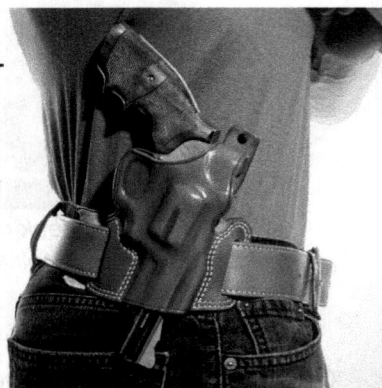

A high ride, holster sample. A tight, arm tuck in suspicious circumstances can start protecting your weapon.

In holster summary

It is not my purpose to turn this chapter into a holster catalog, but to provoke thoughts on the subject. Protecting the belt! There are many such stories. Keep your eyes and ears open for them. And, keep experimenting. Just think about handgun/holster retention. In 26 years in line operations, I have had only five attempts on my holstered pistol. There are many attempts on record all over the world. It happens. Statistically your odds on an attempt may be like one in 40,000? But if it happens to you? It's one in one.

Protecting the Belt: Holster situations, challenges and reflexive solutions.
Are you aware of and prepared for these situations? Consider all of them.

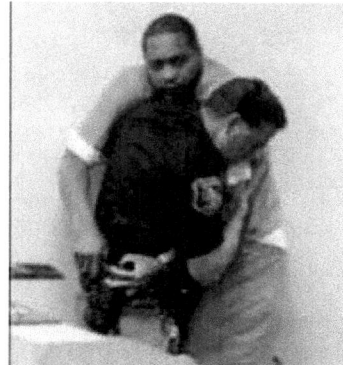

1: Completely trust your retention holster? And use both hands to strike the grabber?
2: Jam your hand on your holstered handgun.
3: His hand atop your holstered handgun.
4: His two hands on your holstered handgun.
5: Your hand atop his hand on your holstered handgun.
6: Your two hands atop his hand on your holstered handgun.
7: Your two hands atop his two hands on your holstered handgun.
8: Your same-side hand on his forearm as his hand on your holstered handgun.
9: Your far-side hand on his forearm, your same-side hand atop his hand, atop your gun.
10: A taken handgun often comes out upside, causing a stall in use?
11: Grabs from the front, right side, left side and rear.
12: All of the above via the common carry sites.
13: Long gun grab off a shoulder carry.
14: Long gun grab off a frontal carry.

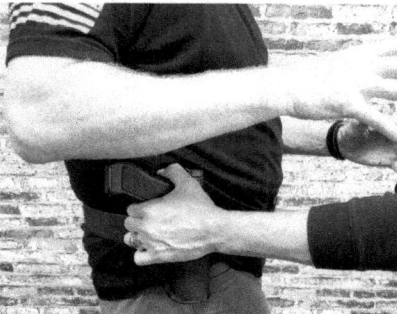
Sample: Completely trust your retention holster and fight on?

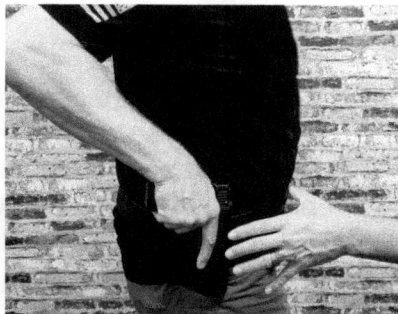
Sample: Your shoving-down hard on your holstered handgun.

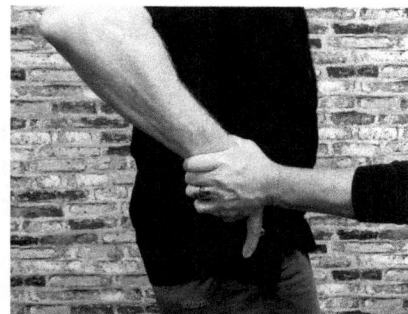
Sample: His hand atop your hand on your holstered handgun.

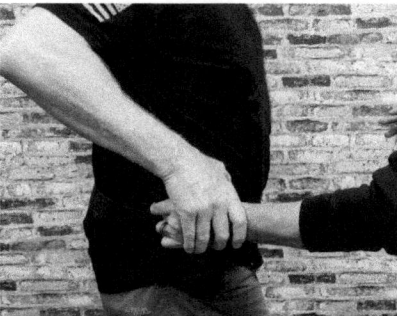
Sample: Your hand atop his hand on your holstered handgun.

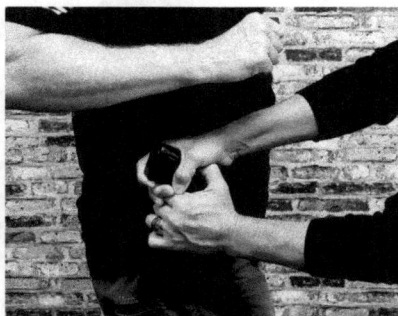
Sample: His two hands on your holstered handgun.

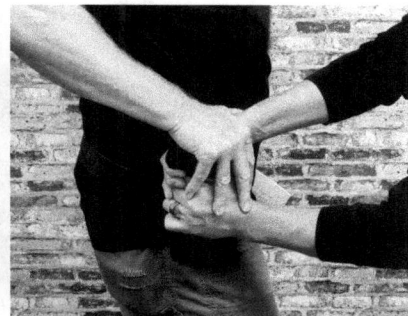
Sample: Your hand atop his two hands on your holstered handgun.

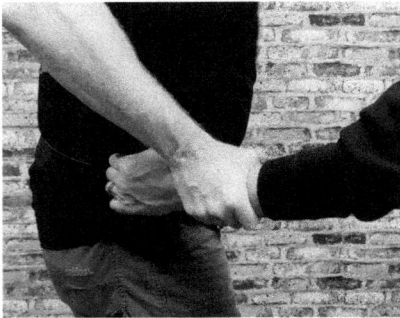

Sample: Your same side hand grabs his wrist.

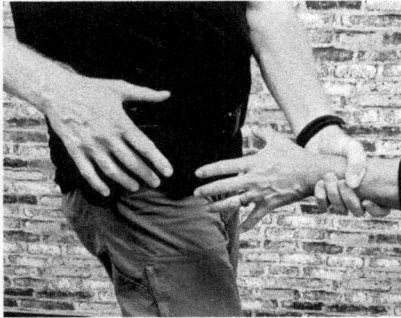

Sample: Your other hand grabs his wrist.

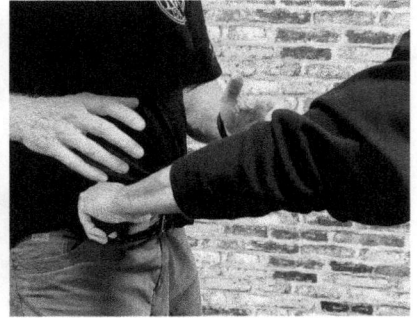

Sample: Both hands grab his grab.

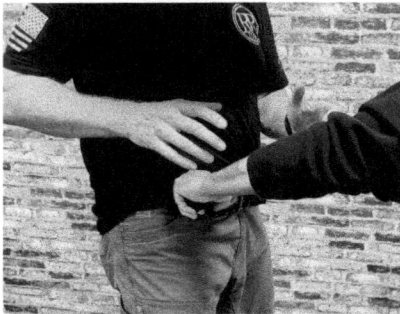

Sample: All of the above via the other carries. Here the appendix carry.

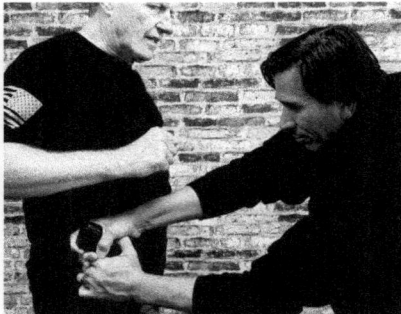

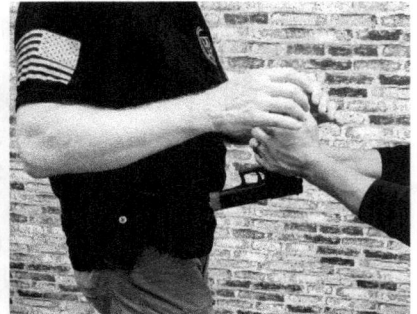

A taken handgun often comes out upside, causing a stall in use?

The upside down, frontal pull

If a bad guy grabs your pistol from a common belt carry, from the front and pulls it out. It will be upside down for him. This is a surprise to him, but I hope not to you. There is a strong chance, he will stall, and think, to upright the gun to use it. Take this time to squash him with all you got. Few practice shooting with an upside pistol.

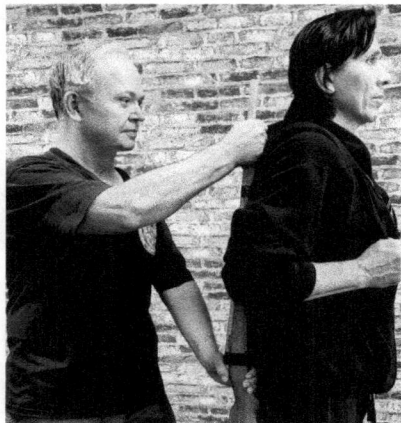

Sample: Grab of long gun off a shoulder carry.

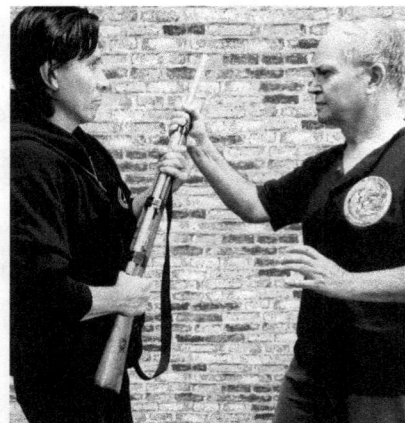

Sample: grab of long gun off a front carry.

Next, let's try and solve some of these...

Protecting the Belt, Gun in Holster Solutions

Universal belt protection retention methods
We discussed gear as being the first step. Body position the next step. Now for some movements. However universal? They probably aren't practiced enough. Here are my suggestions

Protecting the Belt, Gun in Holster 1: The Blocking of Strikes, Reaches and Attempted Grabs

We start in the very beginning. Remember your distance. Remember your footwork. In order to get your gun, the opponent must reach for it. If you see the reach attempt, you may blast it aside. You might use a palm strike, a palm slap, a hammer fist strike, or a forearm.

> Blocking drill 1: Trainer stands before trainee. Trainer lunges for a gun grab with a right hand. Trainee thwarts the attempt.

> Blocking drill 2: Trainer stands before trainee. Trainer lunges for a gun grab with a left hand. Trainee thwarts the attempt.

> Blocking drill 3: Trainer stands before trainee. Trainer lunges for a gun grab with both hands. Trainee thwarts the attempt.

> Blocking drill 4: Trainer stands before the trainee. Trainer tries to strike the trainee's head, and then tried for a gun grab. Trainee thwarts both.

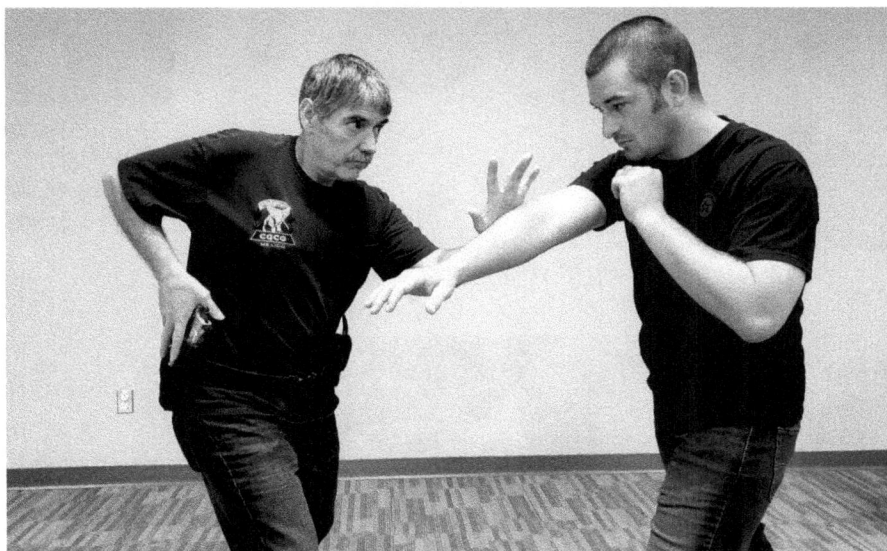

Thwart the attempted grab. Palm strikes, forearm strikes and footwork.

Protecting the Belt, Gun in Holster 2: His Hand Atop Your Hand, or Your Wrist.
My "Step Away from the Gun" scenario. You try to draw, but his hand gets on top of your hand. Or, you see his gun grab attempt and beat him to your gun. Either way, he doesn't have your gun! You do. Often this generic position ignites a frenzy of handgun retention methods that are limited in comparison to what you can do with your two hands free. You let go of your gun, lifting his hand also, as you step away, half of the in-and-out footwork of this level). Slap release and fight on, or you still might draw your pistol if needed?

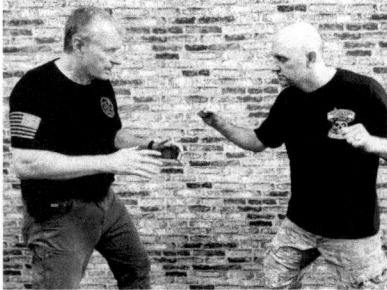

1: A suspect squares off, looking for a fight.

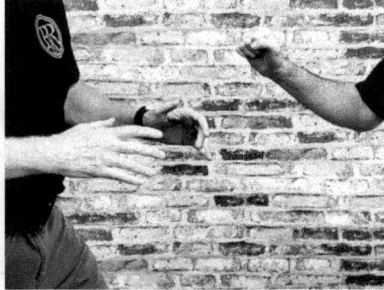

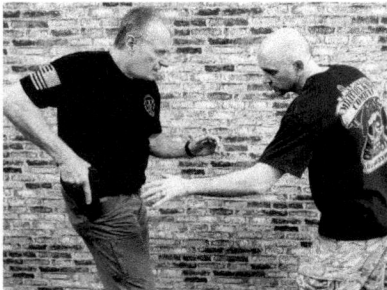

2: He makes a direct move for your gun. You protect your pistol.

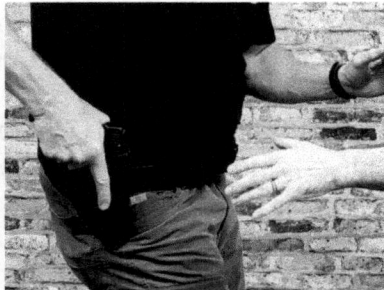

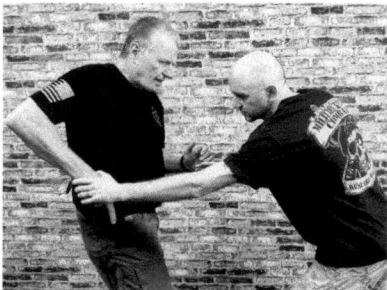

3: His hand lands on top of your hand.

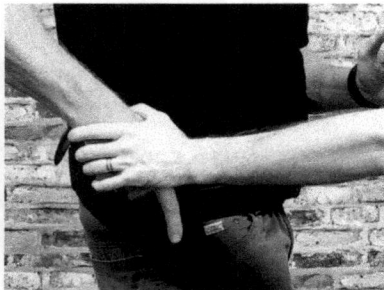

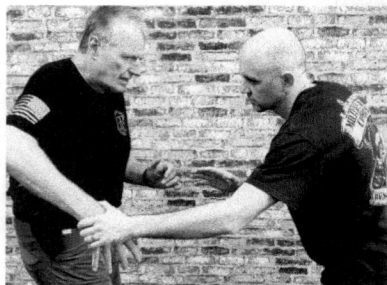

4: He only has your hand! NOT your holstered gun handle.
You let go and step back and away.

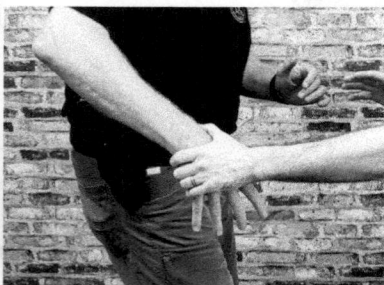

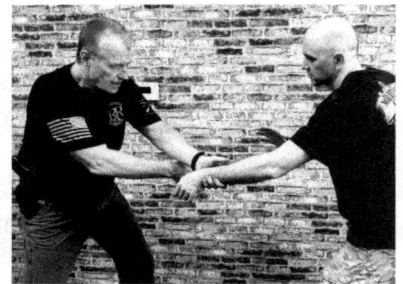

5: You slap release, and fight
on.

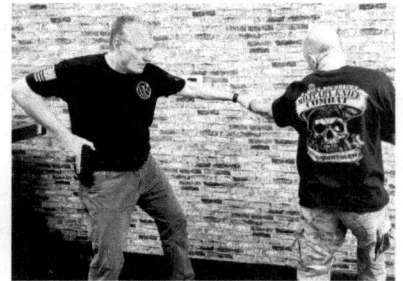

6: Or, you hang on and pull an
arm drag to the side, and
may decide to draw your
pistol anyway.

Protecting the Belt, Gun in Holster 3: Your Hand Atop His Hand.
If the bad guy grabs your holstered pistol, let's review the possibilities:
- with his right hand.
- with his left hand.
- with both hands.
- from the front, back, right-side, left side.
- from above, from below.
- differing carry sites on your body, will alter your response. Customize.

Despite your confidence in your holster's retention tricks, just about everyone reflexively puts their hand on top of his hand and shoves the pistol back into the holster, regardless of the carry site. Or, they grab what they can and that is the wrist or forearm. Or, they put their hand atop his hand and, with their free support hand, grab his wrist or forearm. You have now lost the ability to fight with that one protecting hand, which leads us to the next two vital series of gun in holster work-outs.

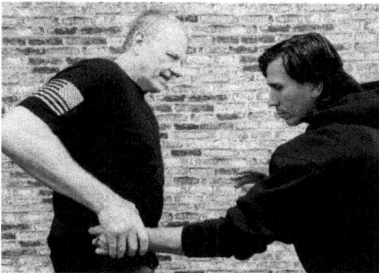

You ram your hand down on his hand to keep your pistol in your holster.

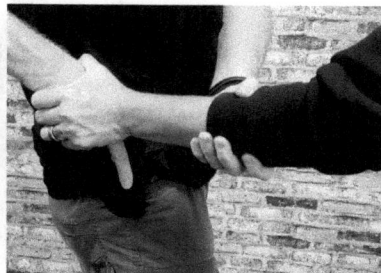

And, your support hand grabs at the best thing at the instant, like the attacker's wrist or forearm.

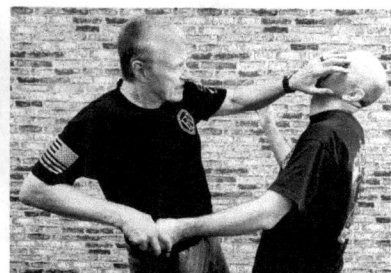

Your free hand grabs his arm to keep your pistol in your holster.Though a reflexive move, something like an eye strike with that free hand might be smarter.

By all statistics this is usually a lethal force, life threatening situation. My first suggestion is to protect your gun with one hand, as you probably, reflexively will, and attack/maul the eyes of the attacker with the other. Next, he probably will, reflexively also, try to stop the mauling with his free hand. Or, release one of his hands on your gun to stop you. Consider this eye attack, from *Training Mission One*, the first step in pistol retention.

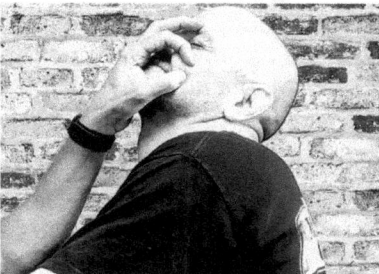

The eye attack and face maul.

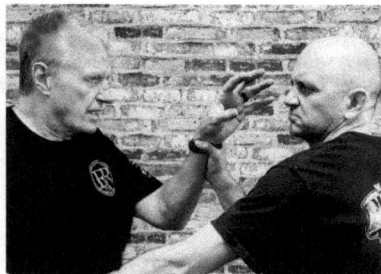

Now distracted, he might grab your attack.

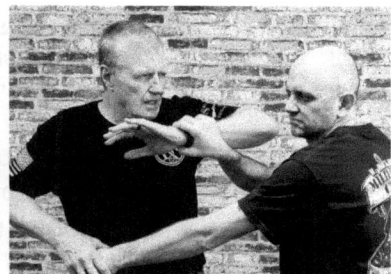

Use a release from this book such as the elbow roll-over to continue the mauling.

Protecting the Belt, Gun in Holster 4: The Body Twist.
Where is your carry site and will a football/rugby power, body twist knock his arms away? In my estimation, the second most popular pistol carry site after a side carry, or hip carry, is the old "pelvis carry," now called the "appendix carry." Despite some objections to this appendix, carry site, even from veterans, it offers an easier draw with the support hand in emergencies, such as when ground fighting.

Anyway, with these body twists, experiment in power, position and direction. Think about how a body twist and arm blast might just "blast" the pistol from your holster! If he has a firm grip on your gun and your holster (and belt) is not up to standards.

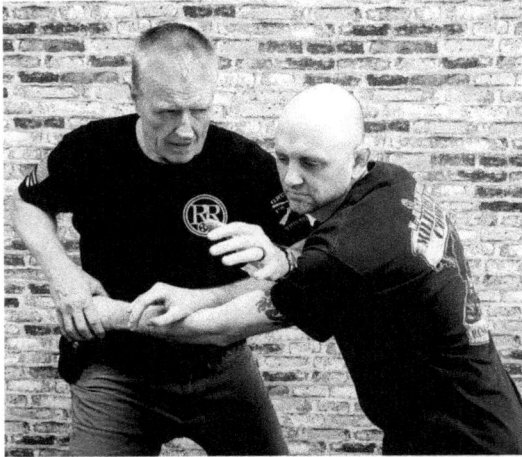

Twisting and arm blasting...

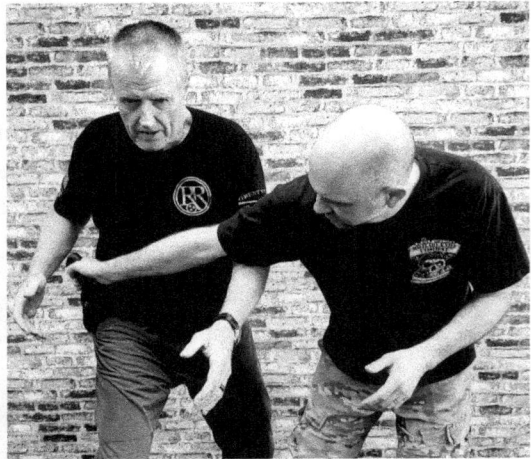

Will your twist and arm blast help him yank out your pistol?

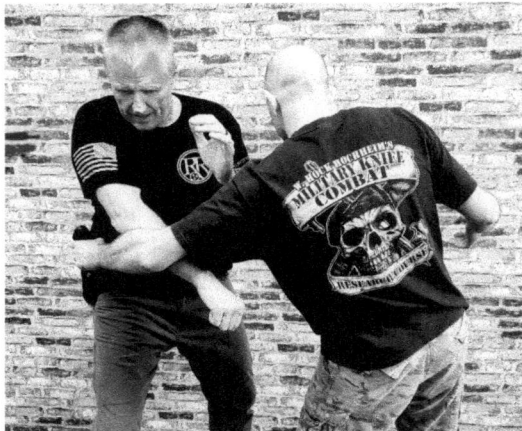

Will your twist and arm blast help him yank out your pistol? Aim your strike well, so as to not help the upward extraction of your pistol..

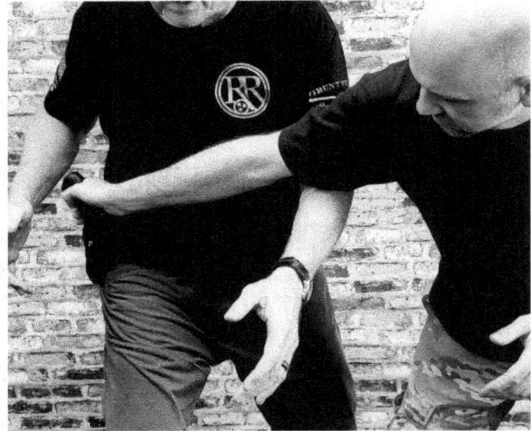

At some point with a body twist you will either hyper extend his elbow? Or let go of your protective grip to get his arm free.

Couple the ramming body twist with the basic releasing methods in this book. The slapping hand, palm strike, as listed here in level 2, *Stop* 2, seems to work well in conjunction with the body ram twists in this predicament. And, at some point, you have to know when to let go of his hand on your weapon.

> - powerful body, ram twists.
> - palm strikes/slaps (and forearms) to the arms.
> - knowing when to let go of your gun hand, after the strike and twist works.

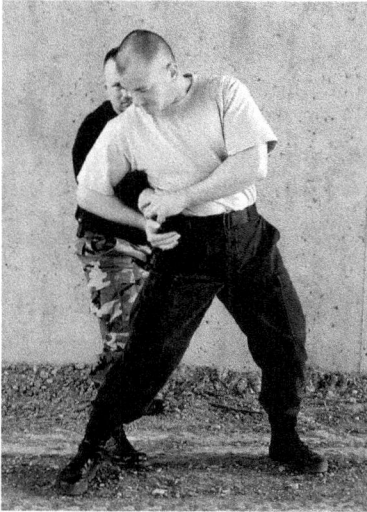

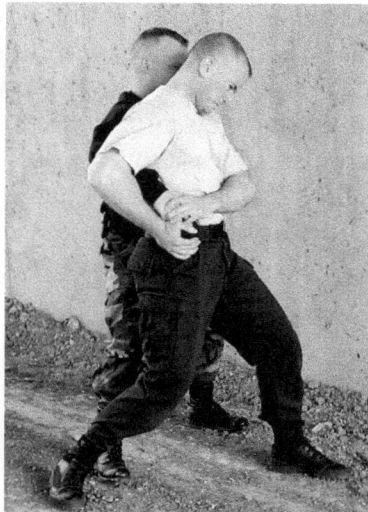

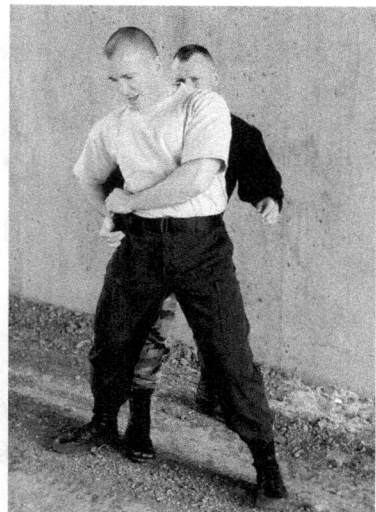

Gun grab from behind. Freeze the pistol in the holster.

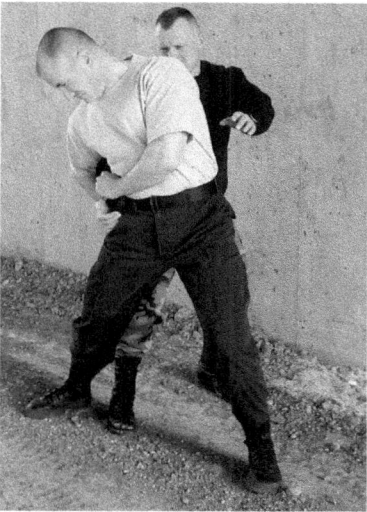

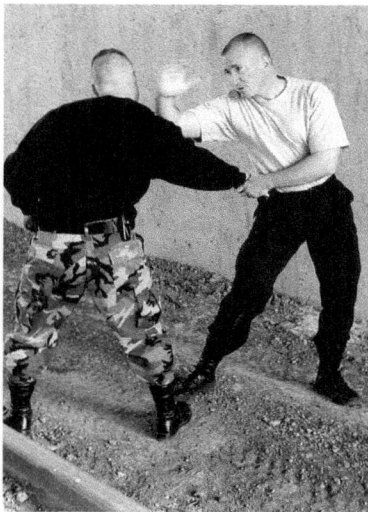

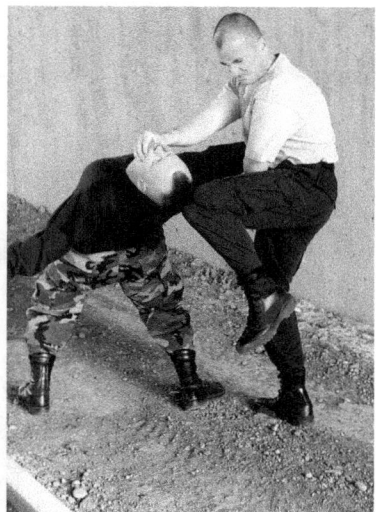

*He hasn't grabbed you anywhere else yet. Turn out on the gun side
and away from the grabber. Beat him and kick him.*

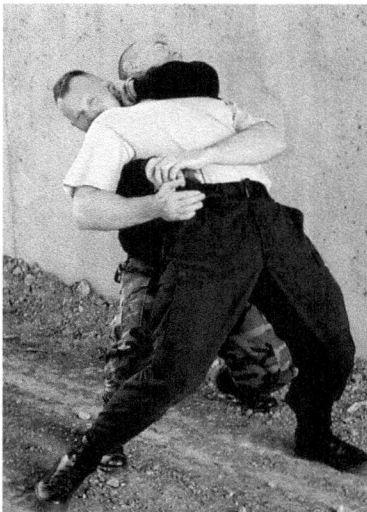

*If he does grab your holstered weapon
and you like this? Oh, no! Bad! But this
is a Stop 4 "bear hug" problem and
we will solve it in Stop 4!*

Protecting the Belt, Gun in Holster 5: Strike and kick sets
You might have to fight like mad to defend yourself and your firearm. Here is a method. The trainer puts his hand on your holstered weapon and he holds a martial arts pad or shield. While securing your gun in your holster with one hand, the other hand practices these striking (blocking) and add kicking sets recorded in this book. The very fact that you are pushing your gun down in your holster will affect your striking power, if you let it. Below is a regular workout list for this situation. Each strike category is further developed in later *Training Mission* books and the *Force Necessary:Hand* course.

- Sets of eye attacks.

- Sets of palm strikes.
- to face and/or throat height.
- to torso height.
- to grabbing arms.

Sets of punches.
- to face and/or throat height.
- to torso height.
- to grabbing arms.

Sets of hammer fists.
- to face and/or throat height.
- to torso height.
- to grabbing arms.

Sets of forearm strikes.
- to face and/or throat height.
- to torso height.
- to grabbing arms.

Sets of elbows.
- to face and/or throat height.
- to torso height.
- to grabbing arms.

Sets of blocks, (trainer needs to throws some strikes).

Sets of closed expandable baton draws and strikes.
- to face and throat height.
- to torso height.
- to grabbing arms.

Sets of baton draws and strikes.
- to face and throat height.
- to torso height.
- to grabbing arms.

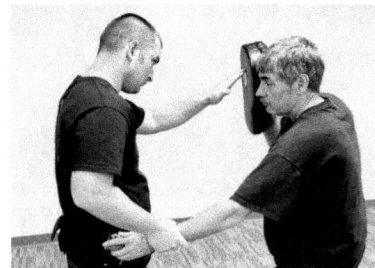
Eye attacks with grabbed gun.

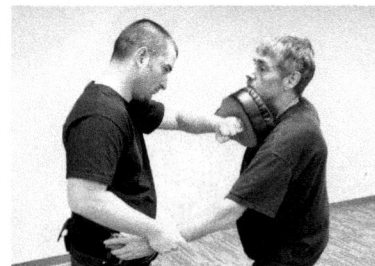
All punches, hammers....

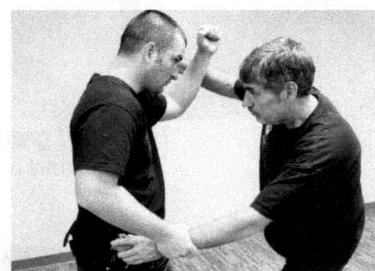
All blocks.

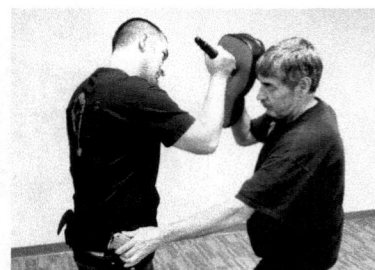
Closed and opened batons. It is likely your first response will be with a hurried closed one.

Sets of closed folder draws and strikes.
- to face and throat height.
- to torso height.
- to grabbing arms.

Sets of knife draws and open folder or fixed blade strikes.
- to face and throat height.
- to torso height.
- to grabbing arms.

Sets of knee to leg and groin.

Sets of shin kicks.

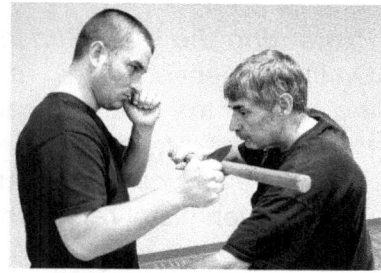

Trainer holds onto gun, trainee pulls dull knife and "cuts" stick.

Protecting the belt striking sample

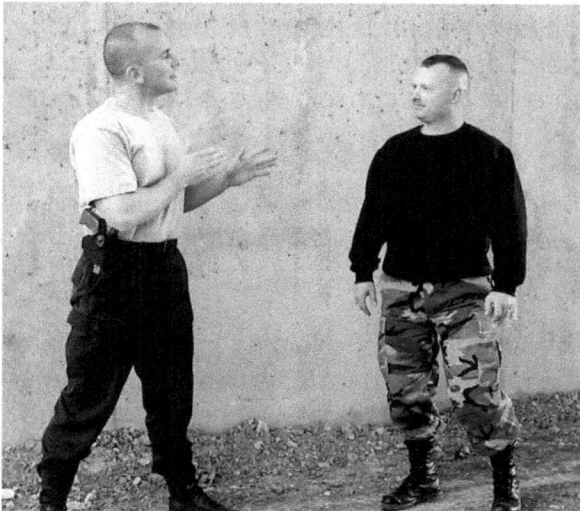

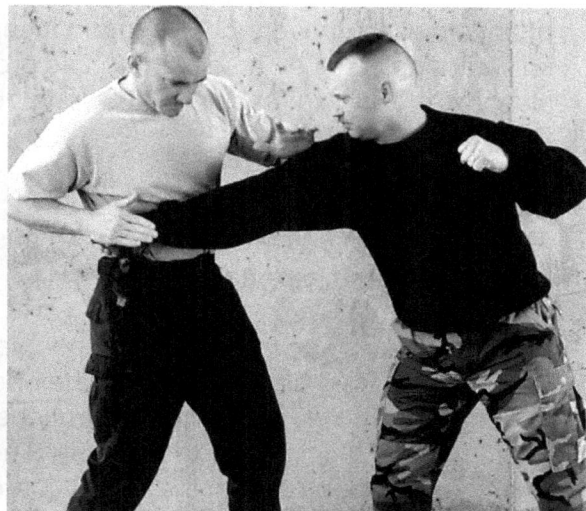

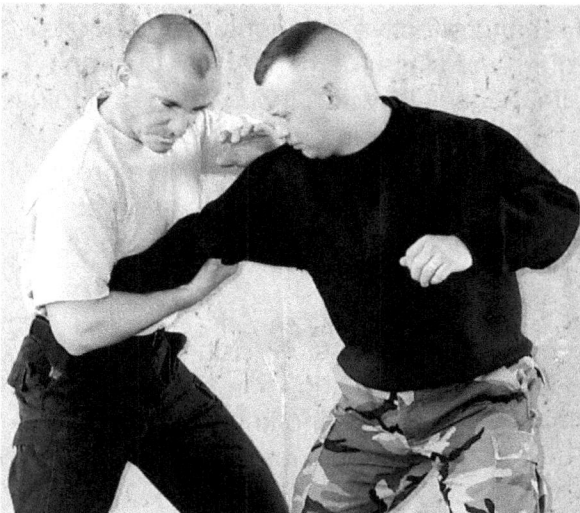

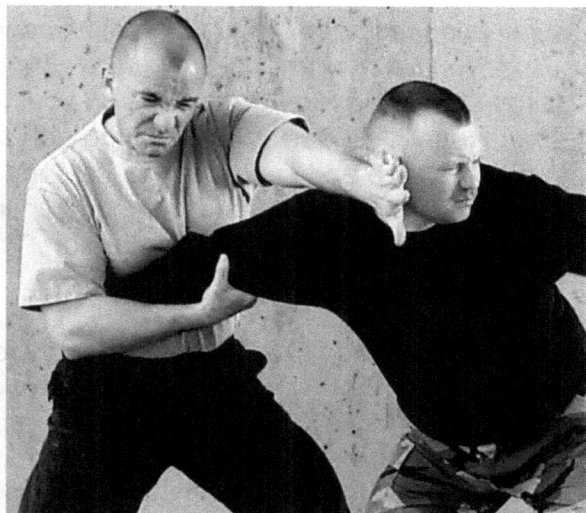

Protecting the Belt, *Gun in Holster 6: More on the Knife as a Pistol Retention Tool?*
On the subject of knives, many folks believe that pulling a knife is
the cure for the retention cancer. But there are many considerations.
Here are but a few:

Knife carry site - is your knife handy enough to be used for
sudden pistol retention?

Knife quick draw - Is your knife a folder? How fast can you open
it? Practice that much? Under deadly stress of losing your gun?

Stabbing - is your knife size significant enough to stop
someone quickly? A majority of knife stab survivors do not
report incapacitating wounds and feel as though they have
only been punched, not stabbed. Many of these small knives
people sell as a solution to this problem, are...well...very small knives. Even multiple
stabs with a small knife may not get immediate results.

Slashing - is your knife size significant enough to stop someone quickly? A majority
of knife slash survivors do not report incapacitating wounds. Many of these small
knives people sell as a solution to this problem, are...well...small. People survive
slashing more than stabbing. How long before he loses consciousness? Bleeds out?
From your slashes?

Do you know where to stab and slash for the quickest results? - Most people don't
realize how ineffective some stabbing and slashing can be with ignorant targeting and
under-estimating adrenaline.

Which knife? - I know a number of people who carry a gun, a folding knife and one of
these small, fixed blade knives on their belt near the belt buckle, with a odd, rounded
knobby handle that is too small to truly be stable and functional. So, he's got a hand
on your gun! Which knife do you pull? The little cute one or the big one that you have
to manage to pop open in the "rugby match," "goal-line-stand," power fight over your
pistol or long gun?

Eye gouge instead? - Do you realize how fast and effective a serious eye gouge is?
And, you have been practicing "opening" your hand since the crib. Also, you won't
drop your hand like you might drop your knife, especially when trying to open a folder
under stress. I hope you will go through some "rough-housing" scenario practice
offered above and see what you can and cannot do. Several years ago, in a group of
police officers, some rather famous gun instructors you might recognize, worked on
the knife vs. eye jab in pistol retention. The eye gouge won out as being much faster
and easier.

My official advice to you - in this deadly force situation of possibly losing your pistol,
and your life, is to seriously attack the eyes with the moves shown in *Force Necessary:
Hand:* Level One. I do want you to experiment with the stick and knife in the drills to
experience the event, the time and effort. But the eye gouge is faster and very effective.

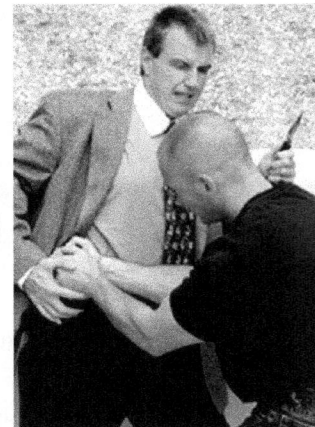

Protecting the Draw Process, Solutions

The next level of retention concern after protecting the belt is protecting the draw. The suspect can attack your weapon while it is being drawn or while it is presented and/or while it is being fired.

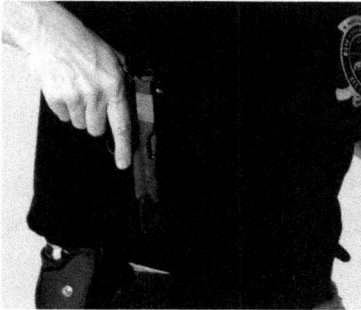

Gun is out. The handgun has left the holster.

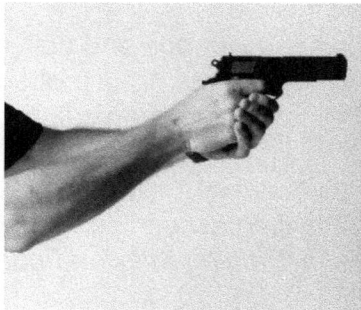

The handgun is up and threatening.

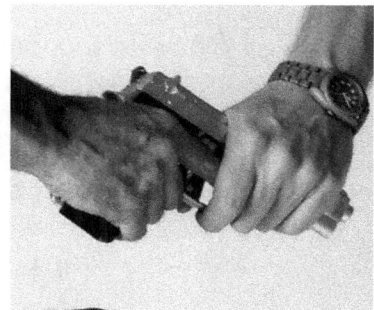

The handgun is firing and someone tries to take it.

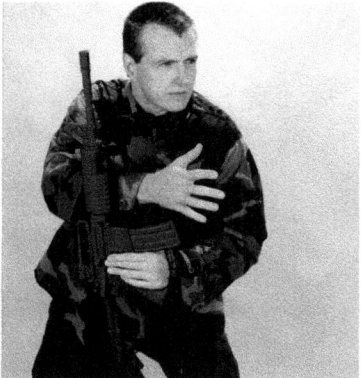

The long gun has left its carry site and is in the presentation process.

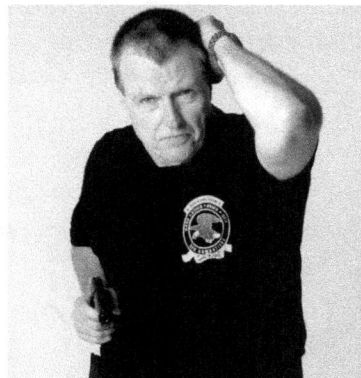

Always protecting your head this way is a mistake. Distances and predicaments are situational.

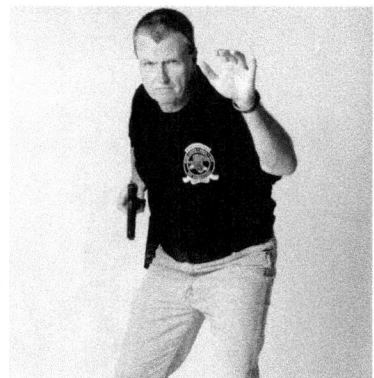

At times this support hand position is practical.

Protecting the Draw Process 1: Getting the Weapon Side Away from the Enemy
You might need a surreptitious or sudden, desperate body twist and step away, along with a protected free, support arm can help the process.

Lots of range shooters mindlessly put their hand or forearm on the side of their head, like in the photo above, when the attacker might not be close enough to worry about this. I fear this will become built-in habit. Use your support arm situationally and wisely.

A habit? A rather famous gun instructor teaches a quick draw with this protected head cover, position, then shoves the pistol outstretched with an extended two-hand grip. If there were such a close suspect as to warrant such tight head protection, it would be foolish to extend out into a two-hand grip. This is shallow, thoughtless instruction from an inexperienced person.

Protecting the Draw Process 2: How Do These Pistol "Death-GripCatches Happen?"
Back in *Training Mission One* we explored two very common paths of a draw from a common hip carry or even an appendix carry. I refer to them as the "bowler/scooper" and the "pivot" or "rib pivot," as the gun comes up rib high, pivots and goes forward.

- the bowler/scooper draws the weapon and delivers it, in one quarter of a circle in some sense, like a bowling ball toss. This probably will lead to a palm down, low arm/hand catch. (We will cover arm wrap catches in *Training Mission Four*.)

- the rib pivot draws up, pivots at a rib (which one?) and delivers the pistol straight forward which will probably be susceptible to a palm up high, hand catch. (We will cover arm wrap catches in *Training Mission Four, Stop 4*.)

- differing carry sites (and stances) and draw stroke/paths will produce differing hand catch results. Make sure to experiment from your chosen site. Have a partner stand before you and see what he naturally grabs as you draw your weapon from your chosen carry site.

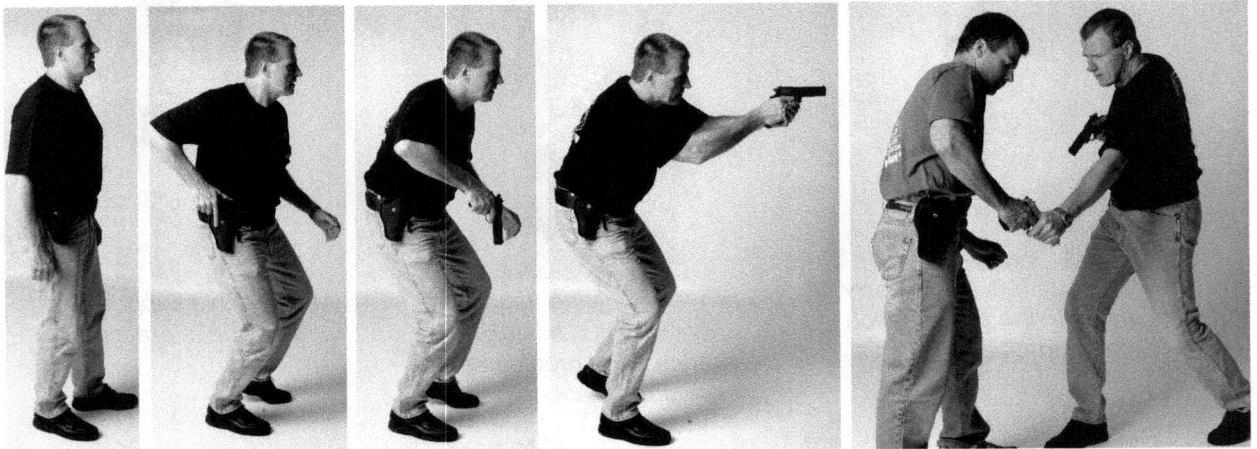

A bowler/scooper from a hip carry or an appendix carry, could lead to a low catch on the arm or gun.

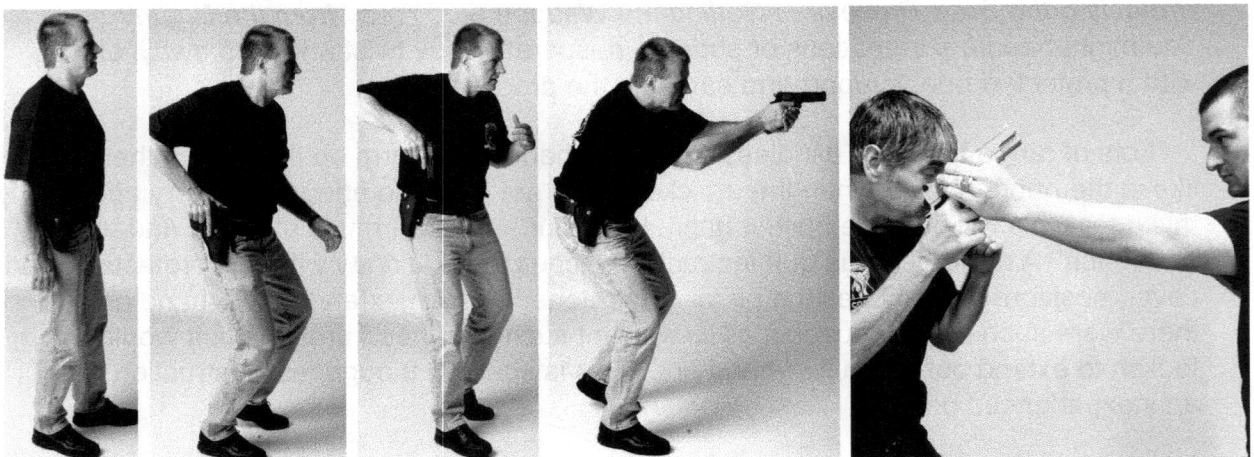

A pull and pivot at rib height, then a thrust forward, might cause a high catch of some kind.

Protecting the Draw Process 3: Pistol Lanyard Options?
Pistol Lanyards. They exist, but there are so many pros and cons, I will not dedicate the required space here to cover them all. Some people consider pistol lanyards similar to long gun slings. I wore one in the military police. Two times they significantly saved an MPs lives in my small world.

For one example, an MP fell down a steep hillside in traffic stop, gunfight one night. The driver bolted out of his car, pulled a pistol and started firing. The MP raced off between the cars trying to draw from his mandatory flap holster.

The hillside was next to them. He hit the curb and went airborne down the grassy hill. He lost his .45. He came to stop, upside down and could see the shadows of the shooter at the top of the hill by the two cars. It looked like the shooter had lost track of the MP and was hunting for him.

"Where's my gun?" he thought. Then he reached for the lanyard hooked to his shoulder and pulled the "lost" pistol in. As soon as the pistol hit his hand, he fired into the air, and tried to upright himself to climb the hill. With the gunshot, the suspect fled in his car.

He had called in the license plate at the beginning of the stop, and we caught the guy next day. That being said, the lanyard attached to the shoulder uniform epilate, as we had to do back then, is more for show than any good. Whereas ones securely fastened to the belt would be better. Built for survival, not show.

Running simulated ammo scenarios, I have seen numerous people running and tripping and losing their pistols. One time, dropping the pistol and kicking it under a car! Two weeks later I saw this happen for real in a news video. A cop dropped and accidentally kicked his pistol under a parked car.

There was once a model that was somewhat popular that extended and contracted like from a belt box, like a tape measure. It reached as far as an extended, two-hand grip. It did not dangle, but it seems the old, "telephone cord" version is mostly for sale now. That cord would just hang off you belt, where the retractable version would rewind inside a carrier box on your belt. A hanging cord may catch on things.

Retention? Well, it would depend on the carrier and the cord, and the distance of the good guy and bad guy. I bring this lanyard topic up here because it relates to retention, and like it or not, use one or not (it's completely up to you) all gun people need to be able to know of and intelligently discuss the topic.

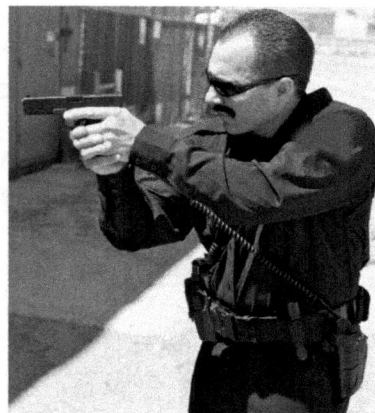

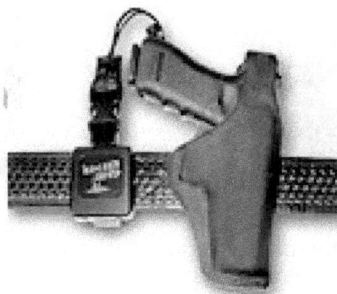

I am not suggesting you absolutely must get one of these, but some people like them.

Protecting the Draw Process : Trigger finger catch
In this *Stop 2* topic, the subject of the trigger finger catch comes up. Depending on where on the body someone carries their pistol. A grab on your hand while drawing the gun, might catch your trigger finger outside the trigger guard. The same is true for your catch on the opponent's hand during his draw. The situation is still quite fluid, but this can happen. You shouldn't be surprised.

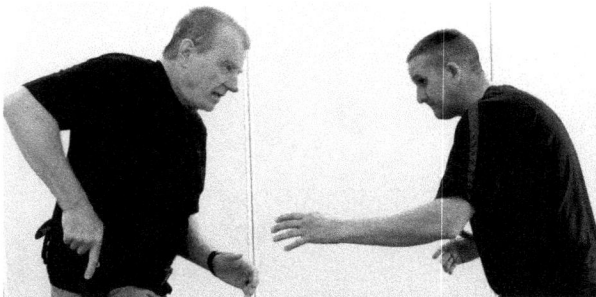

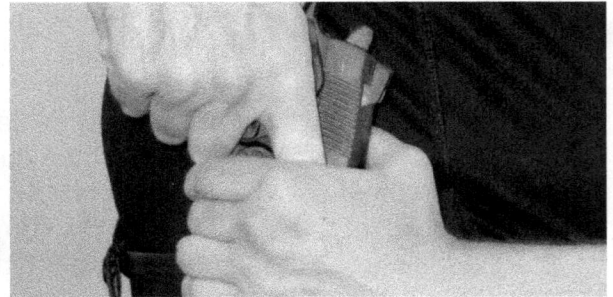

Protect the Draw Process 5: "Knife-hand' strike, "wipe" releases of low grabs
As you draw your pistol he grabs the top of your gun with one hand. Your "knife" hand (the outside edge ot your hand) or your hammer fist, or your forearm strikes down on his hand as you pull your pistol back.
- trainer's right hand grab. Smash eyes, face, throat, hit/wipe grab free.
- trainer's left hand grab. Smash eyes, face, throat, hit/wipe grab free.
- trainer's both hands grab. Smash eyes, face, throat, hit/wipe grab free.

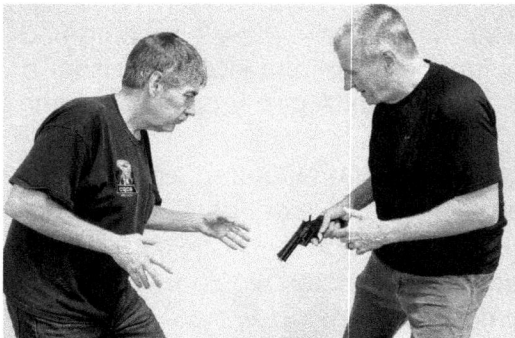

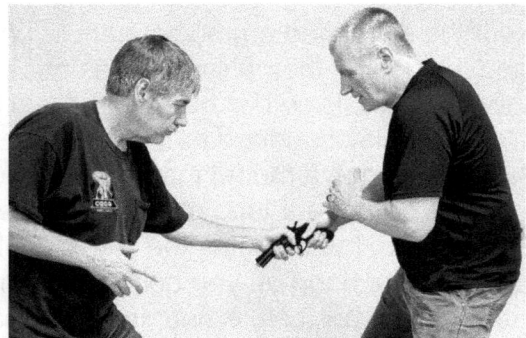

He rushes in to stop your draw. He grabs your forearm, hand or gun.

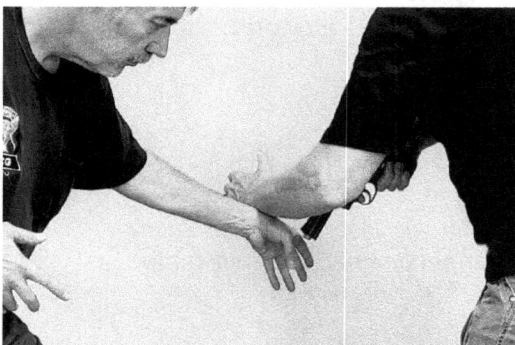

You downward strike his grip, with your knife hand, hammer fist or forearm.

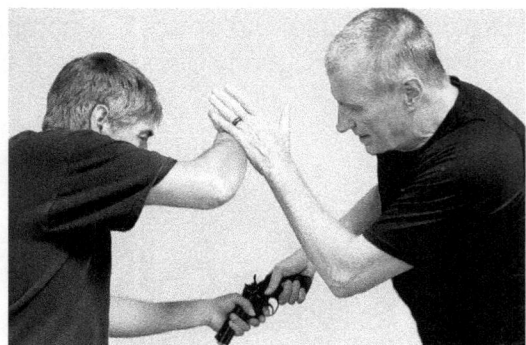

Then do this again after blocking some common punches.

Protecting the Draw Process 6: Pros and Cons of the Shirt Lift
Many carriers conceal their weapons under clothing. The draw process must include getting this clothing out of the way. This clothing clearance is done by the gun draw hand, or by way of the other "free," non-gun hand. These are topics detailed in the prior *Stop One* and *Training Mission One* book. A gun carrier must realize that there are many times when that "shirt-lifting" hand is busy or grabbed.

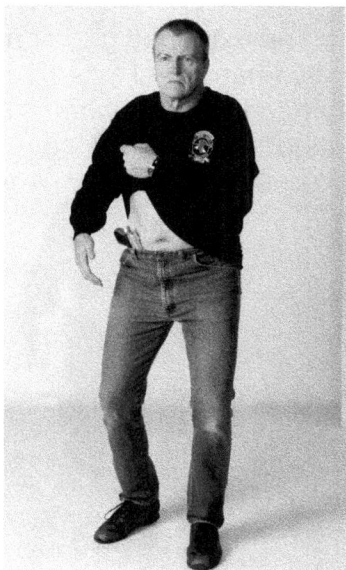

The classic "shirt lift, draw, shoot."

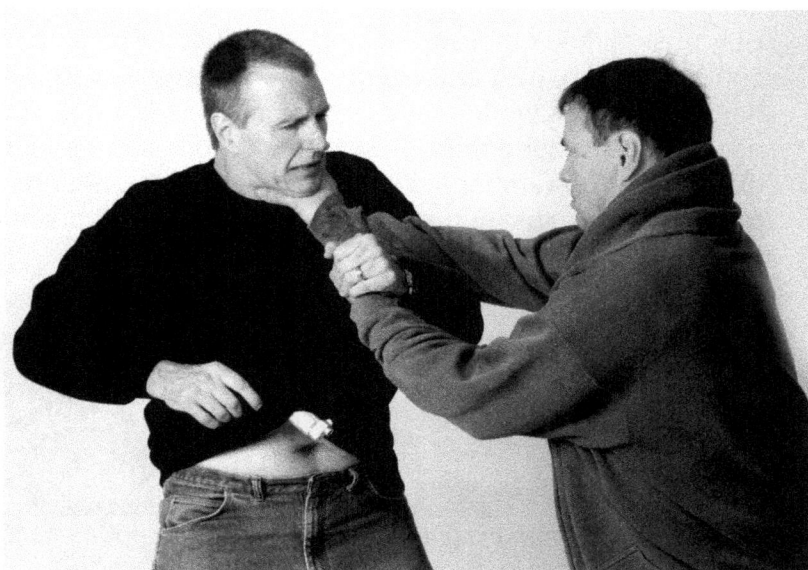

Single-hand, clothing covered draws can be a problem under stress, rendering the handgun to a no-shot, or one-shot operation.

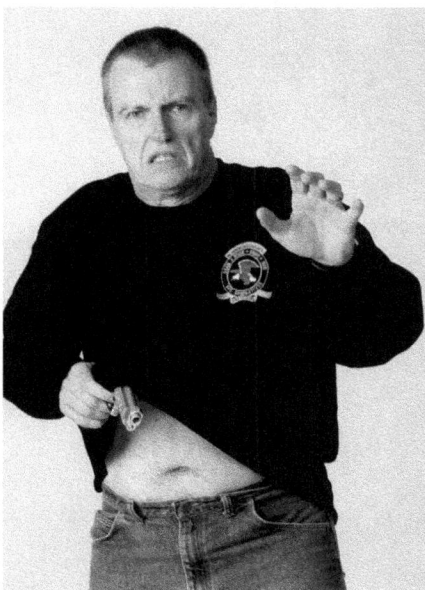

Several years ago, I taught a simulated ammo class to a rather large, police narcotics unit. Their standard operating procedure was to do the old "shirt lift" at the range. Lift. Draw. Shoot. It included my usual amount of interactive, close-up, grappling style scenarios and the "plain-clothes" officers had the usual troubles tying to clear their draw from close quarter attackers. And, their trained, shirt-lifting hands were very busy fighting off the trainers.

At the end of session, the unit commander told me they were going to re-think their carry and draw, as they hadn't considered these other "second-hand problems." Hadn't considered these other problems? I found that statement odd. Narcotics officers are usually patrol veterans and would be aware of close-up, stress draw, grappling problems. And, it's hard to train this without a commitment to safe ammo guns. I am also sure that there are plethora of concealed carry people, also content with lift shirt, draw, shoot, and are not fully cognizant of grappling, reality problems.

The commander decided they needed to broaden the training methods to include these situations with simulated, safer ammo. One solution is to really work on that single-hand, under-the-clothes draw, while that the other hand can fight off an attacker.

Series 3: Protecting the Drawn Gun

Protect the Drawn Gun 1: Do NOT shove your pistol out too close into the reach of a bad guy

This is a **big problem**. Since some 80 percent to 90 percent of live fire practice is done with two hands, so, in reality, people will subsequently, mindlessly draw into a two-hand grip.

But, every time you draw a pistol, you must make a decision on an extended grip or a contracted grip, with one or two-hands. Retention is best with two-hands. All two-handed disarms work against one hand grip, but not all one-handed disarms work against two-handed grips. A two-hand grip is more secure, but not perfect for close distancing. Remember the "two-giant-steps-and-a-lunge" classic, distance advise. And remember how fast someone can cover even that distance.

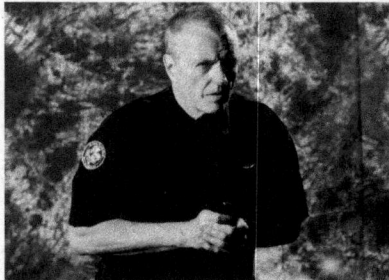

Two-hand grip, contracted.

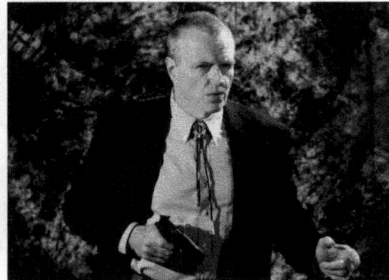

One-hand grip, contracted.

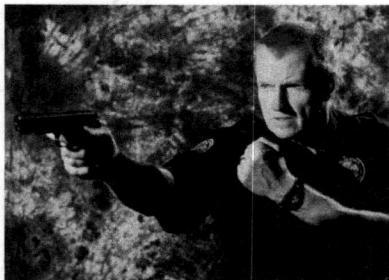

One-hand grip, extended.

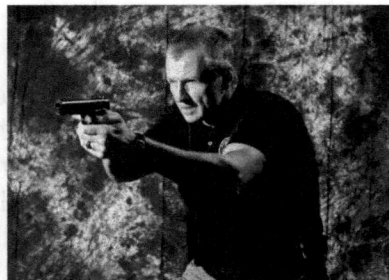

Two-hand grip, extended.

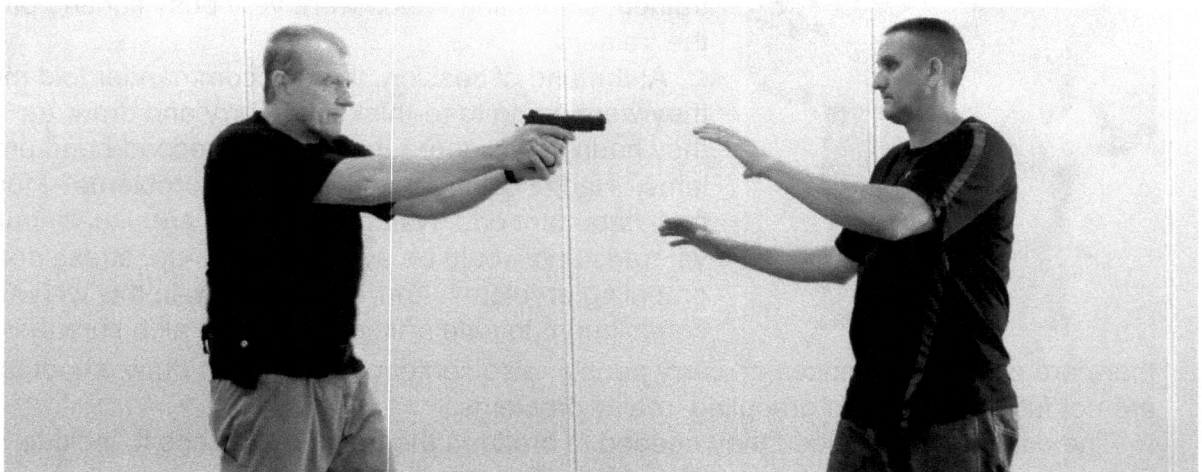

Too close for this distance! Maintain your "anti-social" distancing!

For Your Perusal: The Tokyo Drop!

Many years ago, I learned this from the Tokyo, Japan Riot Police, a SWAT-like group famous for their extreme, hard core training. If they could not get their gun free from a serious grip, they dropped onto their backs and, with this power, yanked back against the grip. It is hard for the suspect to hang on; and if they somehow did, they would be "bicycle kicked," off and away. As with all such position shooting, don't shoot your knees or feet! This is a last resort move, unlike some Brazilian JJ police instructors suggest, who seem to have you drop on your back with a "drop of a hat."

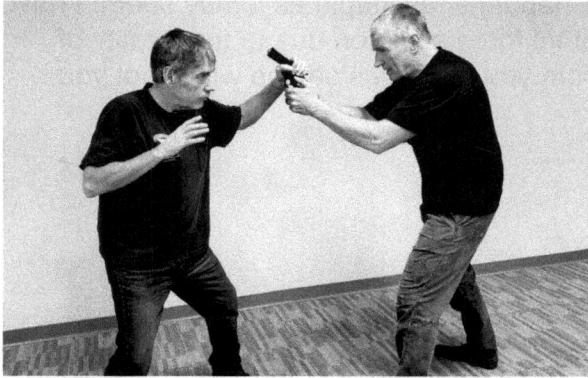
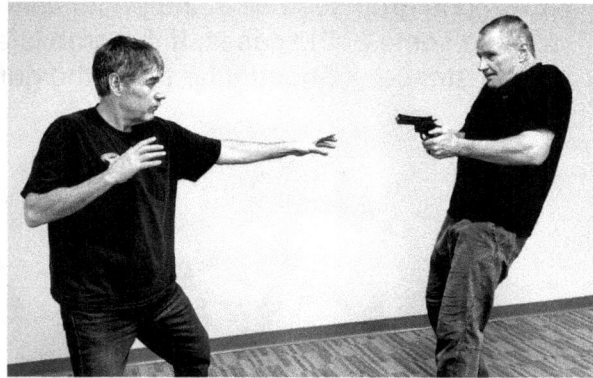

Verus the grab, a powerful yank back and step back might work. But, what if he hangs on still?

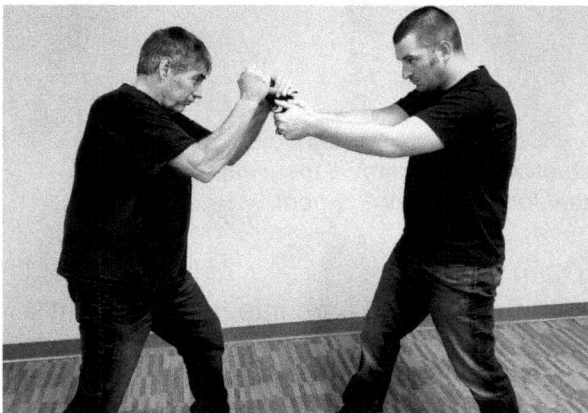
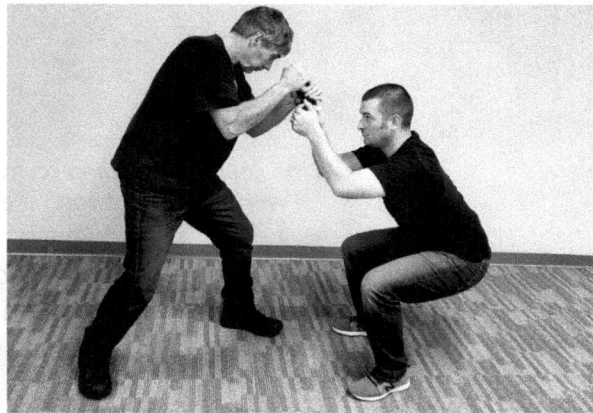

Some experts suggest twisting your gun a bit aids in the yanking free.

In the Tokyo Drop, you use your full body weight and yank back strength to get the release and retention. If such escape force is needed.

Always react legally and accordingly from there. You may not like this, but try it, and at the very least, you know some riot police moves.

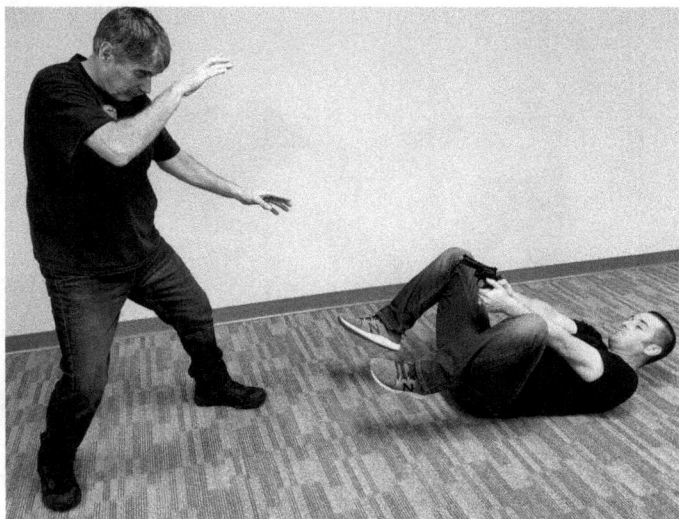

Protecting the Drawn Gun: The Long Gun Sling or Lanyard
An opponent reaches out and grabs your long gun with one or two hands. Must he defeat your sling or lanyard? A sling or lanyard will inhibit rifle grabs and take-away. The long gun can be attacked. If you do have a sling or a lanyard how is it attached to your body? The attachment may save you from a takeaway, yet may be used as a "handle" so to speak to pull you around and/or down.

Protecting the Drawn Long Gun 1: The Long Gun Shoot!
A weapon grab such as in the photo actually happens, as stupid as it may seem. I have worked some of the cases. If the grab is a lethal force situation due to the totality of circumstances? Shoot! If he takes the gun from you, statistics say he will shoot you.

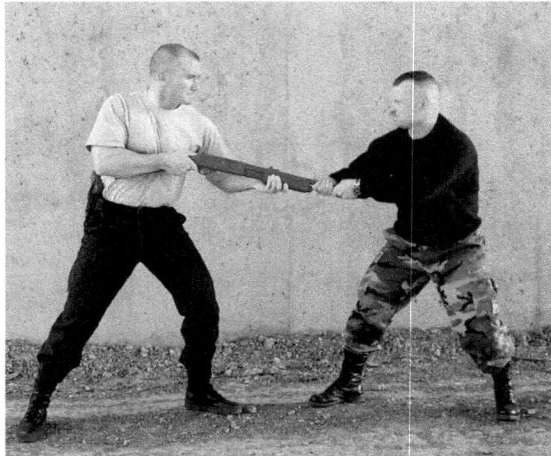

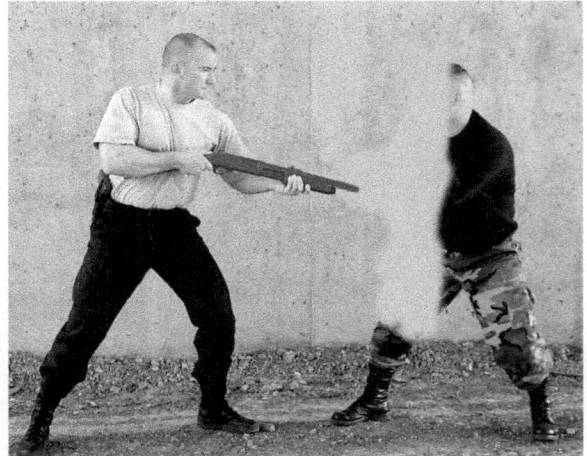

He makes the grab. Depending on the situation you might pull the weapon back with added footwork. If a lethal force situation? Shoot.

Protecting the Drawn Long Gun 2: The Long Gun Shove!
He grabs and you feel as though you can shove the weapon hard into the opponent's chest, which may somewhat open up his grab on your barrel.

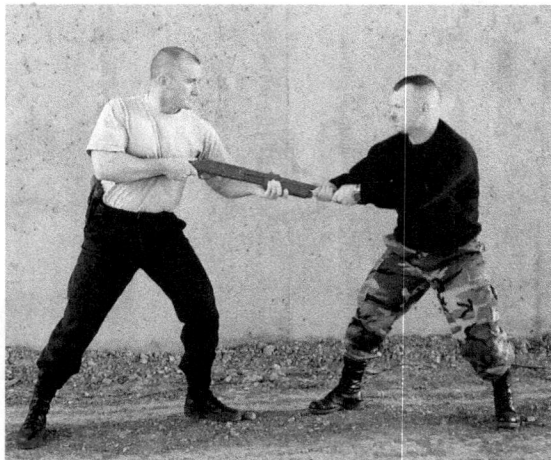

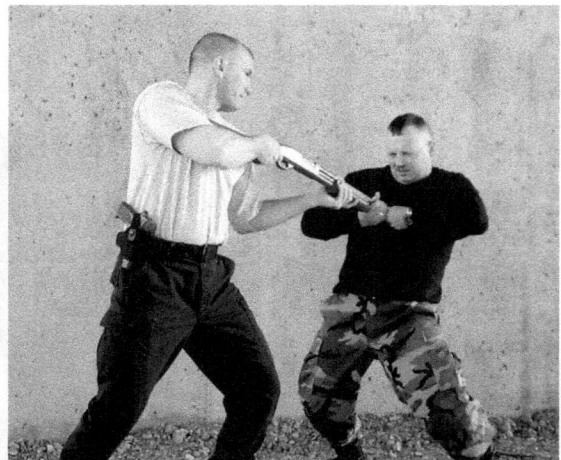

You might ram the long gun forward like a concentrated power strike, and get a release and retention.

Protecting the Drawn Long Gun 3: The Long Gun Thrust - Barrel 1
Due to the grab on the gun, and with your arm strength and the "in and out" footwork of this level. Thrust into the sternum.

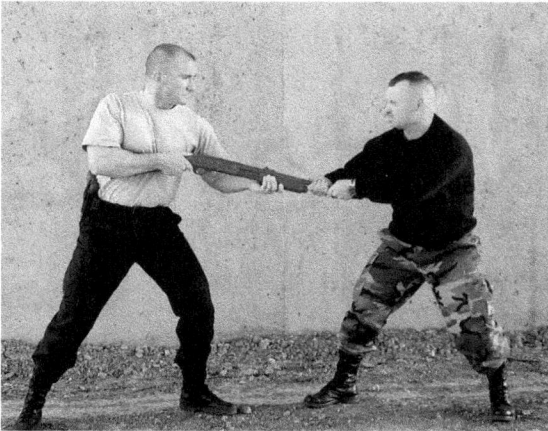

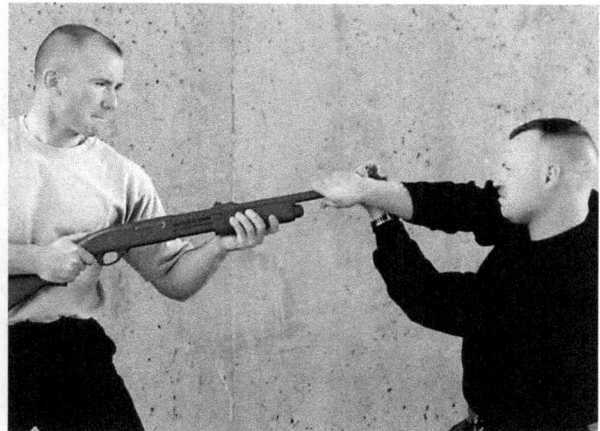

Protecting the Drawn Long Gun 4: The Long Gun Circular Release - Barrel 2

Due to the grab on the gun, and with your arm strength, small circle right or left, get that center lock position on him and push down hard.

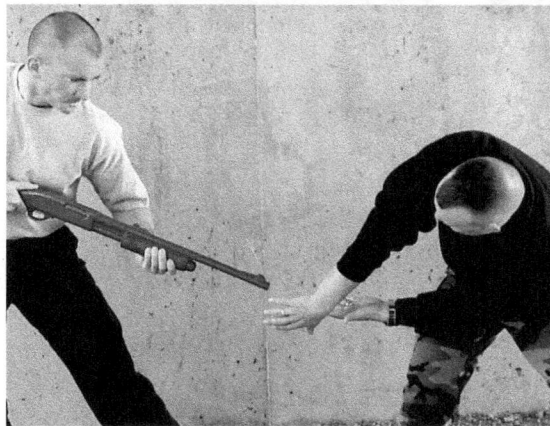

Protecting the Drawn Long Gun 4: The Long Gun "Row" Release - Entire Weapon

The following "row release" is the same Figure 8 motion as used to retain a stick. This motion gets rid of many hand grips on long weapons.

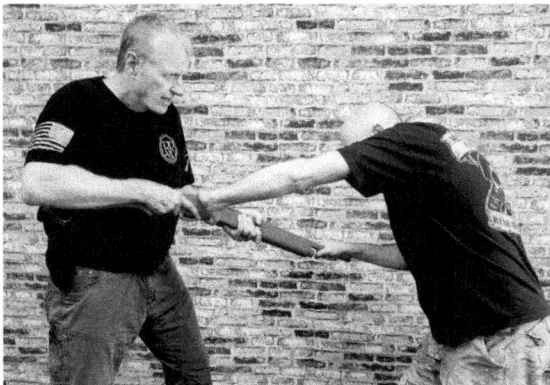

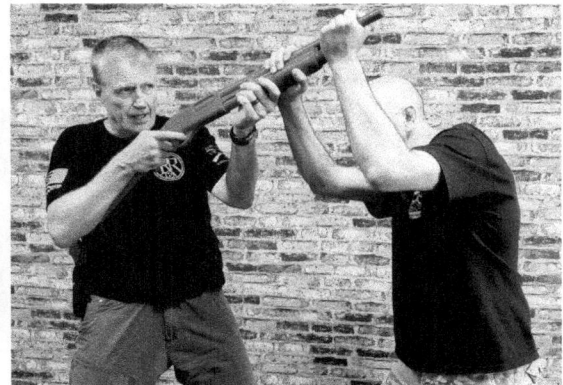

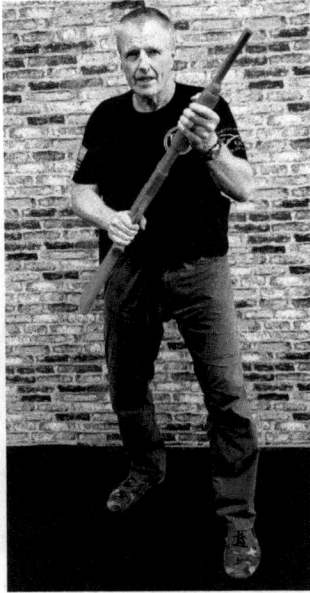

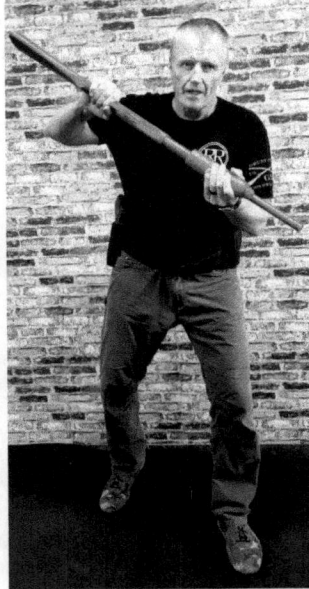

Ready...   Stock up and downward on an angle "over" the hand grab.

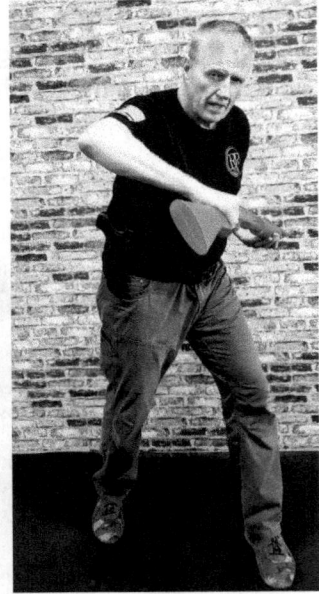

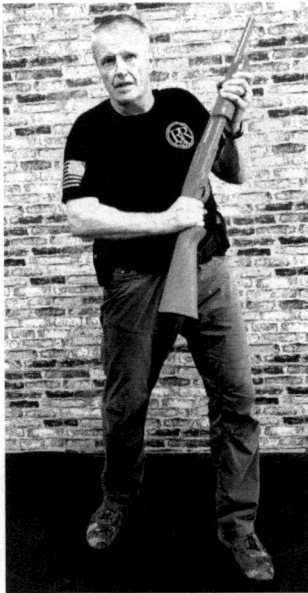

Barrel up and downward on an angle "over" the hand grab.

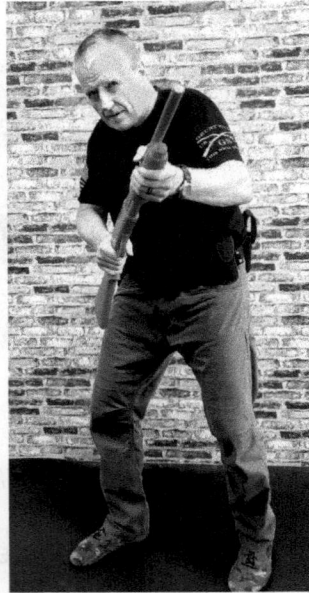

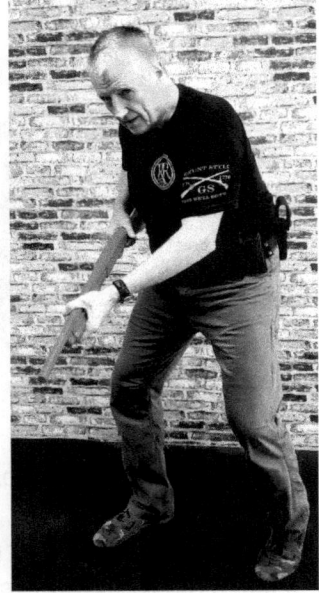

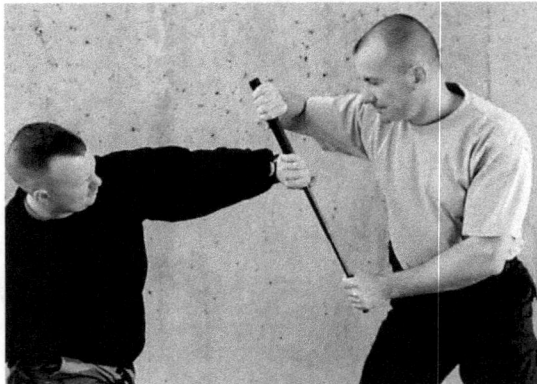

As with the stick, the rowing motion cramps the wrist and can get a release.

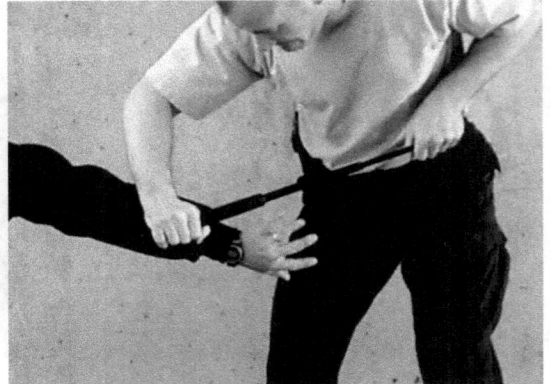

Gun-out basic, core releases

A study of the major releases via the "Pistol Death Grip." Your lower limb/hand gets grabbed. High or low. These work versus one hand and two hand grabs and that appears in *Stop 2* to Stop 6 also. This book only covers *Stop 2*, but you will be asked to remember and review this releasing foundation as the *Stop 6* and *Training Mission* books continue.

Sample 1: The yank-out. Like a hit and retract, use your arm and whole body if need be to get put of this *Stop 2* grab. Same on the low end. Yank out, pull out in the smartest direction. Many experts suggest turning the pistol a bit to get a release.

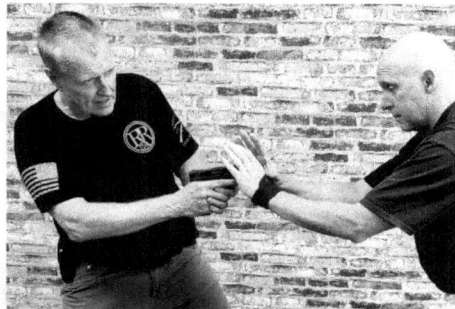
One or two hand yank-outs. Powerful yank-backs with arms and footwork.

Sample 2: The circular release and the joint lock position releases. Rotating your pistol hand clockwise or counter-clockwise can often get a release. It will depend on the grip, high or low. Sometimes a quarter-circle or a half-circle will allow you to use a quicker, joint lock release. At times, a second after the release, you can push the hand away with your saber or reverse grip, freeing a better path to your next attack, else the opponent will simply re-grab your limb. Look for this push-out opportunity in your practice.

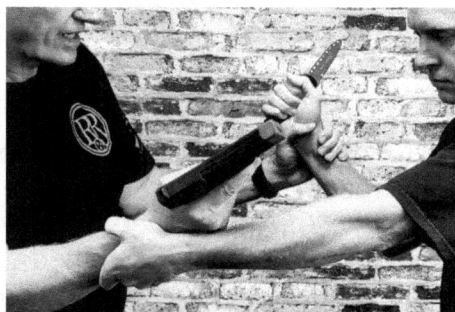
This is an "up and over" circular release.

Sample 3: The elbow rollover. This is also really a joint lock release, but it serves an honorable mention for its easy success. If you can, it's:
1) elbow up.
2) elbow over his forearm.
3) elbow down like a flapping motion. You can accompany that downward flap with a bit of a body drop against very strong grips.

Sample 4: The shoulder release. If you can't get a release from a strong grip? Pull his captured hand out from his body and get your upper torso under his arm, a bit sideways. Hammer your caught hand down as you stand up like a squat. This should get a release. *Take care not to get caught in a head lock range,* by going a bit deeper in and a bit of sideways. Be dynamic after the release to avoid the headlock.

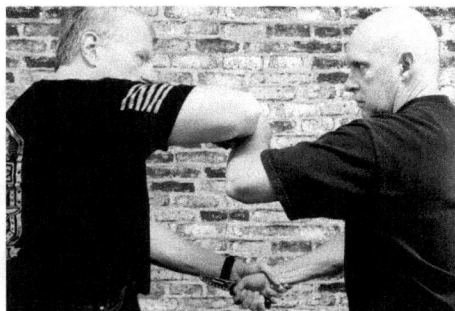
Elbow roll-overs. Elbow up. Elbow over and torso and elbow down.

Sample 5: A knee release. On the low side of the clock, if you can't get a release, and you can judge from prior practice versus various heights, lift and drive you knee against his grabbing forearm, and pull your caught limb back and out.

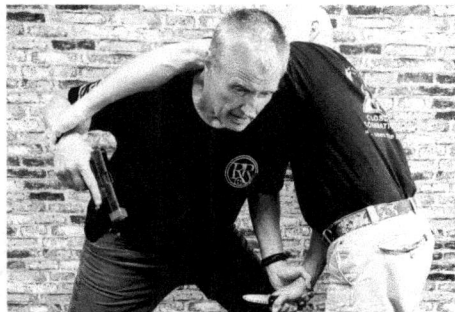
Shoulder releases.

Sample 6: A bite release. If you can't get a release, you can try stepping in and biting his arm, if his clothing makes this available.

Sample 7: Arm rams. Any cross arm catch, or when in a righty versus lefty jam-up, you could try to ram his arm up or down to get a release.

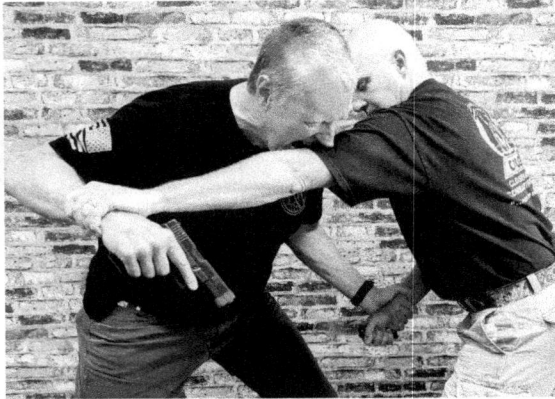

Bite releases.

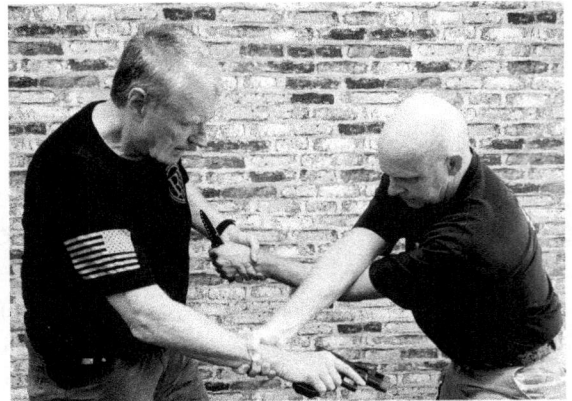

Arm ram releases when righty versus lefty.

Gun-Out: Grabbed? Shoot right away
We must cover the aforementioned releases, for the record, after introducing the common releases, it is important in a life and death situation to immediately shoot the armed attacker. You really need to pull your pistol. It is a life or death situation. Then as soon as your weapon limb is grabbed - shoot. It might be a wrist twist away. This wrist twist could be done when on the "death grip" of each other, versus a knife, any lethal force situation.

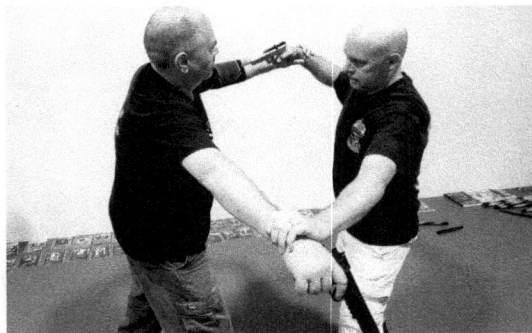

High grab? Twist your wrist inward to shoot right away.

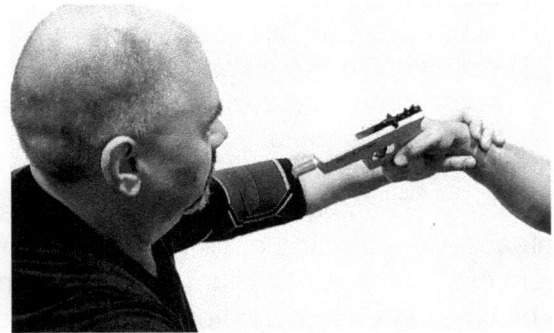

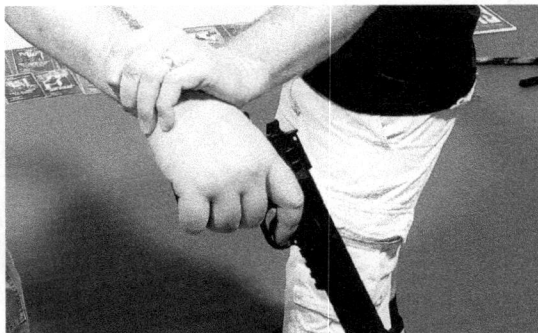

Low grab? Twist your wrist inward to shoot right away. Thigh? Then pelvis? Then higher.

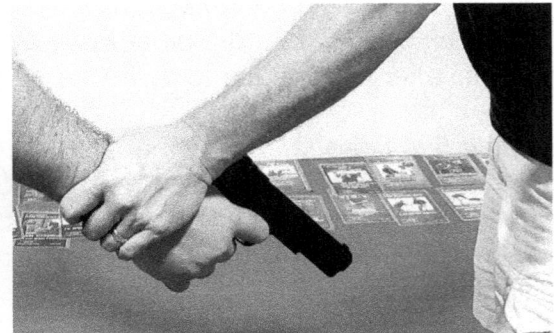

Of important note! If your opponent has a pistol out, he too can wrist twist and shoot you. Totally untrained people have done this, as well as poorly, incomplete trained people also. Since this is a problem, When you grab his pistol wrist, two vital tricks:

- Try to scoot your grab down to get a grip on both his hand and wrist, TIGHTEN! This should restrict his hand a bit from pointing his gun inward. Shoot fast!

- Shove his weapon limb out. This makes his pointing inward at you even harder. Shoot fast!

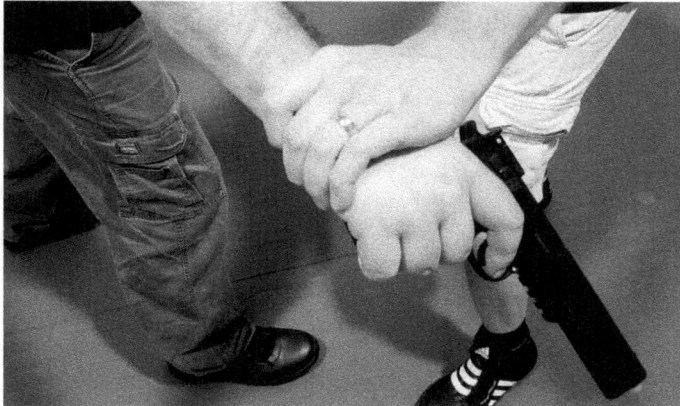

Get that hand/wrist vice grip. Shove his gun hand out and away from you! The higher the grab up the wrist and onto the hand, the harder it is for him to twist the barrel in at you. Limit his chances to wrist twist and shoot you.

Gun-Out: Ride the gun down!
This is another vital, life-saving tip. You are in the, "Death Grip of the Gun!" In each other's clutches. You shoot him. He starts to fall. *YOU CANNOT LET GO OF HIS GUN OR HIS GUN HAND*! You must follow him down and control the gun and gun hand all the way down and keep the barrel off of you. Assess along the way and once down, then yank it out of his hand for a disarm.

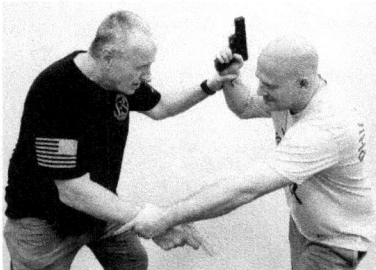

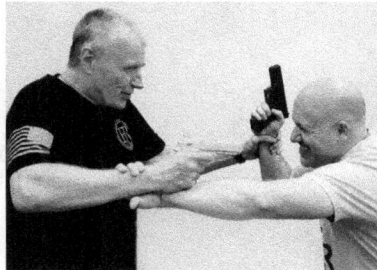

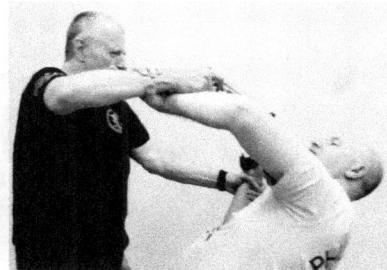

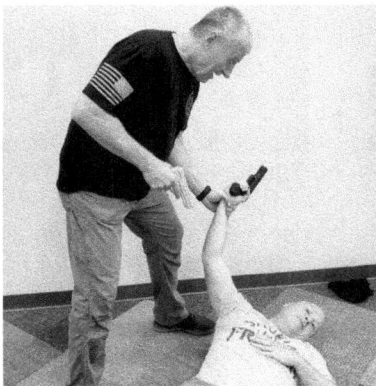

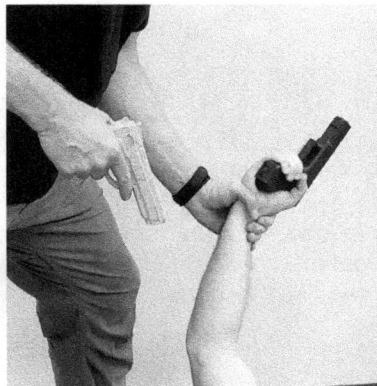

In this example of "riding the gun down," you are stuck in a classic *Stop 2*, mutual grab situation. You counter-clockwise circle and shoot. He's hit and falls. It behooves you to follow the gun grip down so he does not accidentally or on purpose shoot you!

A *Stop 2* Shoot/ Don't Shoot Pistol Exercise

Citizens, police and military cannot get enough shoot/don't shoot practice. Here is one of my favorite scenarios I like to teach. The trainer and trainee tangle up in a *Stop 2* situation. The trainer breaks free and goes for a pistol on his hip, pocket or appendix carry. The trainee realizes that he cannot draw his own pistol in time and he must interrupt the trainer's draw.

A reminder from *Training Mission One* that in close encounter, stress quick draws where you are responding to the cues, tip-offs and motions of a concealed pistol quick draw, given action beats reaction, given the suspect does not fumble a bit, you are hard pressed to see, alert, draw and shoot him before he shoots you.

The trainee dives in with a rear arm-bar hammerlock, emphasizing the elbow for control, NOT the shoulder. This is a successful grapple. This is a lethal force, firearm's situation, the trainee must draw his pistol. The trainee orders the trainer down on the ground, to be controlled and disarmed. The trainer can decide to submit or to reach across his bent body and try again to draw his pistol (or knife). This is a deadly decision as the trainee has no choice but to shoot the trainer. This practice can be done fast, safe and many times with things like wooden rubber band guns. I ask the trainer to:

      1: The first 5 or 10 times to surrender.
      2: The next 5 or 10 times to "cross" reach and draw his pistol.
      3: The next series of times, mix it up. Now the trainee must see and read
         the situation and react. The decision making training begins here.
      4: The next few, the trainer can improvise with a few surprises he has developed.

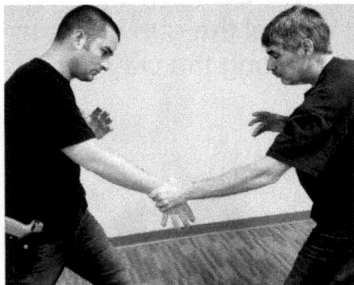

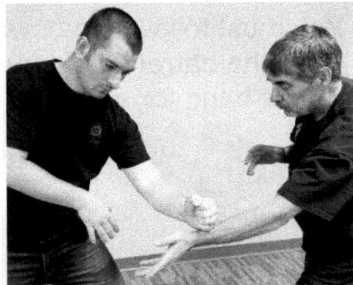

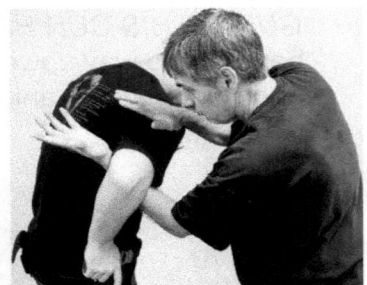

He gets free of the tangle, and drops his hand to a carry site. You leap in for a hammerlock.

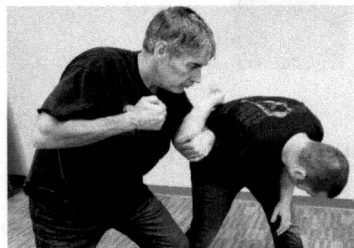

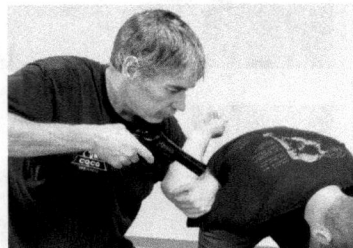

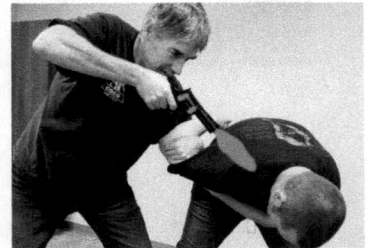

He clearly has a gun (or knife). You pull your gun. You issue surrender commands. Surrendered? A leg sweep takedown ensues. Disarming follows. Capture for the milliary, control for police and competent, confident citizens for arrest, or if you need be? Escape?

You see the cross body reach to get the weapon and must shoot. Take care to get your inside foot and leg out of the way, in case your round fragments off the skull and into your body.

Summary on Weapon Retention in Conjunction with Weapon Disarming
Stop 2 covers stick, knife and gun weapon retention, not necessarily disarming. A complete course of study in weapon retention includes a complete study of weapon disarming. Weapon disarming is a copious amount of material, inappropriate for a Level 2 study progression. Level 2 and *Stop 2* is about essentially about grabbing and releasing with dabblings a little further. We will cover stick, knife and firearm disarming in great detail later in *Training Missions Seven, Eight* and *Nine*. Suffice to say these retention methods listed here cover and counter a vast amount of enemy disarming methods.

The *Stop 2* Ambush, Dodge, Evasion and Grab Pistol Exercise.
As I warned in *Training Mission One*, you will see the Ambush Drill re-appear in various forms as the *Training Missions* continue. Here in *Stop 2* the trainee now grabs the arm attacks. Versus the leg shots, just dodge them with Level 2 "In and out" footwork. The weapon attack is a deadly force situation, causing a weapon response. A trainer stands before you. Close, but not too close. See the steps below. Review the Big 10 hand, stick or knife attacks. We select the knife attack here as a clear lethal force situation.

> 1: A right hand, high, hooking strike from his high right.
> 2: A right hand, high, back-handed, hooking strike from his right hand.
> 3: A right hand, belly high, hooking strike from his high right.
> 4: A right hand, belly high, back-handed, hooking strike from his right hand.
> 5: A right hand, thigh high, hooking strike from his high right.
> 6: A right hand, thigh high, back-handed, hooking strike from his right hand.
> 7: A right hand, low to high hook.
> 8: A right hand, high to low hook.
> 9: A right hand thrust to the stomach.
> 10: A right hand thrust to the face.
> * *Reset, and attack with the left hand.*
> * *Attack with hand, stick and knife.*

The trainee
> Series 1: Dodges *without* footwork, just body elasticity. Review *Training Mission One*.
> Series 2: Dodges *with* footwork and elasticity. Review *Training Mission One*.
> Series 3: Dodges and blocks.
> Series 4: Dodge, blocks and *Stop 2* catches the attacking limb.
> Series 5: Combinations. Trainee dodges the first attack, becomes alert, stops/catches the next one. Draws gun and counter-attacks to a legal finish. *Combinations can be worked.* Dodge the first attack, dodges the second attack as one becomes alert, stops/catches the next one, draws pistol and counter attacks to a legal finish.
>
> The local instructor will decide whether to stop at the *Stop 2* catch, draw and shoot, or catch, draw, footwork and threaten for a surrender. Within the modern framework of less-than lethal options, I suggest this "drop the _____," threat be officially included in the training doctrine.

Note: This Ambush exercise is best be passed onto to you with personal hands-on, instruction, as true, step-by step analysis, might take hundreds and hundreds of photos and a thousand words to document here. I hope what is presented here will inspire you and develops the skills of you and yours in *Stop 2* problems. Each attack is meant to be a solo ambush, produced from a concealed grip or quick draw.

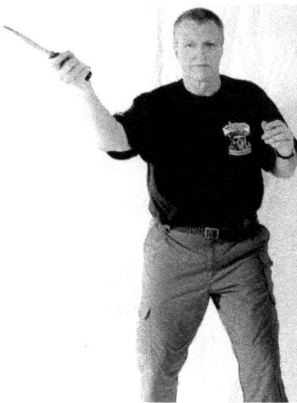

1: High right side slash.

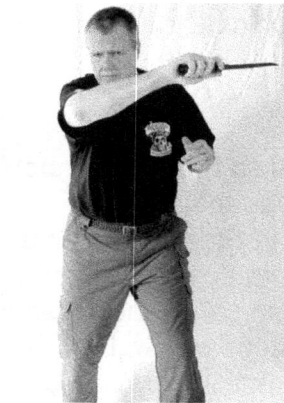

2: High left side slash.

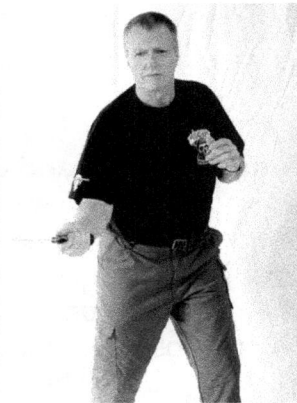

3: Middle right slash.

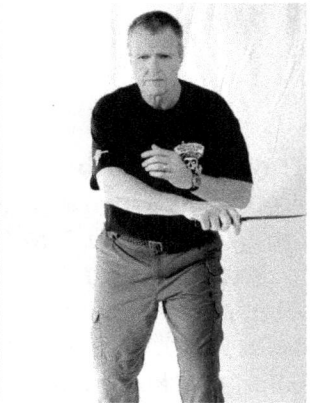

4 Middle left slash.

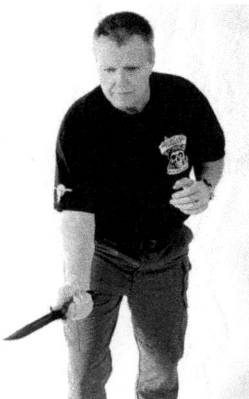

5: Low right leg slash.

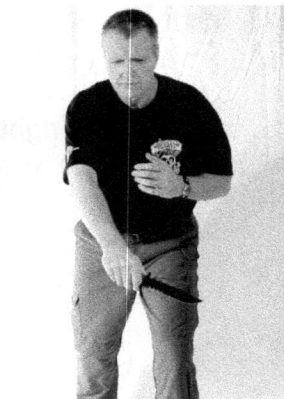

6: Low left leg slash.

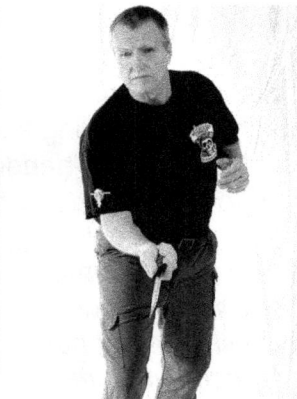

7: Uppercut slash.

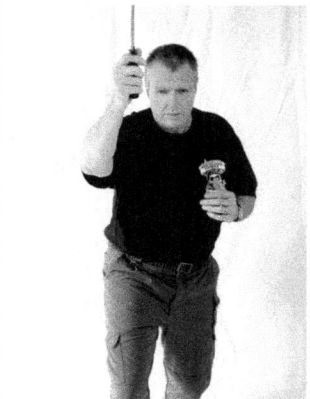

8: Downward slash.

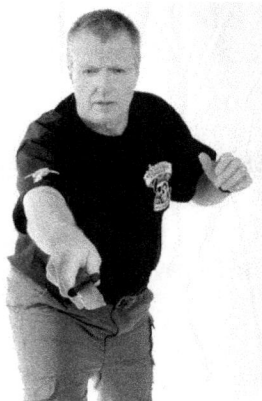

9: Stomach area stab.

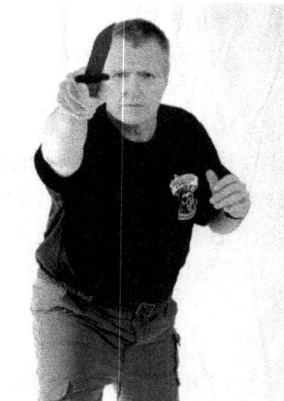

10: Face/neck stab.

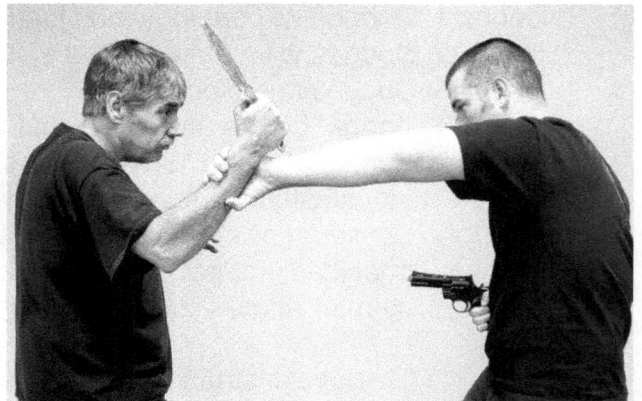

Review the list as a warm-up. Then emphasize the block/stop/grab from the 10 attacks, draw pistol and shoot. Also, experiment with the surrender, "drop the knife" command/threat.

The Level 2, *Stop 2,* Pistol Tangler Exercise

In *Training Mission One*, we pulled our weapon while the armed attacker stalked us. Now in Stop 2 we explore when he hardly stalks and mad rushes in. The trainer stalks, rushes in and only grabs the trainee's pistol hand, or pistol side wrist. Or both grab each others weapon side, hands or wrists. Trainee solves the problem. Instructors should be aware of how well trained and experienced the trainees are when managing scenarios, so as to decide how far into a combat scenario they should proceed. Participants must have safe ammo and protective gear conducive to the level of safe ammo.

These may include two releases. The first release to get a hand free, a second one after the pistol is drawn and that limb is re-grabbed, or you may hand twist your gun into a good aim. In these chaotic scenarios see what happens. Use all the skills and tactics developed in this book.

The Tangler to a Draw Series

    1: This is a special scenario for those who feel as though an unarmed attacker, due to the totality of circumstances is a deadly threat. This must be legally articulated later. Trainer mad rushes in and the empty-handed trainee is "Stop 2 grabbed." Trainee gets a grip release and draws pistol and shoots. Also, rehearses a threatening surrender.
        * one rehearsal of a trainer surrender.
        * several examples of shooting.

    2: Trainer is armed with a knife. The trainer mad rushes in and the trainee is "*Stop 2* grabbed." Trainee gets a release and draws a pistol and shoots.
        * one rehearsal of a trainer surrender.
        * several examples of shooting.

    3: Trainer is armed with a stick. The trainer mad rushes in and the trainee is "*Stop 2* grabbed." Trainee gets a release and draws a pistol and shoots.
        * one rehearsal of a trainer surrender.
        * several examples of shooting.

    4: The trainer mad rushes in while pulling their pistol, and the trainee is "*Stop 2* grabbed" with the trainee catching the pistol itself, the hands, wrist or forearm. Trainee gets a release and draws a pistol and shoots.

    5: The unarmed trainer rushes in as the trainee is pulling a pistol. The trainer grabs the draw process in some manner. The trainee gets a release, pulls their pistol and threatens attacker to surrender.

    6: The unarmed trainer rushes in, pulling their pistol as the trainee is pulling a pistol. The trainer grabs the draw process in some manner. The trainee still shoots the attacker either by a wrist twist or a release.

The Level 2, Stop 2 : "It's On! Exercise"

You are close, maybe too close but the subject has invaded your space. Circumstances happen. In Stop One, *Training Mission One* we established an opponent's weapon carry sites and trained our eyes to alert on hands traveling to those carry sites.

Primary Carry Site 1: Belt line and pockets. Think quick draw.
Primary Carry Site 2: Back-up sites, the layer away from quick draws.
Primary Carry Site 3: Lunge and reach, off the body.

The "It's On" exercise concerns itself with primary carry sites. The suspect will have a gun (or knife):

* 1:30 on the belt line - the so-called appendix carry.
* 3 o'clock-ish on the hip (for rightys.)
* 6 o'clock in the small of the back, the "SOB."
* 9 o'clock hip cross draw from belt.
* 9 o'clock cross draw from the should holster.
* Reverse for lefties.

All the Stop 1 tip-offs might be on your alert mind. "Innocent Hands" are typical hand movements we recognize from everyday life. Often situational gun draws begin with fast movements, concealed movements, prep knee bends, etc., not to mention the situation and the location. The trainer will begin to draw his gun from those carry sites, and the trainee will lunge and grab the wrist of the attempted draw and will draw his or her gun. An effort should be made to identify the true motivation of the trainer's movement and spot the weapon "top." The shoot the trainer with their simulated ammo handgun.

While hope is never a good strategy, the suspect may not practice or have a "Hollywood" fast draw? If you just wrestly with the grab/catch alone, this match will just go on and on until the

A shirt or jacket lift is always suspicious.

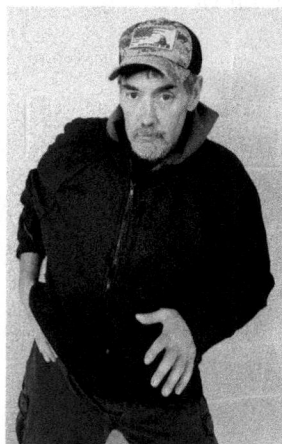

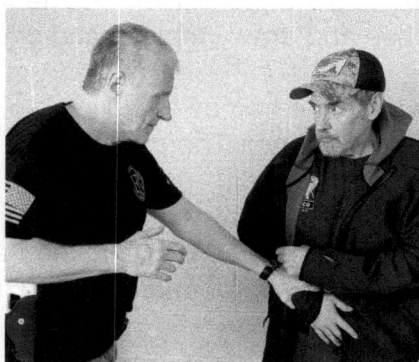

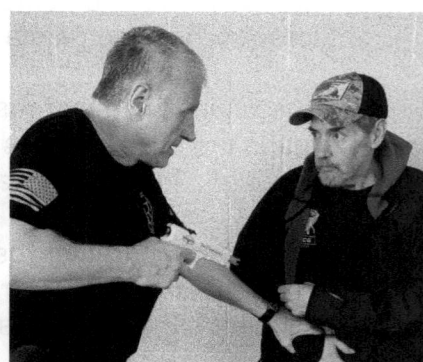

opponent gets his gun free of you. Think of all the retention we have learned thus far.

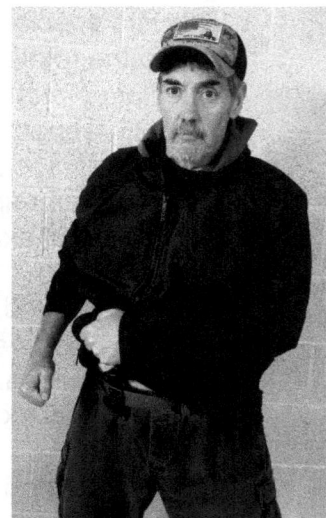

The appendix pull is spotted. Free hand catches the attempt, drives in, pulls and shoots if the suspect has a gun or knife.

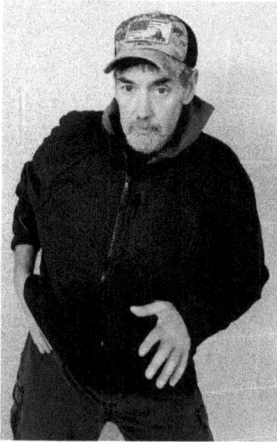

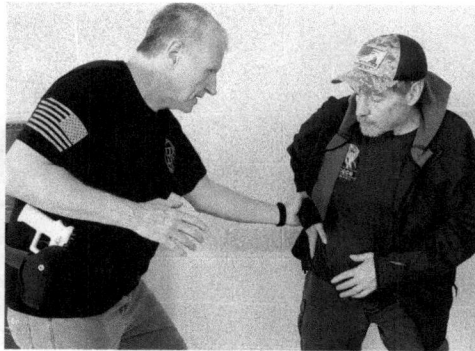

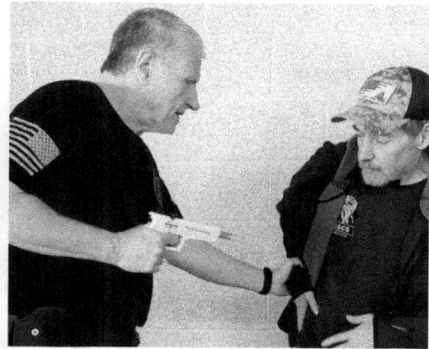

The hip pull is spotted. Free hand catches the attempt, drives in, pulls and shoots if the suspect has a gun or knife.

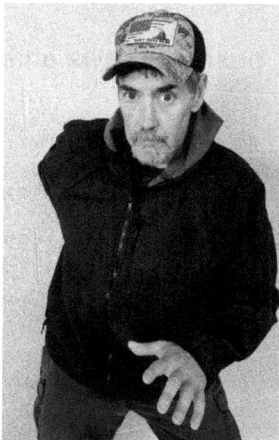

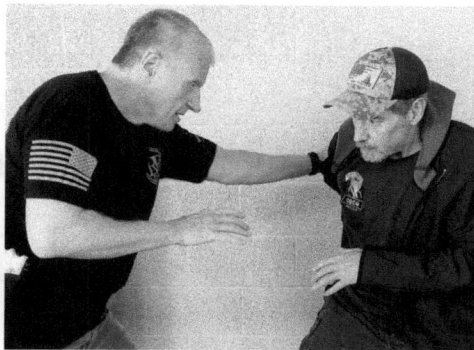

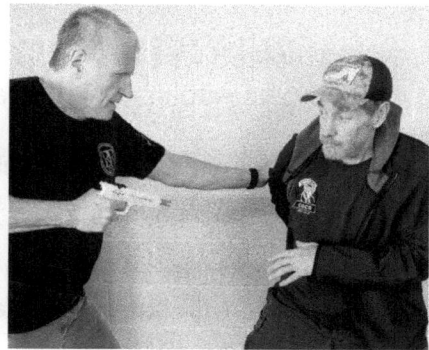

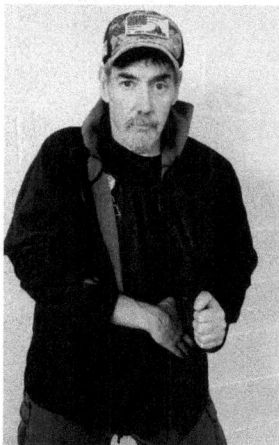

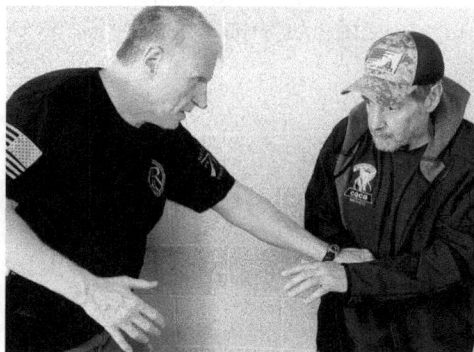

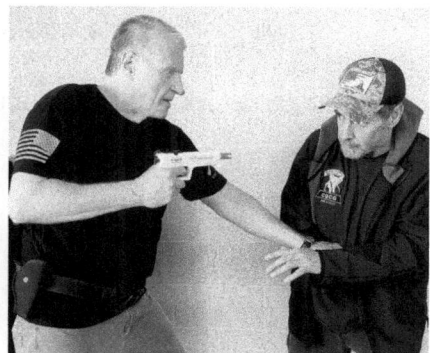

The SOB pull is spotted. Free hand catches the attempt, drives in, pulls and shoots if the suspect has a gun or knife.

The low cross draw pull is spotted. Free hand catches the attempt, drives in, pulls and shoots if the suspect has a gun or knife. Consider where to shoot to stay clear.

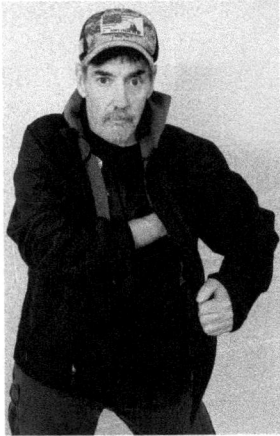

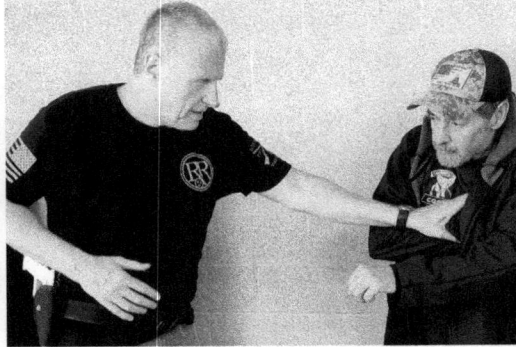

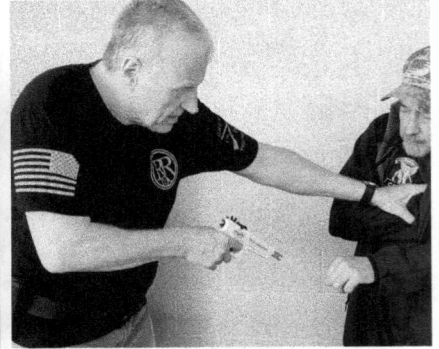

The high cross draw pull is spotted. Free hand catches the attempt, drives in, pulls and shoots if the suspect has a gun or knife. Consider where to shoot to stay clear.

Set 1: Trainer draws from appendix carry. The trainee grabs the draw, pushes, draws and shoots with safe simulated ammo.

Set 2: Trainer draws from hip carry. The trainee grabs the draw, pushes, draws and shoots with safe simulated ammo.

Set 3: Trainer draws from SOB carry. The trainee grabs the draw, pushes, draws and shoots with safe simulated ammo.

Set 4: Trainer draws from low cross draw carry. The trainee grabs the draw, pushes, draws and shoots with safe simulated ammo.

Set 5: Trainer draws from high cross draw carry. The trainee grabs the draw, pushes, draws and shoots with safe simulated ammo.

Note: Work against a lefty trainer.

FN: Gun Addendum 1: The Dropped Gun

(In *Training Mission 2* and *Stop 2*, we worry about weapon retention and dropped weapons, thus this topic is related and important.)

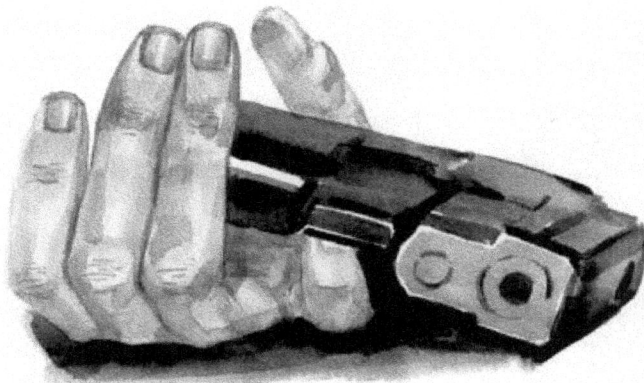

"If I die in a combat zone. Box me up and ship me home." You've all heard that ditty? Maybe you haven't? It comes for most who have as a cadence - a song - we all sang while marching and running in the military. It has been bastardized, or satirized and altered for various messaging. One paraphrased version we don't see much anymore, but old-timers will remember, was popularized on some t-shirts and posters years back. It was about dying in a combat zone and having your gear split up, the words accompanied by art of a rip-shirt, commando. This splitting-up is a very good idea for several reasons, but I don't think the commandment reaches deep enough in citizen and police training methodology.

It is a common theory in shoot-outs that drawing and using a second gun is faster than reloading your first one. This of course depends on where you are carrying that second gun, but the advice is classic and comes from veterans. Did you arrive at this scene with a second gun? Can you find a second gun at the scene? More ammo? More gear? Such is great in a firefight.

There are numerous, vitally important, physical, survival things you cannot and

will not learn or get to do, if you decide to forever shoot on a paper target range and consider that practice to be the end-all to gun-fighting.

One such subject is what to do about a "drop dead gun," or the dropped gun. One dropped by a seriously wounded or dead person. You can lecture on this, show charts, and talk it up, you can put various kinds of guns in various conditions on a bench at the shooting range and make people pick them up, make-ready, load them and shoot them (which has been done forever by clever people by the way), but the true savvy and timing of doing this pick up inside a hot, under-fire, being-hunted situation is hardly practiced on the range.

Technically, this is weapon recovery. Weapon recovery is typically discussed in inner circles when your pistol has been disarmed from you and how you must recover it. You instantly charge in to get it back while the taker is hopefully fumbling with it. Recovering disarmed weapons is a missing link in most martial art systems when students work pistol disarms. Students take the gun from an attacker, the students usually quite oblivious to the fact that a real worl, bad-guy may mad-rush in, to get the gun back at a hundred miles an hour. These students often just take the gun, flip it around, fiddle with it (some instructors demand that the student tap the magazine and rack the side), not expecting the vicious counter attack and weapon recovery.

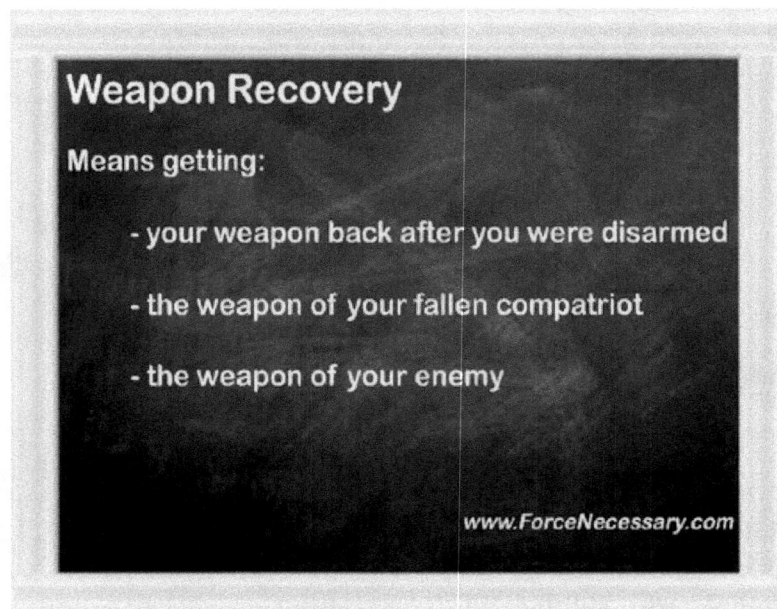

Weapon Recovery

Means getting:

- your weapon back after you were disarmed

- the weapon of your fallen compatriot

- the weapon of your enemy

www.ForceNecessary.com

But weapon recovery is a bigger issue that just disarming and the recovery of your gun. There's the recovery of your comrade's weapon and even the recovery of your enemy's weapon.

Aside from disarming, guns are dropped by accident, taken or dropped/lost in combat. Long guns and pistols are dropped with some frequency in non-combat life, of which we have no stats on, but my hunch is they get dropped from time to time. I can't recall dropping mine in some 45 years, but I've seen my friends/co-workers drop theirs a time or two. And we see them drop on YouTube videos. We also see photos and hear about such fumbles in both normal and stressful times. We see them dropped in simulated ammo scenario training. We even see them dropped at live fire ranges.

What about a fumble during a draw or inside a grappling fight? Back in the 90s, when I first started teaching safe ammo, interactive shooting methods. I once saw a range master, and trophy winner cop, standing before an armed training partner in a scenario. Both with gas guns. The draw! And the vet lost his pistol in the air. He had never drawn right in front of an armed man with a pain-delivering gun before him.

I can say with some accuracy that four common things happen when someone holding a firearm is shot. The person:

1: Drops the gun, or
2: Convulsively fires the weapon, or
3: Aims and shoots back, or
4: The gun does nothing. Remains unfired in the hand.

So, what about the dropped weapon of a shot, severely wounded, dead compatriot or enemy? A drop dead gun, just laying there. This year, 2020 marks the 24th year that I have routinely, almost weekly, created and supervised simulated ammo shooting scenarios of some sort. Some are short and involve two people. Some are much longer and involve numerous people, in numerous situations and locations. In the short or longer shootouts in buildings and on the streets, open areas etc., people get shot by whatever simulated ammo we get to use for the training session. In a briefing, I ask the people, once "shot," to evaluate their wounds when hit. If shot in their shooting limb, then they switch hands. If shot in the leg, they limp on for a bit. If they take two serious shots, or shot in the head, I ask them to drop right where they are and essentially…"they be dead." Playing this part is important, as you will soon read...

As the organizer, overseer of these scenarios, as the "ref" if you will, I see so many things in all of these shoot-outs. I see things people really do when in various predicaments. These occurrences, these experiences are quite remarkable and extremely educational. And one of the many things I consistently see is teammates, running past and around their deeply wounded, still or dead, yet still armed partners. Whatever kinds of weapons we are using, Airsoft, gas, markers, Simuntions, whatever I can get wherever I am, these guns run out of ammo, gas, power or break down at the damndest instances. I want to advise, "pick up that gun!" as they run by their fallen compatriots. Sometimes they have the time to do so. But, I do not want to bark orders or suggestions to interfere in the middle of the firefight exercise. I've see many folks run right by other available guns and ammo. I wait until the after-action review to bring the subject up, and still they forget to do it the next time.

Once in a while I see a practitioner who instantly knows to snatch up his dead buddy's gun. Either, it is something trained and remembered, or they are just that naturally gun-and-ammo-hungry to simply know this and do this instinctively. They swoop down and snatch up the weapon as they go by. This is an event that never happens in live fire range training, but rather could and should happen in real life, and bolstered in simulated ammo, scenario training whenever possible.

I might add quickly here, that weapons are sometimes attached to people by lanyards and slings, something that can be very life-saving for the original holder, but also may flummox your partner's attempt to get your weapons once you are down and out. Know your partner's gear. Look them over.

Different gear? Different guns? Different ammo? In many organizations such as with the military or police, certain weapons are mandated for all in policy for good reason. If we all have the same gun, we all have the same ammo, magazines and we can pick up, exchange, provide, etc., weapons. It can make for good sense. I am not advocating for the "one-gun, one-ammo" policy, I am just reporting on it. There is something to be said too for personalized guns.

When military people move into policing jobs, they often and should carry with them these overall concept. Well, I mean, if you were an Army "clerk," you might not take this to heart, but people trained for dangerous jobs and have experienced danger are better carriers of this idea.

So often, citizens minus this background, police management, etc. may not consider this, or not have the deep heartfelt, burn, understanding of the concept. Shooting instructors of all types may never even know to suggest this topic.

Minus police and military experiences, If you just teach or do live fire on a range, essentially that being that "clerk," with no emotional attachment to experience, you must realize that you might be missing huge chunks of important tactics, topics, subjects and situations. You might begin to dwell deeper and deeper into repetitive "gun minutiae" within your teaching. (Haven't gun magazines really been publishing the same redundant information, redone and re-shaped for decades now? Why? Why, do they stick in this redundancy when there is so many more-diverse combative situations to dissect and train about?)

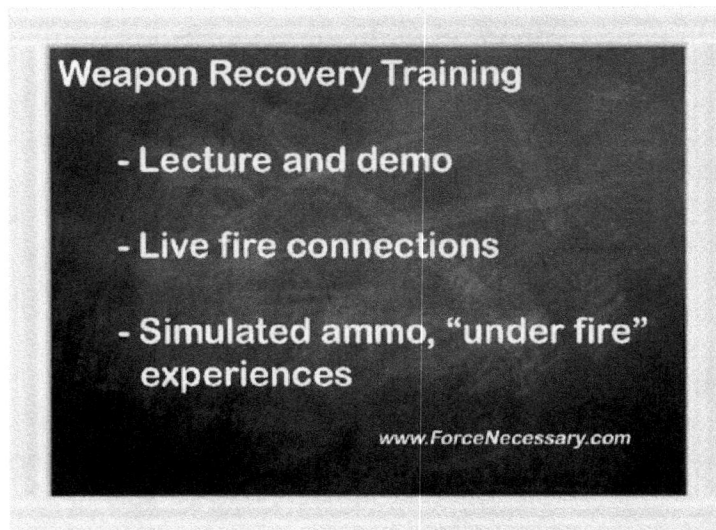

Weapon Recovery Training

- Lecture and demo

- Live fire connections

- Simulated ammo, "under fire" experiences

www.ForceNecessary.com

Two answers to these teaching and training problems. One is to continue educating yourself on real experiences. What precisely has happened to your friends? Your teammates? Your neighbors? Victims? Cops? Military? Learning second or third-hand is better than not learning at all. Who can possibly experience the common spectrum of such problems? No one. We all must keep this education up. Second? Simulated ammo scenarios. Simunitions or likewise, otherwise, at some level. Take your "power point" tips and your segmented, live fire examples and move them into physical experience with safe ammo. Move them over into a stressful, interactive, situational scenarios with simulated ammo. Such are psychologically and neurologically proven better learning experiences. The experts call it "deep learning." In other words, simply put – get off the range and do these interactive shoot-outs.

There has been something of a newer concern and movement in this "pick up" subject, as people contemplate the active shooter problem and consider picking up the guns of shot police, downed security, etc. This concern has manifested in a slight increase in related speeches and some abstract, live fire exercises. Martial arts instructors, ones who appear to have no gun experience or limited gun backgrounds, have also organized some active shooter response classes. But when working out and testing the unarmed methods, the attendees all bum-rush a stunt man in a helmet holding a rubber gun. I would wish that they, at least once, let the actor carry in a sims-ammo, (could be with very safe ammo) machine gun and let him cut loose on the crowd so that the attendees could truly experience the hideous, quick, devastation one can do with such firearms to a group. Perhaps this might be too demoralizing?

Also, remember when you pick up another pistol, you don't know how many bullets are left in it. And by the way, in certain crime and war circumstances, when citizens pick up the dead bad guys gun and the police arrive? Do I need to remind you? You look like the bad guy. You could be shot. Act, surrender accordingly.

But, be it that sort of "mass shooting," or a crime or in war, in the case of the drop dead gun training and simulated ammo training, a prep speech can first be made about the weapon recovery from downed and dead rescuers or teammates. It has been my experience that once suggested in this briefing, many people do think of it when the action starts and the possibility arises. The more they do it? The better.

The gun may be dropped, but it ain't dead. So, the next t-shirt or poster rant and chant?

**"If I die in a combat zone? Get my ammo, guns
and gear and...continue to kill the enemy."**

(...And, a quick note, if you pick up a dropped pistol, the sights may be ajar, or...gone?)

FN Gun Addendum 2: The Sam Elliott Decision, To Treat or Not To Treat?

Years ago, I saw a western with Sam Elliott. I can't remember the name of the western. Two guys came to kill him at a woodsy cabin. He shot them. One survived, and Sam immediately hauled him into the cabin and started treating him for his gut-shot wound. I realized I had a nickname for a situation that might help people remember an aftermath element all gun people need to consider more and more these days...

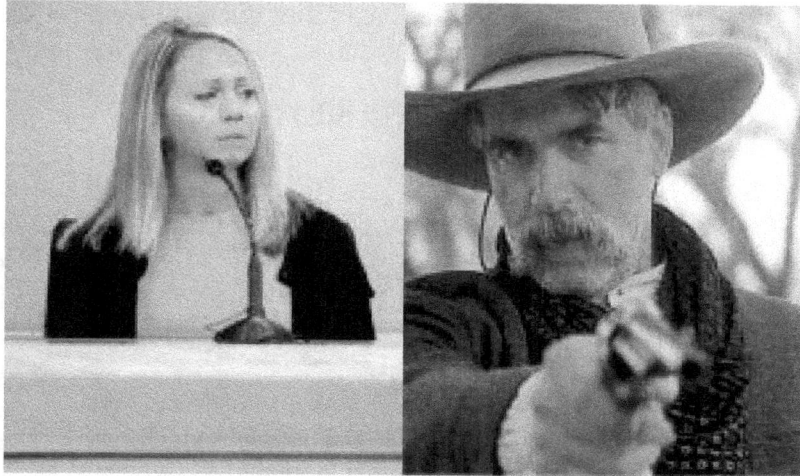

Years ago, then and now former Dallas PD Officer Amber Guyger, came home late at night from a 12 hour shift, drove into and walked through her dark apartment building, a place where some 15 percent of residents have reported going to the wrong apartment. Call it bad "forensic architecture." She entered an unlocked door, saw a guy in "her" living room and shot him dead. It's was a big deal in Dallas and hit the national and even international news media. A big deal because the poor victim watching TV on his couch was by all accounts, a terrific young black guy. And we were smothered with Black Lives Matter agitators here in North Texas and controversy. So, it's was a terrible mistake, and she paid. She was eventually found guilty of murder and got a 10 year sentence.

She testified! Which is an oddity. Under prosecution questioning and in her testimony was the fact that she did not apply any tactical medicine methods to the save the guy. And she had some very handy too in a police backpack she was carrying. She did call 911, etc. but didn't do much for the dying right away. This received many grimaces in court. It suggests a negativity. An uncaring intent. A secret racism is claimed. It fortified a guilty verdict and then a prison sentence. This is just one example of what I am talking about.

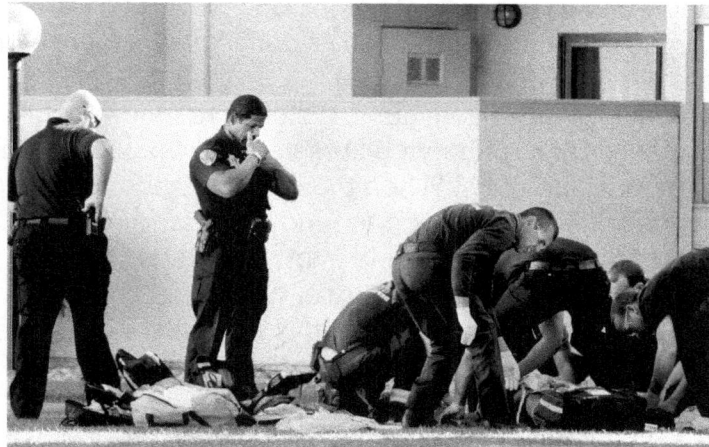

Even the military can suffer from this. Think about Navy SEAL Gallagher recently accused of war crimes and killing off a wounded teenager-combatant for one example. One of the contentions was he did not treat the wounded enemy teen properly. (Read about it in his *The Man in the Arena* book.)

Trouble for the military, the on-duty and off-duty police officer. But, in a criminal or civil court what then for a citizen? Aside from off-duty Amber, it is becoming more and more apparent to me through the years that if you shoot someone in self defense, the "law," be it civil or criminal, the carefully selected jury, the media, is going to ponder in a later calm and cool courtroom and want to know, want to ask you why you did or did not try to save their life after you shot them. Could you? Should you? Would you? Can you articulate why?

Past training for the police? We in the business have always had some medical and first aid training, however simplistic and poor, as far back as my involvement starting in the early 70s. Not much was said about situations and who deserves what kind of treatment. And when? The practice was that the wounded (or dead) bad guy had to be handcuffed. His weapons collected-secure. We had to close in, guns up and take care of this business. I have done this dozens and dozens of times, (more with prone, "unshot" suspects) but it's dangerous, and I cannot expect citizens to do this all the time. An ambulance was called. Not much medical attention, if any, is given to the grounded, dying criminal. We had to and still must "make the scene safe," and we couldn't let the EMTS in close without securing the body and the scene.

44 MINUTES IN NORTH HOLLYWOOD

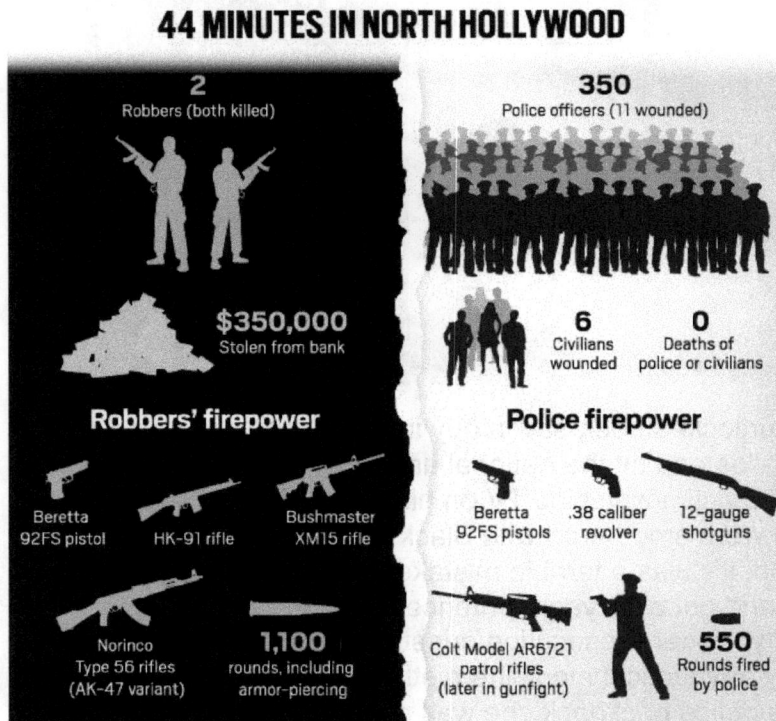

2 Robbers (both killed)

$350,000 Stolen from bank

Robbers' firepower

Beretta 92FS pistol

HK-91 rifle

Bushmaster XM15 rifle

Norinco Type 56 rifles (AK-47 variant)

1,100 rounds, including armor-piercing

350 Police officers (11 wounded)

6 Civilians wounded

0 Deaths of police or civilians

Police firepower

Beretta 92FS pistols

.38 caliber revolver

12-gauge shotguns

Colt Model AR6721 patrol rifles (later in gunfight)

550 Rounds fired by police

Anecdotally, in the 80s we shot an armed robber of a restaurant one night. Now, it being 35 years ago, I do not remember if he was dead yet, but we took his rifle and handcuffed him behind his back, and...let him be. Ambulance called. Neighbors watching complained that we let the guy die. His mother sued the department for not treating her kid. Nothing much came of it because it was Texas and 35 years ago. If the city settled? I don't know. I can safely say, none of us thought of treating the guy.

This "no treat concept-decision," was more publicly challenged after the infamous Los Angeles bank robbery decades ago, in the 90s, by the two guys tacked-out, vested and with machine guns. When the second robber was shot, there was news footage of the aftermath. The cops stood around. The family of that robber sued LAPD for ignoring their son's treatment after being shot. Due to the carnage they wrought, there wasn't much sympathy at all. But, of course, LAPD settled $$$.

This official scene-securing is not a civilian requirement. In a way, in a biological, psychological way, I think we all can understand how people shooting a robber/attacker, are reluctant to help them.

"The SOB might get kicked rather than get a tourniquet!"

"Well he was trying to rob me, so F____ him."

That works at the bar, or the buddy BS session. And while I certainly really do appreciate gallows humor, your words might not hang well with the grand jury, the criminal court, or the civil court.

Police, military, citizen or otherwise, nowadays, serious gun owners spend a lot time on tactical medicine, but for whom exactly? Medical technology improved so much, so quickly, in the last few decades. I remember the wonders of QuickClot! But think about it for a moment. The general thrust of these courses had been to heal yourself, family and co-workers. Not really, not ever the criminal. But, is it sometimes safe to move in, kick the bad guy's gun away (or pick it up) look the bad guy over, and maybe...do something for him? Do nothing? Don't care to? Too scared to look? Don't care to look? Are you alone? Mad, scared or caring?

Think about it. Sometimes, under some situations and circumstances, church or school, wedding or workplace shootings to name just four, you are the "man", or the "woman," and you may have to move in and step up. Do something. Sometimes you can't or shouldn't . And sometimes you need to evacuate.

Anyway, my message is, if you shoot someone, lest of all kill Hannibal Lector himself, later somewhere will be looming around - prosecution, defense, lawyers, families, political groups - trying to torture you for not immediately performing a heart transplant to save him. I don't think this reality has fully hit total ground zero with all the gun people in the USA just yet. Just calling 911 and running and hiding out in the parking lot behind a car as suggested by some trainers for *ALL* shooting situations, may not be enough anymore in *ALL* situations. It is VERY situational.

Some of my smartest gun trainers and legal beagle friends say they teach rescue care. As far as medical treatment, some more thoughtful ones suggest -

 * **treat yourself first, then,**
 * **family, comrades, friends, then,**
 * **third, consider the shot bad guy.**

So for some, the wounded criminal is somehow on the medical list to at least think about. As a professional cop or soldier, you have to monitor him anyway. You have to get close to get his weapons away from him, anyway, we have to cuff him, anyway. Again, that's situational. What should a citizen do? It's also situational.

I am not laying out a mandatory list. I am just making a point for all people to think about ethics, the interpretations of law and post-shooting problems. Should every citizen shoot and run away as suggested by numerous self defense instructors? Always? Do you shoot a school shooter in a crowd or a church shooter in a crowd, or mall shooter in a crowd should shoot and immediately head for the hills? Is the bad guy dead? Stunned? Wounded? Up again and skulking around still? What constitutes closure? What constitutes closure in this or any situation?

Get ready for more enforcement institutions to mandate more of this. I first wrote this essay in 2019. Since then, I've seen numerous body cam videos of police rushing in to save the lives of the people that they just shot (black or white). They have to now! It seems everyday in the US, legal systems are becoming more "liberal." More suspect-driven. Prosecutors are becoming more and more liberal (thank you Darth-George-Soros-Vader).

In many places it appears that that's a movement to turn mere gun ownership into a sin and common sense, self defense into vigilantism! (Never mind the laws of other countries. It's too late for most).To treat or not to treat? This is a legal (and moral?) question. Lots of my friends and police say this emergency medical treatment is far too dangerous. No way will they. Citizen, police or military, you should be able to articulate why you did or did not choose to treat the shot person these days. But proclaiming you will leave every one to die, every time, all the time, no matter the circumstances is just not smart legalese, nor smart instruction What I am saying now is for everyone, what of a "Sam Elliott Decision?"

You should or will have to articulate at some point, with understandable, common sense, why you did or *did not* do something medical to and for a bad guy, if just to your lawyer so they know as you prepare your defense strategy. I am confident that at least your mindset and then your possible attempts can be beneficial to your defense.

We have spent a lot of time and effort to remind police and citizens to message:

"I shot to stop him, not to kill him."

This is just a further manifestation of that messaging. There will be situational reasons for or against helping the dying suspect. But, you'd better think about it, this... "Sam Elliott Decision." To survive the civil or criminal follow-up, it is much wiser to be the type of person who:

* **Thought about helping.**
* **Who wanted to try and help, but couldn't or shouldn't.**
* **Who tried and did do something.**
* **Rather than someone whose doctrine totally, always condemned the concept.**
  (I think this mindset could be troublesome, especially in the future, for the person or the subpoenaed gun teacher. Can you hear the questioning? "So you teach that you should simply let everyone die, no matter the circumstances? Is that what you teach?)

CHAPTER 25: LEVEL 2 TEST REQUIREMENTS

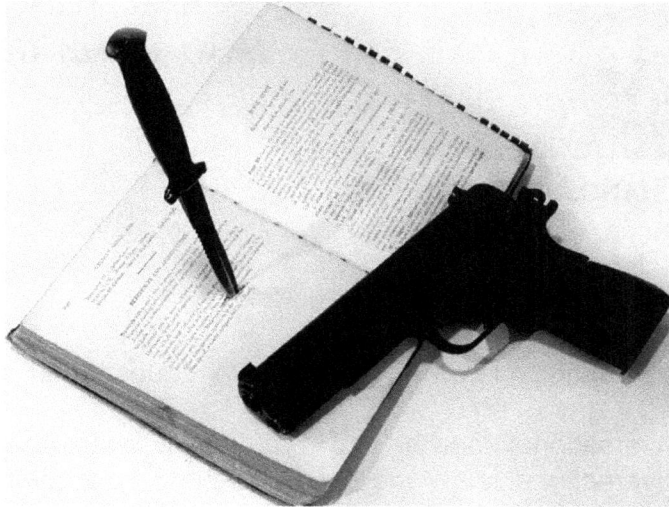

TESTING REQUIREMENTS FOR:

FORCE NECESSARY HAND: LEVEL 2
FORCE NECESSARY STICK: LEVEL 2
FORCE NECESSARY KNIFE: LEVEL 2
FORCE NECESSARY GUN: LEVEL 2

CLOSE QUARTERS CONCEPTS GROUP LEVEL 2

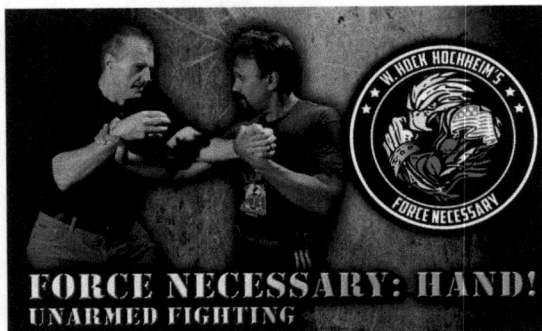

HAND VERSUS HAND
HAND VERSUS STICK
HAND VERSUS KNIFE
HAND VERSUS GUN THREATS

FORCE NECESSARY HAND: LEVEL 2 TEST

12 more hours experience working on these Level 2 materials. Time and grade in similar themed systems may also count, upon approval.

Knowledge and Understanding
* A working and conversational knowledge of the *What* question as it relates to unarmed fighting.
* A working and conversational knowledge of *Stop 2* as it relates to unarmed fighting.
* A working and conversational knowledge of the all the *Stop 2* commonalities.

Physical Accomplishments
Level 2 Palm Strikes
* Demonstrate on pads and people, and explain the universal palm strike.

Level 2 Stomp Kicks
* Demonstrate on pads and people, and explain the universal stomp kick.

Level 2 Grappling
* Demonstrate and explain 5 applications of the wrist manipulations, catches and takedowns.
* Demonstrate one wrist/crank lock flow (minimum 3 locks/cranks).
* Demonstrate the core basic releases from *Stop 2* grips and catches.

Level 2 Footwork and Maneuvering
* Demonstrate the "in and out" footwork on the Combat Clock. Right and left leads.

Any Local Instructor Additions.
Test fee $100.

FORCE NECESSARY: STICK!
BATON & "STICK" FIGHTING
Stick vs. Hand - Stick vs. Stick - Stick vs. Knife - Stick vs. Gun

STICK VERSUS HAND
STICK VERSUS STICK
STICK VERSUS KNIFE
STICK VERSUS GUN THREATS

FORCE NECESSARY STICK: LEVEL 2 TEST

12 more hours experience working on these Level 2 materials. Time and grade in similar themed systems also may count upon, approval.

Knowledge and Understanding
   * A working & conversational knowledge of the all the *Stop 2* commonalities.
   * A working & conversational knowledge of the *What* question, as it relates to batons.
   * A working & conversational knowledge of *Stop 2* as it relates to impact weapon fights.

Physical Accomplishments
   * The in and out footwork while holding a stick, on the Combat Clock.
      - while holding a one hand grip.
      - while holding a two-hand grip.

   * Demonstrate the Tangler basic releases from *Stop 2* grips and catches on your stick carry site and stick drawn catches on your hand/wrist or forearm.
      - 2 releases from belt line grabs.
      - 2 releases from single hand grabs on your stick.
      - 2 releases from double hand grabs on your stick.
      - 2 releases from a double-hand grab, one on your stick, the other on your wrist.

   * Demonstrate the Level 2 Stick Tangler Exercise
      2 stress draws vs. an unarmed attack.
      2 stress draws vs. a stick attack.
      2 stress draws vs. a knife attack.
      2 stress draws vs. a pistol rush.
      2 attacks vs. an unarmed attacker, stick drawn.
      2 attacks vs. a stick attacker, stick drawn.
      2 attacks vs. a knife attacker, stick drawn.
      2 attacks vs. a pistol pulling attacker, stick drawn.

><

Remember to include a few with a closed baton.

Any Local Instructor Additions.
Test fee is $100.

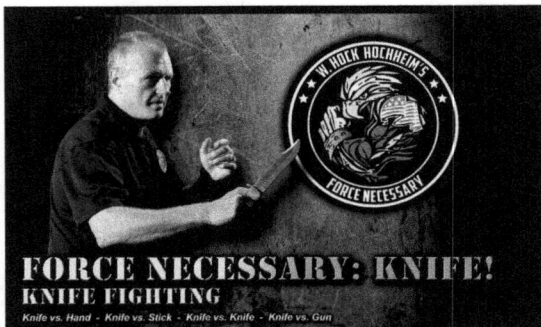

FORCE NECESSARY KNIFE: LEVEL 2 TEST

12 more hours experience working on these Level 2 materials. Time and grade in similar themed systems may also count, upon approval.

Knowledge and Understanding
  * A working and conversational knowledge of the all the *Stop 2* commonalities.
  * A working and conversational knowledge of the *What* question, as it relates to the knife.
  * A working and conversational knowledge of *Stop 2* as it relates to the knife.

Physical Accomplishments
  * The in and out footwork while holding a knife, on the Combat Clock.
    - Saber and reverse grip. Add slashing and thrusting.

  * Demonstrate the "Death Grip of the Knife," Tangler problem solutions.
    - 1 release from a pocket carry grab.
    - 1 release from an appendix carry grab.
    - Any 6 knife vs *Death Grip of the Knife* Releases.

  * Demonstrate the Level 2 Knife Tangler Exercise
    2 stress draws vs. an unarmed attack.
    2 stress draws vs. a stick attack.
    2 stress draws vs. a knife attack.
    2 stress draws vs. a pistol-pulling rush.
    2 attacks vs. an unarmed attacker, knife drawn.
    2 attacks vs. a stick attacker, knife drawn.
    2 attacks vs. a knife attacker, knife drawn.
    2 attacks vs. a pistol-pulling attacker, knife drawn.

><

Remember to include a few with closed folders.

Any Local Instructor additions.
Test fee is $100.

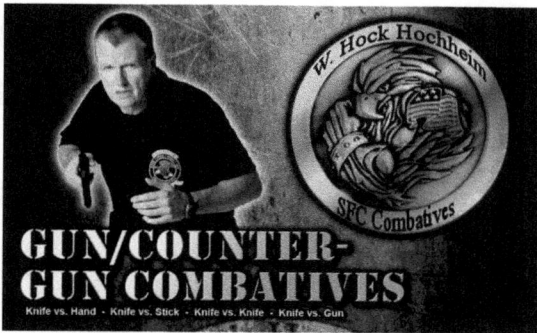

GUN/COUNTER-GUN COMBATIVES
Knife vs. Hand · Knife vs. Stick · Knife vs. Knife · Knife vs. Gun

GUN VERSUS HAND
GUN VERSUS STICK
GUN VERSUS KNIFE
GUN VERSUS GUN THREATS

FORCE NECESSARY EXTERNAL FOCUS GUN: LEVEL 2 TEST

12 more hours experience working on these Level 2 materials. Time and grade in similar themed systems may also count, upon approval. Practitioner must have attended one more live fire gun course.

Knowledge and Understanding

* A working and conversational knowledge of the all the *Stop 2* commonalities.
* A working and conversational knowledge of the *What* question, as it relates to a firearm.
* A working and conversational knowledge of Stop 2 as it relates to a firearm.

Physical Accomplishments

* The in and out footwork while holding a pistol and while holding a long gun.

* Demonstrate the Level 2 Firearm Tangler Exercise.
    2 stress draws vs. an unarmed attack.
    2 stress draws vs. a stick attack.
    2 stress draws vs. a knife attack.
    2 stress draws vs. a pistol-pulling rush.
    2 gun drawing vs. gun drawing Death Grip of the Gun attacks.
    2 releases from long gun grabs.
    2 "It's On! Gun draw interruptions.

Any Local Instructor Additions.
Test fee is $100.

CLOSE QUARTER CONCEPTS LEVEL TWO SUMMARY OF REQUIREMENTS CHECKLIST

Level 2 Time, Understanding and Experience
____ 12 more hours experience on Level 2 related unarmed material.
____ 12 more hours experience on Level 2 related stick/impact weapon material.
____ 12 more hours experience on Level 2 related knife material.
____ 12 more hours experience on Level 2 related gun material.
____ A working and conversational knowledge of the *What* Questions concept.
____ A working and conversational knowledge of Stop 2 of the Stop 6.
____ A working and conversational knowledge of Stop 2 commonalities.
____ Have a working understanding of self defense laws.

Level 2 Footwork
____ The *In and Out* footwork around the Combat Clock, when unarmed.
____ The *In and Out* footwork around the Combat Clock while holding a stick.
____ The *In and Out* footwork around the Combat Clock while holding a knife.
____ The *In and Out* footwork around the Combat Clock while holding a pistol.
____ The *In and Out* footwork around the Combat Clock while holding a long gun.

Level 2 Basic Releases
____ Demonstrate the core releasing moves while unarmed.
____ Demonstrate the core releasing moves while holding a stick.
____ Demonstrate the core releasing moves while holding a knife.
____ Demonstrate the core releasing moves while holding a pistol.

Level 2 Unarmed Physical Requirements
____ Hand: Demonstrate the palm strikes on gear, standing and on the ground.
____ Hand: Demonstrate 5 combat scenarios involving palm strike attacks.
____ Hand: Demonstrate the stomp kicking series on gear.
____ Hand: Demonstrate and explain the 5 main wrist directional cranks.
____ Hand: Demonstrate 5 wrist attacks vs. hand, stick, knife and gun threat attacks.
____ Hand: Demonstrate 3 counters to wrist cranks.
____ Hand: Demonstrate one wrist/crank lock flow (minimum 3 locks/cranks).

Level 2 Stick/Baton Physical Requirements
____ Stick: Demonstrate the core basic releases from *Stop 2* grips and catches on your stick.
____ Stick: Demonstrate the Tangler basic releases 2 releases from belt line grabs.
____ Stick: Demonstrate 2 releases from single hand grabs on your stick.
____ Stick: Demonstrate 2 releases from double hand grabs on your stick.
____ Stick: Demonstrate 2 releases from a double-hand grab, one on your stick, the other on your wrist.
____ Stick: Demonstrate 2 stress draws vs. an unarmed attack.

____ Stick: Demonstrate 2 stress draws vs. a stick attack.
____ Stick: Demonstrate 2 stress draws vs. a knife attack.
____ Stick: Demonstrate 2 stress draws vs. a pistol rush.
____ Stick: Demonstrate 2 attacks vs. an unarmed attacker, stick drawn.
____ Stick: Demonstrate 2 attacks vs. a stick attacker, stick drawn.
____ Stick: Demonstrate 2 attacks vs. a knife attacker, stick drawn.
____ Stick: Demonstrate 2 attacks vs. a pistol pulling attacker, stick drawn.

Level 2 Knife Physical Requirements
____ Knife: Demonstrate 1 release from a pocket carry grab.
____ Knife: Demonstrate 1 release from an appendix carry.
____ Knife: Demonstrate Any 6 knife vs. *Death Grip of the Knife* Releases
____ Knife: Demonstrate the Level 2 Knife Tangler Exercise.
____ Knife: Demonstrate 2 stress draws vs. an unarmed attack.
____ Knife: Demonstrate 2 stress draws vs. a stick attack.
____ Knife: Demonstrate 2 stress draws vs. a knife attack.
____ Knife: Demonstrate 2 stress draws vs. a pistol-pulling rush.
____ Knife: Demonstrate 2 attacks vs. an unarmed attacker, knife drawn.
____ Knife: Demonstrate 2 attacks vs. a stick attacker, knife drawn.
____ Knife: Demonstrate 2 attacks vs. a knife attacker, knife drawn.
____ Knife: Demonstrate 2 attacks vs. a pistol-pulling attacker, knife drawn.

Level 2 Firearm Physical Requirements
____ Another live fire course.
____ Gun: Demonstrate 2 stress draws vs. an unarmed attack.
____ Gun: Demonstrate 2 stress draws vs. a stick attack.
____ Gun: Demonstrate 2 stress draws vs. a knife attack.
____ Gun: Demonstrate 2 stress draws vs. a pistol-pulling rush.
____ Gun: Demonstrate 2 gun-drawing-vs-gun-drawing, Death Grip of the Gun attacks.
____ Gun: Demonstrate 2 releases/retentions from long gun grabs.
____ Gun: Demonstrate 2 "It's On! Gun draw interruptions.

TM 2 Addendum - Skill, Speed and Flow Exercises

Note: If you do not like what ignorant knuckleheads call "dead drills," please stop here. The following is an important, isolated, speed, skill and flow exercises for the development of grabbing and counters to grabbing. Remember, that in order to grapple with someone, in order to stop a weapon draw, in order to seize a weapon, you have to first grab. In this Stop 2 *realm, the grab is around the lower forearm, wrist, hand and fingers.*

The Stop 2 Windmill Skill Developer

I learned this in the Philippines and it was described to me as truly root, historical and foundational exercise. You both make big "wheels" and later little wheel motion. Your free hand starts out by cupping and pulling down his downward, stick (or knife) wrist. There are many versions and angles to this exercise, but since this is not a Filipino book, but a study in the *Force Necessary, Stop 2* realm, I will only cover a few basics.

      Basic 1: The big circle.

      Basic 2: The small circle.

      Basic 3: The centerline, horizontal "chain saw."

      Basic 4: All down with:
                 * knife.
                     - saber grip.
                     - reverse grip (more conducive to the movement).
                 * stick
                 * hand (the hammer fist is very conducive to the movement).
                 * unarmed versus weapons.
                 * knife versus open or closed baton.

      Basic 5: Inserts and interruptions.
                 * the block.
                     - this also moves into the block, pass and pin drill.
                 * the "c-clamp" catch.
                 * rear arm bar hammerlock.
                 * hits with hands and weapons.

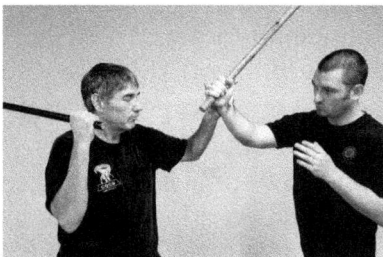

| Done with stick pommels and closed batons. | Done with knives and baton and knife. | Done with hand, or hand versus weapons. |

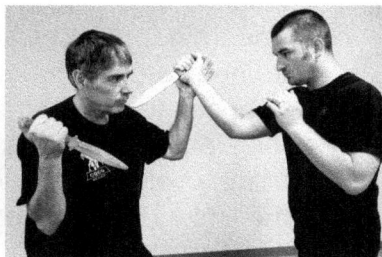

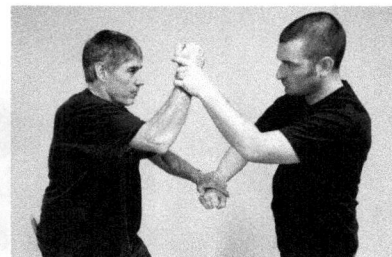

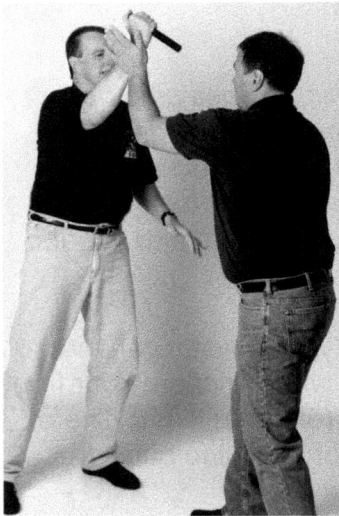

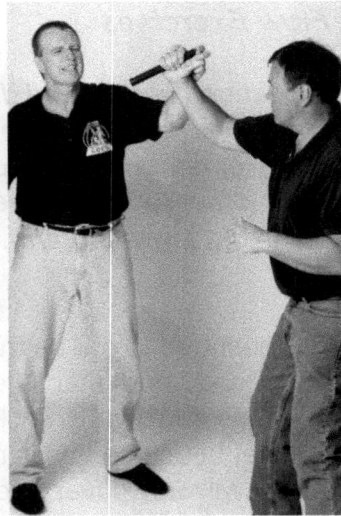

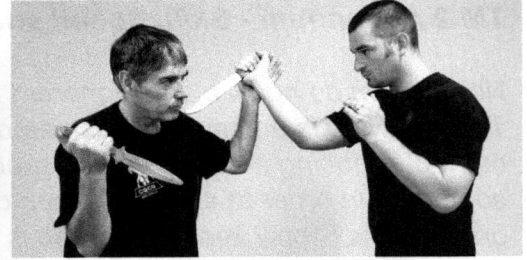

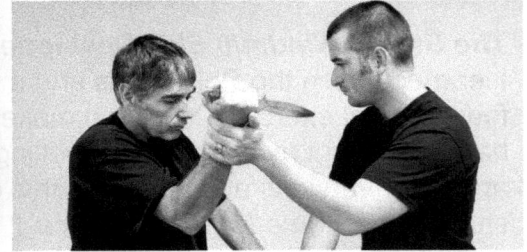

A big downward circle. The weapon hand is hooked and pulled away off target, also with a bit of body-dodging twist.

Small Windmill. A small circle, knife tip aimed at the cutting side of the neck.

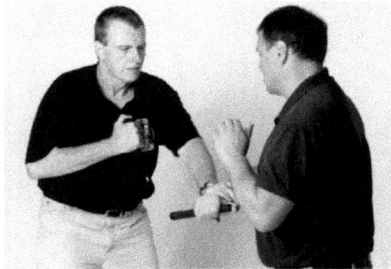

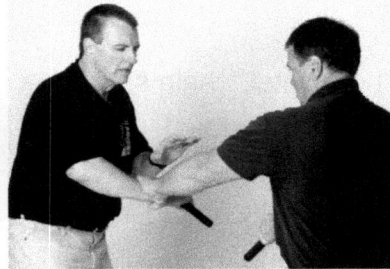

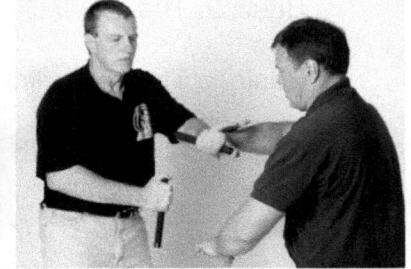

The horizontal, center line circle, nicknamed The Chain Saw.
The target is a stomach stab below the sternum.

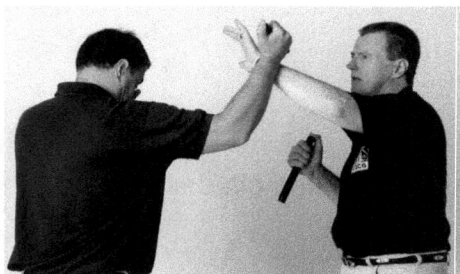

Inserts - Forearm block inserts
The trainer does a forearm block interrupting the windmill pattern. The trainer blocks. The trainee then blocks the trainer and then trades blocks back and forth until the trainer doesn't block but sweeps the attacks back into the windmill circle. Try this hand, stick and knife.

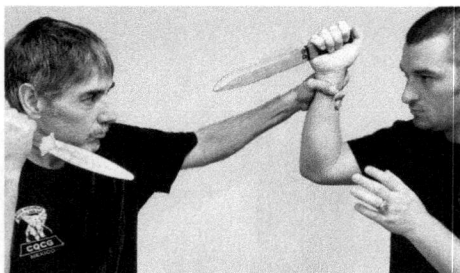

Inserts - The Stop 2 "C clamp" catch.
The trainer catches the attacking forearm. The trainee catches the attacking forearm. There are nuances to this that are best shown in person, but the clamping catches fails, and countered with trainee yank-outs, back and forth until it truly seizes the limb. The concepts is a Filipino grip test. Again, hand, stick, knife.

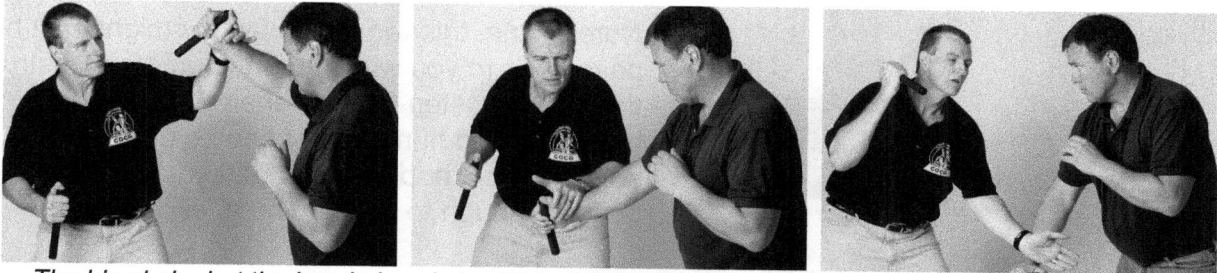
The big circle, but the hand also circles the wrist in prep for grappling. His arm must be positioned.

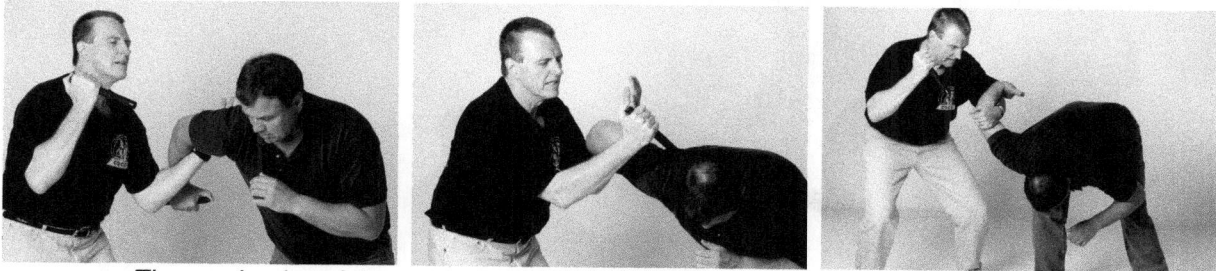
The mechanics of the rear arm bar hammerlock, helped by the reverse grip knife.

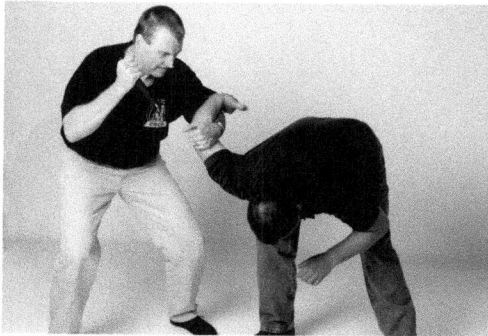
Any legal finish.

Inserts - The rear arm bar hammer lock.
The big circle, but the hand also circles the wrist in prep for grappling. His arm must be positioned. The mechanics of the rear arm bar hammerlock.

This hammer lock will be detailed in *Stop 4, Training Mission Four* which highlights "grappling arm bars," if you are new to the move? Learn it in a class. Again, with hand, stick, knife.

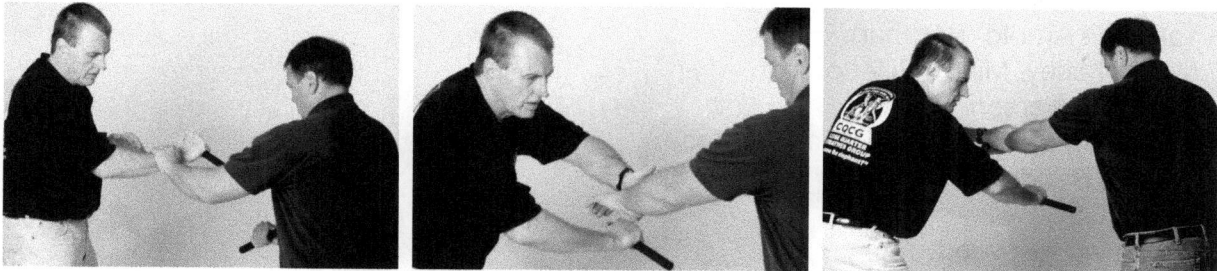
From the chain saw - a push pull release, stomach stab.

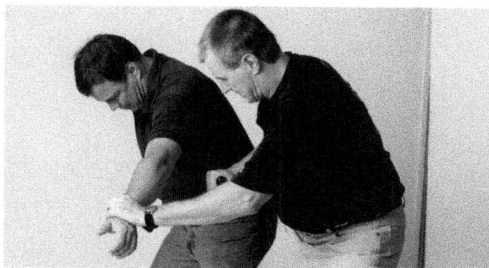
...with a step aside and cutting stomach rip.

Inserts - Release and stomach stab, stomach rip.
From the chain-saw circling, a push-pull release, stomach stab, with a step aside and cutting, under the ribs, stomach rip. And an arm bar frontal takedown. This requires a fast release and grab and a dynamic leap inwards.

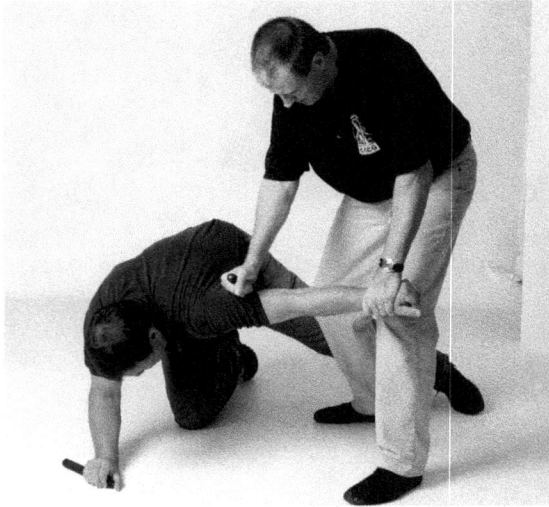

Note: Again, this windmill exercise might best be passed on to you with personal hands-on, instruction, as true, step-by step analysis, might take hundreds and hundreds of photos and a thousand words. I hope what is presented here will be just enough to inspire you to experiment.

"And now, the end of Training Mission Two *is near and I face the final curtain. My friends, I'll state my case, of which I'm certain..." (with apologies to Paul Anka.)*

Special thanks to:
 Jane Eden
 Scott Pedersen
 Rawhide Laun
 Kevin Bradburt
 Mark Lyons
 Eric Piper
 Cliff Munson
 Steve Lowery
 Snake Blocker
 Tom "the Arnold" Barnhart
 Mikey, Mikey, Mikey Gillette
 Randy Roberson
 The Dean of Kajukenbo, Dean Goldade
 William Badders
 Jason Gutierrez
 Big Dawg Kerwood
 Ronny Young
 Mike Frazier
 Alan Cain
 Dominique O Navarrete
 Tim Llacuna
 Mike Belzer
 Jethro Randolph
 ...and all others who helped with this book!

W. HOCK HOCHHEIM'S FORCE NECESSARY
TRAINING MISSION THREE

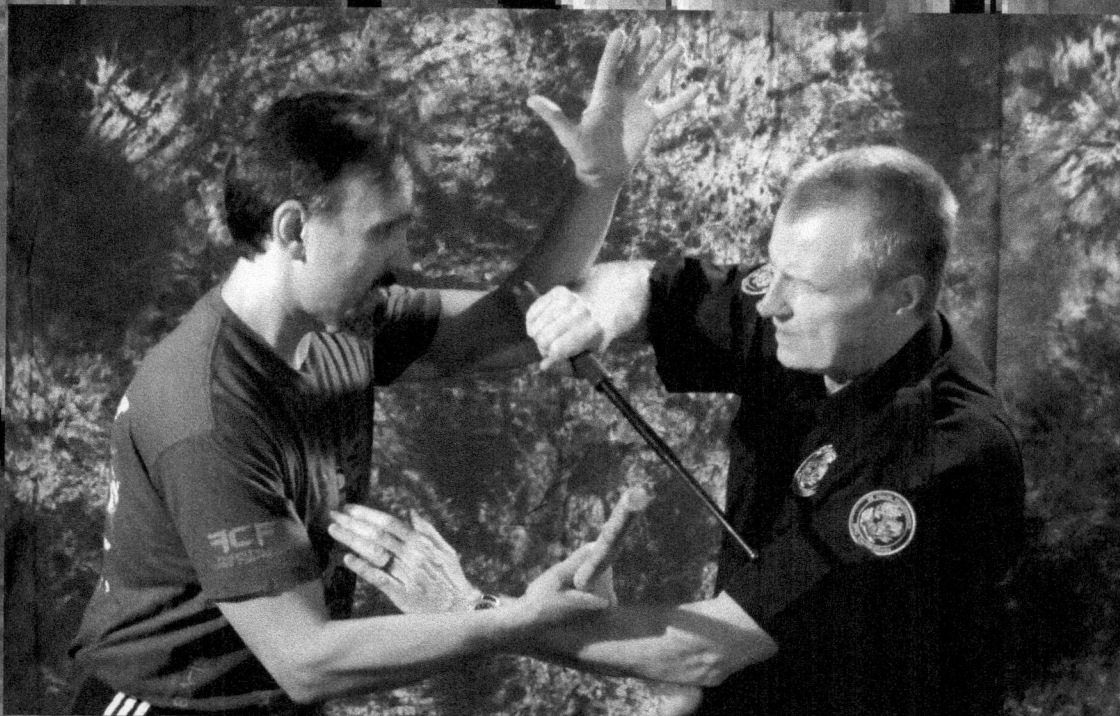

HAND 3
STICK 3
KNIFE 3
GUN 3
STOP 3

LAURIC PRESS

Get the next book in the progression!

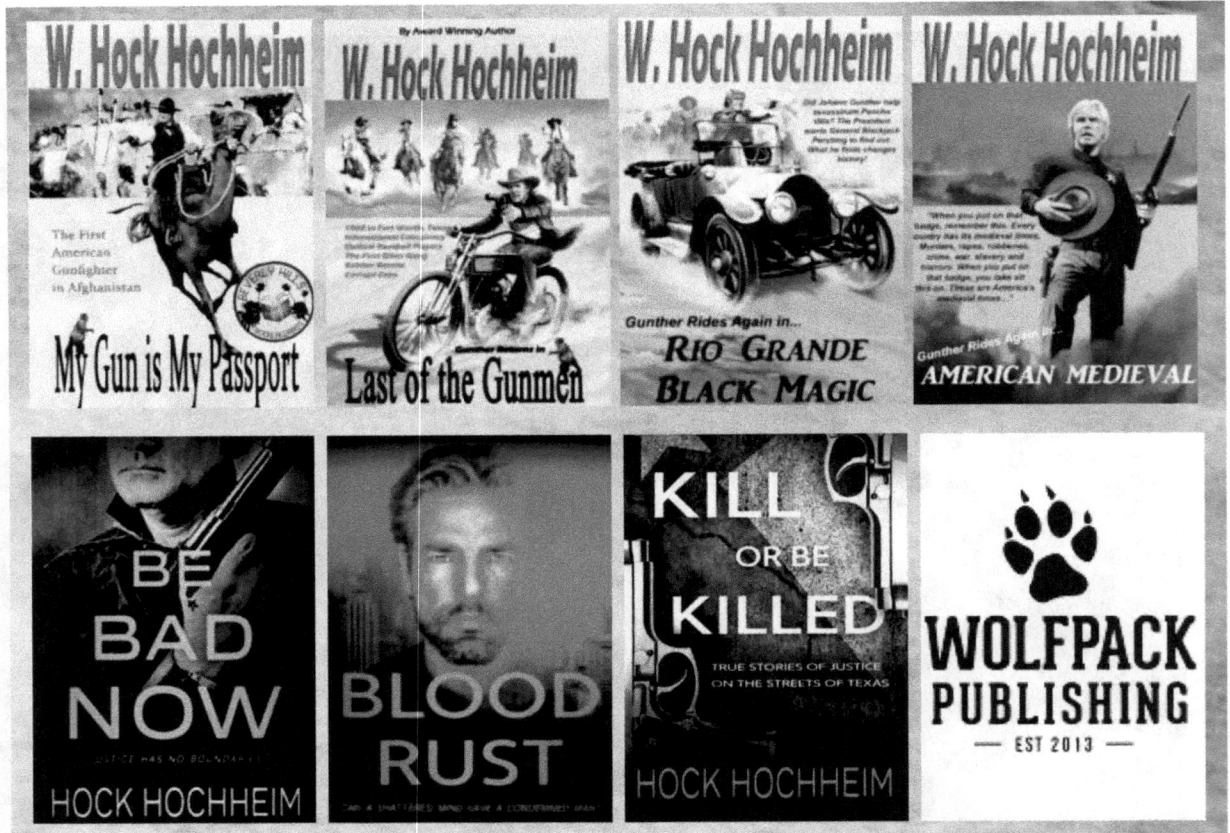

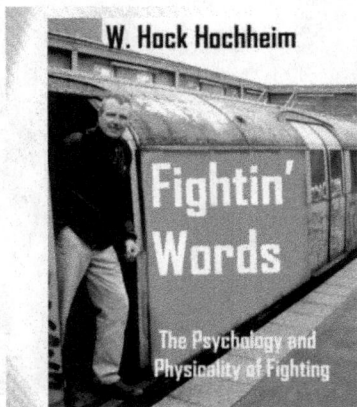

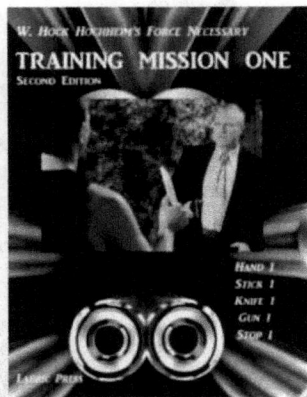

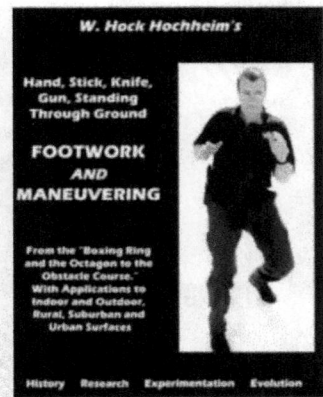

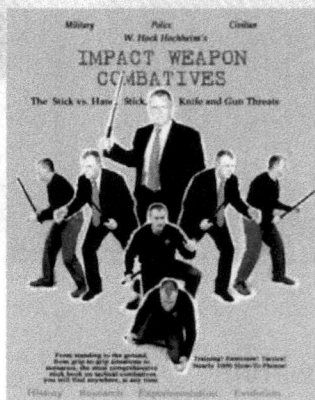

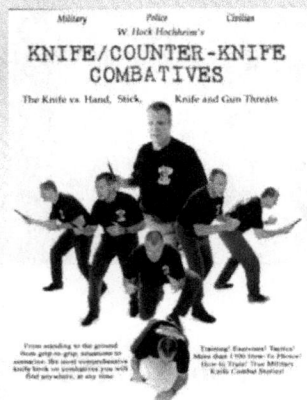

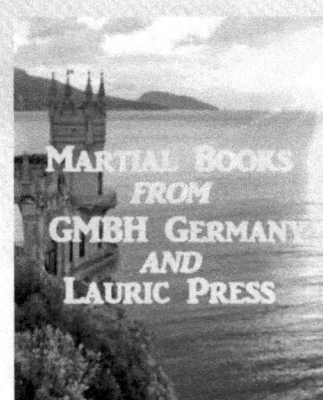

www.ingramcontent.com/pod-product-compliance
Lightning Source LLC
Chambersburg PA
CBHW052110020426
42335CB00021B/2698